The Beginning Psychotherapist's Companion

The Beginning Psychotherapist's Companion

Jan Willer

ROWMAN & LITTLEFIELD PUBLISHERS, INC.
Lanham • Boulder • New York • Toronto • Plymouth, UK

ROWMAN & LITTLEFIELD PUBLISHERS, INC.

Published in the United States of America
by Rowman & Littlefield Publishers, Inc.
A wholly owned subsidiary of The Rowman & Littlefield Publishing Group, Inc.
4501 Forbes Boulevard, Suite 200, Lanham, Maryland 20706
www.rowmanlittlefield.com

Estover Road
Plymouth PL6 7PY
United Kingdom

British Library Cataloguing in Publication Information Available

Library of Congress Cataloging-in-Publication Data:

Willer, Jan.
   The beginning psychotherapist's companion / Jan Willer.
      p. ; cm.
   Includes bibliographical references and index.
   ISBN-13: 978-0-7425-6416-9 (cloth : alk. paper)
   ISBN-10: 0-7425-6416-9 (cloth : alk. paper)
   ISBN-13: 978-0-7425-6417-6 (pbk. : alk. paper)
   ISBN-10: 0-7425-6417-7 (pbk. : alk. paper)
   ISBN-13: 978-0-7425-6393-3 (electronic)
   ISBN-10: 0-7425-6393-6 (electronic)
   1. Psychotherapy. 2. Psychotherapy—Practice. I. Title.
   [DNLM: 1. Psychotherapy—methods. 2. Practice Management. 3. Professional-
Patient Relations. 4. Psychotherapy—organization & administration. WM 420 W712
2008]
   RC480.W55 2008
   616.89'14—dc22   2008009695

Printed in the United States of America

Contents

SECTION II   GETTING STARTED WITH PSYCHOTHERAPY

SECTION IV   CRISIS READINESS

SECTION V   CARING FOR YOURSELF AND YOUR CLIENTS

APPENDICES

Acknowledgments

First, I'd like to thank my husband, Mark Osing, for his unwavering support—both emotional and financial during the process of writing this volume.

In gratitude for his bravery in signing me to this book contract and his many thoughtful comments and excellent advice, I'd like to thank my former editor, Arthur Pomponio, Ph.D. I'd also like to thank my current editor, Ross Miller, for his assistance in finishing and producing the work. Three anonymous reviewers and Dr. Shona Vas provided many helpful insights and suggestions, and I am very grateful to them.

In gratitude for sharing their suggestions, input, comments, therapeutic insights, and other assistance that was helpful to the conceptualization of this volume, I'd like to thank the following: Steve Batten, Ph.D.; Cyndy Boyd, Ph.D.; Mary Ellen Bratu, Psy.D.; Jennifer Caldwell, Ph.D.; Grayson Holmbeck, Ph.D.; Leah Horvath, Ph.D.; Zoran Martinovich, Ph.D.; Matthew Mills, M.D.; John Mundt, Ph.D.; Amberly Panepinto, Ph.D.; Anne Updegrove, Ph.D.; Vicki Seglin, Ph.D.; Suzette Speight, Ph.D.; Rick Volden, Ph.D.; Lou Weiss, Ph.D.; Joy Whitman, Ph.D.; and Kathy Zebracki, Ph.D. I'd like to give thanks to the following friends and colleagues who helped me get the various client and therapist names right throughout the book: Akira Motomura, Ph.D.; Jod Taywaditep, Ph.D.; Shona Vas, Ph.D.; and Louis Weiss, Ph.D. Any errors made in naming the clients and therapists throughout the book are mine alone.

I'd also like to thank all the psychology interns who have taught me so much over the years, in chronological order: Felicity Laboy, Eric Roth, Linda Strozdas, and Mark Woodward (1995–1996); Kathryn Doheny, Jeff Lanfear, Aaron Malina, and Zoran Martinovich (1996–1997); Tim Belavich, Kristin Flynn Peters, Theresa Kiolbasa Campbell, and Beth Summerfeld (1997–1998); Charan Ranganath, Melisa Rempfer, and Delany Thrasher (1998–1999); Beth Mauer,

Sherry Pagoto, Brian Ragsdale, and Donna Zaorski (1999–2000); Rodney Benson, Kim Cooper, Caroline King, and Brian Leahy (2000–2001); Sabrina Baril Young, Patricia Espe-Pfeifer, Dawn Lindsey, and Malia Richmond (2001–2002); Alia Ammar, Samer Effarah, Mark Schneider, and Daniel Zomchek (2002–2003); and Beeta Homaifar, Renanah Lehner, Sarah Keedy, Amberly Panepinto, and Anne Wiley (2003–2004). Thank you all for your insights, your curiosity, and your feedback.

Thanks are also due to three supervisors I had in graduate school and internship who taught so much: Marilyn Robie, Ph.D., who encourages confidence and insight so well in her students; Bill Megan, Ph.D., who taught me how to think more clearly about client problems; and Bill McFall, Ed.D., who trusted me to experiment and find my own style.

I'd also like to thank all my colleagues at the Jesse Brown VA Medical Center who have taught me so much over the years, including the library staff, who were so supportive of my many requests.

Thanks to my family for their encouragement and support throughout the years: Judy Abel, John Albright, Ann Willer, Bill Willer, Dave Willer, Fred Willer, Patricia Willer, and Robb Willer.

And finally, I'd like to thank Deb Smith for asking a very important question back in July 2005.

Introduction

I'm afraid that I don't remember either the face or the name of my first client. But I clearly remember getting ready to go into the therapy room to meet her and feeling terrified. I remember sitting down with the client and being wholly preoccupied with my own fears. Despite the best efforts of the teaching faculty, I felt that I didn't know anything when I actually met her—a real live client. I had no idea how to guide the client through the psychotherapy session. I didn't know how to assess the client's problems or prioritize them. And I was utterly unprepared to deal with crises.

That first therapy session scares me even today but for a different reason. I now know much of what I was ignorant of that fateful day in 1986. If the client had a mental illness that is difficult to diagnose, like bipolar disorder or attention-deficit/hyperactivity disorder, I undoubtedly missed it. I didn't know anything about psychotropics, so if she could have benefited from a referral, she didn't get one. If the client came in feeling suicidal, I would have had no idea what to do. I didn't know anything about charting, and who knows what errors I made about what to include and what not to include in the chart. I doubt that anyone, myself included, told the client anything about confidentiality or informed consent. These reasons are why that session scares me now.

Uncertainty, fear, and lack of knowledge can still exist among beginning psychotherapists today. Friends who supervise beginning therapists tell of students coming into their offices and asking, "But what do I *do*?" These students know a lot about theoretical orientations. They have been taught reflective listening skills. They know about legal and ethical issues in psychotherapy. But how to start seeing a client still eludes them because there has been no one source for all the most basic information they need to know before they start seeing clients.

Often, beginning therapists have no idea how to greet a client in the waiting room or what appropriate professional boundaries are. They don't know how to deal with clients on the phone. They may have to screen new clients but not know much about how to make a diagnosis and what disorders are commonly missed. Beginning therapists (like all therapists) have a lot of emotions about doing therapy, but beginners tend to feel bad about having these feelings (Brody & Farber, 1996), and they don't know what to do about them.

Extreme differences in theoretical approaches can leave the beginning therapist confused. However, it is my belief and my hope that we are moving toward theoretical integration and balance. My focus in choosing my references for each chapter was not theoretical orientation—instead, it was clinical utility—and different theoretical approaches have different clinical strengths. I have tried to draw on the strengths of different traditions to integrate them into a whole that will be useful to you.

I'm sure that it is impossible to take away all the fears of beginning therapists. However, I believe that it should be possible for you, the beginning therapist, to feel less confused and uncertain about what to do with your clients. That belief inspired me to write this book.

This is not really a book about how to *do* psychotherapy. Instead, it is a book about how to *start* psychotherapy. My goal in this volume has been to provide a well-rounded review of important topics that any beginning therapist should know *before* seeing a new client. In addition, I have included some material about the emotional complexities of doing psychotherapy for the psychotherapist. Research (Leiter & Harvie, 1996; Pearlman & Mac Ian, 1995; VanDeusen & Way, 2006) has shown that beginning psychotherapists are more often overwhelmed by their emotional reactions, and this is a topic that is not typically addressed in most books about doing psychotherapy.

There are many helpful resources that provide guidance about the complexities of psychotherapy. I have done my best to find and summarize these resources for you. Since this book is only a starting point for your lifelong learning about psychotherapy, I include a list of recommended readings for most chapters.

In many important areas, however, there is little research or professional guidance available. For example, I could hardly find any articles about the attire of health care professionals in general, much less mental health professionals. Almost everyone is strangely silent on providing guidance about how much you can tell your partner, family, and friends about your clinical work, although my utterly unscientific survey suggests that most therapists do talk about their work, at least a little, with their partners. I know that you will wrestle with these issues, so I have done my best to address these topics nonetheless. The afterword lists some questions that, perhaps, future research may answer.

I have supplied a multitude of appendices that I hope will provide guidance in many common but very specific clinical matters. They are not included for you to memorize but instead for your reference as needed. Depending on the population you are working with, you may need some of these appendices now; later, at another training site, others may be more helpful. I have also attempted to introduce you to commonly used professional jargon throughout; these terms are generally in italics. I hope that this book will be a helpful reference for you now and in the future.

Note that none of the therapists or clients in the vignettes contained in this book actually exists as written. Some vignettes are composites, some have been altered to mask all identifying information, and others were made up simply to illustrate a point. Thus, the names of these therapists and clients are in no way meant to describe any real person, living or dead, and any resemblance is purely coincidental.

Because my expertise is with adults, that is the focus of this volume. In addition, I must emphasize that I am not specifying in this book any legal standards of care that all mental health clinicians should be held to, only some guidelines based on current practice at the time this book was written.

As I was writing this book, I had to wrestle with the vastness of the professional literature about many topics. I felt like the proverbial "jack-of-all-trades, master of none." As someone who is not the master of these subject areas, I may have missed important literature on some of these subjects. For that, I apologize in advance. If you, the reader, have some important information I have missed, your kindness in contacting me would be appreciated. I also welcome any comments that readers might have about this volume. Feel free to send them to me in care of my publisher, or you can find me on the Web at www.drwiller.com.

I sincerely hope that my efforts will help you cope with the anxieties and uncertainties that are inherent in becoming a psychotherapist and help you move forward to appreciate the wonderful opportunity you have to make a positive impact on the personal life of another human being.

Section I

THE THERAPIST'S SELF
AND RELATIONSHIPS

Chapter One

The Therapist's Self

The carpenter has a hammer, the surgeon has a scalpel, the therapist has the self.

(Hayes & Gelso, 2001, p. 1041)

You probably had (or have) anxiety, even dread and terror, of your first-ever psychotherapy session. I remember that clearly myself. I knew a decent amount of theory by then, but I had no practical knowledge whatsoever. This first chapter is to help you think about how you will present yourself to the client during that first session, including how to present yourself professionally. I will talk about coping with the anxiety of beginning therapists. I will also discuss some of the changes—in self-concept and those that are interpersonal, cognitive, emotional, behavioral, and even spiritual—that you may experience as you become a psychotherapist.

Being a therapist will change you and accelerate your personal growth. I was at a symposium once, many years ago, about therapist self-care. I remember one of the presenters asking the audience whether becoming therapists had changed them. Everyone in the audience agreed that it had. When he asked us, we also agreed that we had not anticipated this. This process of personal growth and change will be ongoing throughout your career.

YOUR SELF-CONCEPT AS
A MENTAL HEALTH PROFESSIONAL

Carlos Rivera is a mental health trainee. He doesn't care for the stuffy role that he feels he has to assume. He is working in a partial hospitalization program and is assigned to help with socialization of the patients. He plays pool with them and uses curse words when he doesn't make a shot. He chats casually with patients when he is smoking with them outside. He talks about marijuana use in such a way that all the patients think he uses it regularly.

Everyone acts differently in different relationships. For example, you may act differently with your siblings, your parents, your friends, and your teachers. A challenging aspect of becoming a therapist is developing that new element to your personality. You want to be yourself, but, as with other situations you find yourself in, it is a particular version of yourself.

Your therapist self should project professionalism. As you can see from the example of Carlos, some people struggle with this to one degree or another. Eventually, you may see some differences in how you might talk and relate to others as a professional. Hopefully, you will find that your professional self can project a certain quiet authority. This is a normal progression.

INTERPERSONAL CHANGES
AND PROFESSIONAL DEMEANOR

You come to medical school like anyone else [. . . then] things happen that differentiate you from everyone else you know. . . . You ask private and socially inappropriate questions of people, and they answer you. (Montross, 2007, p. 120)

As a mental health professional, you will interact differently with your clients and colleagues than you do with your family and friends. Like the medical students discussed in the previous quote, you will learn to talk openly and matter-of-factly about subjects that many people find distressing, embarrassing, or socially inappropriate. You will learn to ask clients questions that you might never dream of asking anyone else—and you will understand why these questions are necessary.

You will need to balance authenticity and empathy with a certain professional reserve. I recommend that you attempt to integrate an especially respectful and gracious manner with clients into your professional self. You should err on the side of being respectful yet empathetic to the client rather than overly familiar. Being too familiar with a client has a risk of leading to therapeutic boundary crossings (see chapter 4). You will learn not to share many personal details of your life in professional situations (especially with clients—see the section on self-disclosure in chapter 4 for more information). Depending on the client population, consider referring to the client by last name (e.g., Mr. Brown or Ms. Williams), use your best manners, and use "sir" and "ma'am" as appropriate. This type of self-presentation can often help allay client fears of being disrespected. In addition, this will ensure that you are not inadvertently inappropriate or overly familiar to a client from a more traditional cultural background.

Your professional self may be more assertive with professional peers than you would generally be with your friends. Even if you never choose the restaurant when you are going out with friends, your therapist self will need to develop a decisiveness that you can employ for your client's benefit as needed. For example, if you find yourself with a potentially suicidal client, you must be decisive and provide appropriate guidance.

Sometimes beginning therapists complain that they feel that they can't be themselves with clients if they are editing out so much of their own personal material when they talk. I suggest that you be yourself (albeit a somewhat edited version) through your *process* with the client, for example, the questions you ask, how you react, and what you focus on. As McWilliams (2004) states, "Being in a role is not the same thing as playing a role" (p. 53). But you should leave out most of your personal *content*, for example, the details of your personal life.

PRESENTING YOURSELF AS A PROFESSIONAL

Megan Edwards, a mental health trainee, is interviewing with her potential practicum supervisor, Dr. Larry Cook. The practicum entails working with low-functioning schizophrenic clients, primarily in individual and group therapy and more informally in a clubhouse setting. Megan dressed carefully for the interview and feels that she looks great. However, during the interview, Dr. Cook can't help noticing that Megan is wearing 4-inch heels and has a low neckline and that her skirt has ridden high on her thighs when she sat down. He wonders if she understands that the clients are low functioning and have poor impulse control. He is concerned that she will experience uncomfortable and inappropriate remarks from the clients. He also wonders about her professional judgment since her attire seems more sexy than professional. However, he feels uncomfortable bringing up the subject with Megan. Another applicant ends up being matched to the practicum site.

Joshua Collins is a mental health student who has been working in a pain management clinic in a regional medical center in a mostly rural state. He went to college in a major metropolitan area and, like most of his friends, obtained a number of colorful tattoos during that phase of his life. He has prominent tattoos on his left forearm. The temperature is in the 90s, and it is very humid. Up to now, Joshua has been wearing long-sleeved shirts to the clinic. He wears a short-sleeved shirt today. After he interviews an elderly client, the client goes into the physician's office for the rest of her evaluation and tells the doctor that Joshua "looks like a thug."

Business self-help books generally recommend that you look at what your peers and your superiors are wearing and then dress similarly. Thus, observe the licensed mental health practitioners who you know. Also observe other health care professionals in your setting. You should dress as they do.

Generally, more conservative dress is most appropriate (Morrison, 1995). Research has shown that patients prefer their physicians to dress more formally (Lill & Wilkinson, 2005; Menahem & Shvartzman, 1998). In fact, one study found that, at least for physicians, formal attire increased patients' perceptions of their friendliness, trustworthiness, and even attractiveness (Brase & Richmond, 2004). It is reasonable to assume that the same conclusions would apply to mental health care professionals.

Of course, the therapeutic context must be considered when choosing appropriate professional clothing. What a clinician might wear doing case management with the homeless is not what he would wear when doing smoking cessation with businesspeople. A good general guideline is to wear business casual attire when in less formal settings but to consider wearing more formal business attire if you are working in a particularly formal setting, such as a medical center that serves middle- to upper-middle-class patients. In almost all treatment settings, neither men nor women should wear jeans or tennis shoes. Slacks and a collared shirt are generally appropriate for men. More casual slacks such as chinos or corduroy slacks are usually fine.

Female psychotherapists have more wardrobe flexibility. Unfortunately, this means that the possibility of problematic wardrobe choices is greater. A recent research study indicated that women who are dressed in a sexy manner (more makeup, tousled hair, low-cut blouse, tight skirt, and high heels), with high-status jobs, are seen more negatively and as less competent and less intelligent (Glick, Larsen, Johnson, & Branstiter, 2005). While, as psychotherapists, we do not want to cling to negative and/or sexist stereotypes, we also understand that the focus needs to be on our clients' needs rather than our own attire. In summary, it is wise for women to avoid revealing clothes, tight or form-fitting clothes, very high-heeled shoes, and skirts at or above the knee (as they will reveal much more when you sit down).

We also need to consider our clients' potential reactions to clothing choices. Women who work with predominantly male populations, especially populations that may have poorer judgment or poor impulse control, often find that they prefer to minimize their sexual stimulus value. In any setting, certain clothing choices can result in greater therapeutic time spent on the client's sexual attractions to the therapist and less attention to whatever issues may have brought the client to therapy originally. Psychotherapists should never wear perfume or cologne on the job. According to the American Lung Association (2006), many asthmatics are triggered by perfumes, which can precipitate wheezing or an asthma attack. Perfumes can also trigger migraines (R. W. Evans, 2006).

Tattoos and piercings are becoming more common, but they are still considered daring—at best—by many people, such as Joshua's client mentioned previously. Over 80% of human resource managers and recruiters surveyed see persons with tattoos negatively (Swanger, 2006), so prominent tattoos may have a negative impact on your future career. In addition, Newman, Wright, Wrenn, and Bernard (2005) found that emergency department patients saw physicians with facial piercings (nose, eyebrow, or lip) as inappropriate and would decrease their assessment of competence and trustworthiness. The patients were not affected by an earring on a male physician.

If you are a younger therapist, you may have difficulties getting respect from older clients as it is. My informal discussions with other professionals reveal nearly universal opinions that obvious body art is unprofessional. For that reason, I recommend that all tattoos be concealed by clothing and that you not get any new tattoos in any areas that would be bared by business casual clothing in the summer. As for piercings, I would advise no more than two earrings per ear for women and no more than one earring for men. In more conservative areas, or with older populations, men might consider not wearing earrings in professional settings. I would also advise no other obvious piercings, for example, nose or eyebrow. A tongue piercing, especially, would be inappropriate in a therapy setting because of sexual connotations.

COPING WITH ANXIETY

Kendra Hayes, a mental health trainee, is about to have her first session with a client. The clinic coordinator has already done an intake with the client, so Kendra will be starting therapy with the client. She is very anxious and can't help thinking how little she knows. She worries that she won't be able to help the client. She worries that he will see how anxious she is. She fears that her mind will go blank.

Kendra's fears are normal. It is natural to feel anxious when first doing psychotherapy. I hope that you already know how to cope with your own anxiety in other circumstances. Use that knowledge. For example, before a therapy session, you might be able to get in a workout, a walk, meditation, or some deep breathing. Remind yourself that you know how to use active listening skills and that you can be concerned and empathetic; this alone can be healing.

When you feel anxious, try to refocus on how your client will feel during the session. The client will probably be new to therapy and may be worried and fearful about what will happen during therapy. The client may be worried about having a mental illness and how you will react when symptoms are shared with you. The client may be feeling worn down, lonely, and worthless because of extended struggles with problems. The client is probably fearful and concerned about whether you will be understanding and compassionate. The client may be feeling that coming to therapy shows weakness, failure, and lack of character. Your anxiety may, to some extent, be an empathic response to the client's anxiety.

Putting yourself in the client's shoes naturally leads to some conclusions about how to act in the first therapy session. You will want to provide guidance and structure about how the session will go (which will be discussed further in chapter 12) so that the client feels that something can be done to help. You will want to be gracious and respectful so that the client feels respected and worthy. You might want to compliment the client's wisdom or courage in coming to therapy so that the client may begin to think of coming to therapy as showing the strength to face problems head-on. You will want to be empathetic so that the client feels comfortable and nurtured.

Talk to your supervisors and more advanced peers about your concerns. If your anxiety remains distressing, it would be wise to seek therapy for yourself—but I recommend this for all mental health trainees, anyway—as does Yalom (2002), among many others.

COPING WITH CONFUSION

Kevin Alexander, a mental health trainee, meets with his client, Joe Martin. Joe talks about going to the hardware store and feels helpless and tearful when there. This has happened to him several times before at the same hardware store. "What does it mean, doc?" asks Joe. Kevin has no idea. He feels confused and uncertain about how to respond to Joe. Joe is clearly having distress about the issue, and Kevin wants to help right now. Kevin feels that he should be able to come up with a brilliant, insightful interpretation of Joe's distress about the hardware store on the spot, yet he was utterly at a loss. He feels stuck. After a long pause, "What do you think it means?" is what he resorts to. When Kevin later meets with his supervision group, they provide a multitude of interpretations: "He is conflicted about his masculinity." "The tools represent a sense of personal agency, and he has not been able to accomplish what he wanted to in his life." "Going to the hardware store is one of the few times he is away from work and his family; maybe this distress is a sign of underlying depression that he can be distracted from in other settings." "Maybe he was sexually abused in a tool shed." Kevin is more confused than ever.

This example (which is inspired by Kottler, 2003), illustrates some of the confusion that you, the beginning therapist, are likely to feel. Your clients will have personal problems that you feel you should understand and know how to solve, but you don't. Their situations and emotions prompt intense emotions in you, but you don't know how to interpret all these feelings. Sometimes you will feel so stumped in therapy sessions that you may not even know what to say. If your mind feels "blank" during a session, one helpful strategy is to summarize what the client has just been telling you.

The good news is that as you learn more, you will feel less confused and have more of an idea about how to work with your clients, understand their problems, and manage all the emotions in the room. Here's a little secret: You don't have to know all the answers. It's okay to not know what something means and even to admit that to your client. You and the client can use the process of therapy to figure it out. Thus, Kevin could have said this to Joe, "Joe, I don't know what your feelings in the hardware store are about, but I'm sure that if we continue to explore it together, we will figure it out."

COPING WITH SELF-DOUBT AND FEELINGS OF INADEQUACY

Brittany Hall is a mental health trainee at her first training placement. She is seeing Whitney Clark, a 34-year-old single mother of four. Whitney is in transitional housing with her children and is struggling to maintain her 90-day abstinence from alcohol. She is in therapy for depression and post-traumatic stress disorder (PTSD) and is attending job retraining courses. Whitney relocated to the city she lives in now after a natural disaster destroyed her uninsured home and all her personal possessions. Brittany is impressed by Whitney's strength of character and dedication to her children in the face of so many personal difficulties. She doubts how she, a 22-year-old single woman from a relatively privileged background, can help Whitney.

At the start of the year, in his opening speech, an associate dean warned us that we would each feel ill-equipped at times over the course of these years, that we would wonder whether we are up to the challenge, whether we belong. But when these moments of intellectual disorientation and feelings of inadequacy overtake us, we are nonetheless unprepared. We know we are fraudulent. We see that our peers are not struggling in the same ways. Other students ask us to explain things to them, which we do. But we think that those are the easy things, the concepts they would figure out in another second on their own. I think, "It is this really tough stuff, which they are breezing through, that I simply cannot comprehend." (Montross, 2007, p. 145)

What he or she [the client] does in terms of changing in therapy is not an index of whether I'm doing my job right or not ... sometimes when I do things very very well, the patient doesn't change at all. Other times I might be doing a half-assed job and the patient, because of being in a very good space, picks up whenever I'm into, adds a great deal of his or her own stuff and makes excellent progress, from his or her point of view. I find that to do the best work, I have to free myself from anxiety about the results. A kind of Karma yoga position, I guess. So the change is partly more respect for the patient, less arrogance about myself and more detachment about what's going on. (Kopp, 1977, p. 6)

As a beginning therapist, you are likely to struggle often with feelings of inadequacy and incompetence, and experienced therapists can suffer from these feelings as well (Betan, Heim, Conklin, & Westen, 2005). You wonder whether your clients will get better, and you fear that they will not improve. You may feel that the client's improvement is your responsibility. This feeling of being responsible for the client can get out of hand and feel overwhelming; when it does, consider carefully what Dr. Kopp stated previously.

As the therapist, your responsibility is doing the best job being a therapist you possibly can, given where you are emotionally, physically, and cognitively that particular day. If your client is not getting better, it is your responsibility to seek greater insight into how to help her. We should strive to do the best we can with each client and to solve any therapeutic roadblocks that arise. But, at the same time, it is not your responsibility to make the client "get better." No one can do that but the client herself.

COPING WITH CLIENTS' SUFFERING

Jesse Blackhawk is a mental health trainee working at a center that treats survivors of torture. Jesse's client endured 2 years of jail and torture before being released and then sponsored to come to the United States by relatives here. Before his incarceration, Jesse's client, a journalist, was under house arrest for 5 years and feared for his life every day. The client suffers from severe nightmares every night, hypervigilance, and lack of trust. The client admits to hoarding food at home, even though he knows that his relatives would never let him go hungry. Jesse feels overwhelmed by the pain of his client's suffering. He is starting to have religious doubts. He wonders how his faith can explain why innocent, well-meaning people, such as his client, endure such terrible suffering.

Helping others with their suffering is not easy. Even experienced therapists can feel overwhelmed by their clients (Betan et al., 2005). Coping with clients' suffering is a complex emotional, cognitive, and spiritual task. The feeling of being overwhelmed is often an indication that you are being particularly empathetic to the client; almost certainly if you are feeling overwhelmed, the client is feeling the same thing. Knowing that this feeling emanates from your empathetic response to the client can help you cope with it: first, by reflecting the feeling back; and, second, by knowing that even though you and the client may feel overwhelmed right now, that does not mean that the situation is actually hopeless. Reevaluating the situation cognitively can help both you and the client escape from the trap of feeling overwhelmed.

Your client may have experienced many horrible life events: child abuse, torture, rape, domestic violence, and more. These can result in great suffering. Witnessing this pain is not easy. Treating clients with PTSD can result in you developing vicarious traumatization (see more on this topic in chapter 23). You may start to wonder about this pain from a spiritual perspective. If you think that may be likely, you may wish to begin the process of seeking a deepened spiritual understanding of suffering.

RECOMMENDED READING

Kaner, A., & Prelinger, E. (2005). *The craft of psychodynamic psychotherapy*. New York: Jason Aronson.
The authors provide much helpful advice on how to address common therapeutic challenges experienced by beginning therapists.
Kottler, J. A. (2003). *On being a therapist* (3rd ed.). San Francisco: Jossey-Bass.
Written for the beginning therapist, Kottler gives examples of the personal and professional struggles of a psychotherapist.
Yalom, I. (2002). *The gift of therapy: An open letter to a new generation*. New York: HarperPerennial.
While you may or may not agree with some of Yalom's thoughts about treatment and the therapeutic relationship, he thinks carefully and deeply about these issues. His insights will help your own thought process move to the next level.

EXERCISES AND DISCUSSION QUESTIONS

1. What coping strategies can you use to cope with the suffering of your clients?
2. How do various religious and humanist traditions explain and address suffering?
3. What other feelings, besides anxiety and self-doubt, do you anticipate being problematic when you first see clients?

Chapter Two

The Supervisor–Supervisee Relationship

Your relationships with your psychotherapy supervisors will be some of the most important professional relationships of your career. Your supervisors will guide you in the process of becoming an independent mental health professional. My goal in this chapter is to orient you to the process of supervision. I also discuss some cases in which supervision goes awry and make recommendations about how to cope.

THE SUPERVISION MEETING

Your supervisor's goal is to help you improve your clinical skills. You will discuss how you are working with your client. In the course of these discussions, you may listen to audiotapes of the sessions, watch videotapes, or just report what has happened during the session in summary form. Your supervisor will help you understand the client and formulate effective interventions. Depending on your supervisor's theoretical orientation, you may focus more on dynamic issues, such as transference and countertransference, or you might focus more on progressing through particular behavioral and cognitive tasks that would assist your client. Unless you are adhering to a strict treatment protocol, your supervisor will generally not tell you exactly what to do in each session. Instead, he or she will help you discuss a number of interventions and interpretations that you can use with the client as appropriate in upcoming sessions.

Your supervisor may also assist you with your professional development. Supervision meetings are an appropriate forum to discuss concerns, worries, or frustrations that you may have with clinical work or agency bureaucracy. Some supervisors may take a mentoring role with you, so you can discuss career and professional issues, as needed, with them.

THE SUPERVISOR'S RESPONSIBILITIES

The first job of your new supervisor is to help orient you to your clinical work at the site. Your supervisor will guide you to learn about the clients' presenting problems and diagnoses at the site. Your supervisor will help you learn to navigate the administrative structure of the site and introduce you to other staff you need to know. Your supervisor will educate you about the necessary documentation. Ask for help and information anytime you need to know about any of these topics. I have summarized a number of the questions that you might want to ask your supervisor when you begin at a new site in appendix 1.

You and your supervisor will fulfill some requirements regarding the number of supervision hours that you meet per week. Your supervisor will give you a set time for supervision every week. The supervisor will set this time aside and not let other matters encroach. Unless a client is having an emergency, your supervisor should not answer the phone, respond to e-mail, or be otherwise distracted and unfocused during the supervision hour. Additionally, your supervisor should be available for "spot supervision" as needed between meetings and will let you know who will provide backup supervision if you have a client crisis when he or she is not available or not in the office.

An effective supervisor establishes a climate of trust and honesty (Walker & Jacobs, 2004). Good supervisors are supportive, instructional, interpretive, collegial, and respectful (L. A. Gray, Ladany, Walker, & Ancis, 2001). Your supervisor may talk about his or her own experience with clinical challenges, and what the impact and lessons of these challenges were.

THE SUPERVISEE'S RESPONSIBILITIES: GETTING THE MOST FROM SUPERVISION

Your approach to supervision will influence how much you grow as a psychotherapist (Berger & Buchholz, 1993). Your supervisor is more experienced than you are and will identify issues that you missed. This is normal. Try not to be defensive about it. Few things are more difficult for a supervisor to cope with than defensiveness in a supervisee. Be open to suggestions and new ways of conceptualizing your clients' problems.

Show your supervisor that you are responsible and motivated. Be on time to supervision meetings. If you have to cancel or reschedule a meeting, contact your supervisor well in advance. Think about what clinical issues you would like to discuss with your supervisor and be prepared with questions. If your supervisor has asked you to review your audiotapes or videotapes before the session, do that. Be sure you have finished any reading that was assigned. Write a draft of your progress notes before the supervision meeting so that your supervisor can see them and cosign them during the meeting. Complete any other paperwork that your supervisor needs to see for the work you have done that week. Finish your paperwork at the site on a timely basis so that your supervisor does not have to ask you about it. Keep in mind that you might want to ask your supervisor for letters of reference for you in the future.

When you first start out, your supervisor is likely to want a brief summary of the progress of each client during the supervisory session. You may need some guidance with each client on a weekly basis. As your skills increase, you and your supervisor can devote more time to focusing more closely on any clinical interactions or concerns that you might have with a particular client. Talk to your supervisor about how to allocate time between discussion, tapes, review of progress notes, and other tasks during the supervisory hour.

Be proactive about your learning process. If you recognize that you need to learn more about relevant clinical issues, ask your supervisor to recommend readings. Increasing your knowledge will help allay your anxieties about becoming a competent psychotherapist. Be open to learning about clinical work from different theoretical perspectives. Learn how to apply research findings to clinical practice while maintaining the flexibility to tailor the treatment to the needs of each particular client.

Try not to be rejecting if your supervisor gives you some difficult feedback. Instead, agree to think about it, then discuss the issue with friends, classmates, mentors, your therapist, and/or any other persons you think could give you a helpful perspective. However, later, after you have given the issue sufficient thought and gotten feedback from others, if you feel that your supervisor is wrong, discuss the issue again and ask for further clarification.

HAVE REALISTIC EXPECTATIONS OF YOURSELF

Graduate students can be perfectionistic and want to do well in all their endeavors. However, the reality is that you will need much coaching and support before you are an effective independently practicing psychotherapist. Your supervisor knows that you will be anxious about starting a new clinical experience. Your supervisor is aware of your level of training and does not expect you to completely understand how to implement therapeutic techniques that you have not yet used. Ask questions that will help you understand the clinical setting and the client population and, hence, that will allay your concerns.

Try to have realistic expectations for yourself. A good student will not be a flawless psychotherapist (and, in fact, no one is a flawless psychotherapist). Instead, as a good student, you will be open to learning, sincere, hardworking, and accepting of your limitations. It will help if you realize that as long as your skills are commensurate with your experience, you are doing fine. It is unrealistic to expect to be an excellent therapist immediately. However, with good supervision, you will be competent, which is good enough.

You will make clinical errors, and you need to accept the inevitability of this. Some of the vignettes in the volume were inspired by clinical errors that either I or other professionals and trainees have made. Generally these will be minor errors of empathy, insight, and so on. In almost all cases, your clients will survive these minor errors just fine. The caring and rapport between you and your clients will carry you through most rough spots. When you think you may have made an error, bring the issue up with your supervisor and/or play the audiotape of this section of the session. If you were confused as to what to do, talk to your supervisor. A good supervisor will respect you for identifying your clinical challenges and for wanting to work on them.

If you realize that you have made a more serious error, find your supervisor and talk it over immediately. For example, perhaps your client was much more depressed, but you did not think to ask if he was feeling suicidal. Your supervisor can help you sort out the problem in a timely manner.

EVALUATIONS

You are probably anxious about being evaluated by your supervisor. This is normal. Perhaps learning more about the evaluation process will help allay your fears. Your supervisor can show you the evaluation forms; just ask if you are curious. Whenever you would like feedback about your progress from your supervisor, ask for it.

Often students suffer silently, worrying that they might get a bad evaluation. However, no student should ever reach the end of a training experience and be surprised by a poor evaluation. Instead, if at any time your supervisor thinks that you are having difficulties, the supervisor should work out a remediation plan with you so that you have a chance to work more intensively and improve in time to get a better evaluation.

PERSONAL ISSUES IN SUPERVISION

Amanda Nakamura, a 28-year-old mental health trainee, had just experienced the prolonged and painful death of her father. One medical issue had led to another, and her father had been on a ventilator for 3 months, before dying. Their relationship had been very close. The whole process had been very traumatic for all involved, and her father died only a week before the start of her next clinical placement. Amanda calls the training director to let him know about this. After some discussion, they agree that she will not be working with high-risk clients to start and that she will not be assigned any clients with loss issues until she feels she is ready.

James Green, a 24-year-old social work intern, is devastated. He learned that he did not get the scholarship he had applied for. He discusses this issue with his supervisor and is very self-critical. The supervisor attempts to point out that these decisions are very subjective and that James is an excellent student nonetheless. James continues to verbalize harsh self-criticism. The supervisor suggests that psychotherapy could help James cope with his perfectionism. James insists that he does not need therapy and is offended at the suggestion. They do not discuss it again.

One of your supervisor's responsibilities is to help you become more self-aware by recognizing when your personal issues are negatively impacting the therapeutic process (Vasquez, 1992) and your professional development. The student in the first example is already demonstrating her self-knowledge, and she is using it effectively. Amanda is setting realistic expectations for herself by recognizing her own emotional distress and how it could negatively impact on client care. She has ethically taken appropriate steps to address this by contacting the training director.

Your supervisor will not and should not be your therapist. However, personal issues inevitably will affect your work and your professional development, and these personal issues may arise in supervision. In order to preserve appropriate boundaries, while continuing to ensure your professional growth, your supervisor may recommend that you discuss the details of your personal issues with a therapist. Even if you cannot understand why your supervisor recommends therapy or you disagree, personal therapy is still beneficial for any mental health trainee, if for no other reason than it gives you a greater understanding of your clients.

SUPERVISOR–SUPERVISEE BOUNDARIES

Jenna Harris is a mental health trainee who feels very comfortable with her supervisor, Jaqui Robinson, who is actually the same age as Jenna. They are both single, heterosexual women. Jenna asks Jaqui to go out to drinks and dinner with her. They do so and enjoy each other's company but at the same time feel awkward. Next week, they both realize and agree that they should not do this again while they still have a professional relationship.

Your relationship with your supervisor should be supportive and collegial. Your supervisor may be friendly and interested in your professional development. You might have lunch or coffee at work sometimes, or your supervisor may invite you and your fellow students out for lunch or dinner once or twice. All these are appropriate interactions.

On occasion, supervisees and supervisors become friends after the supervision is over. However, it is not appropriate for supervisors and supervisees to have an intimate friendship while supervision is ongoing. So supervisors and supervisees should not engage in friendship activities, such as one-on-one social outings, while supervision is ongoing or if supervision is expected to resume. They should not engage in any joint business ventures. And it is unethical for a supervisor and supervisee to have a romantic or sexual relationship (Vasquez, 1992).

SUPERVISOR–SUPERVISEE MATCHING

Lisa Anderson, a mental health trainee, is meeting with her supervisor. The supervisor has a psychodynamic orientation, while Lisa's training program trained her in cognitive-behavioral interventions exclusively. Lisa is having difficulty understanding her supervisor's reasoning when he suggests that she interpret the client's transference. Lisa feels that the client's maladaptive cognitions are the best place to start therapy.

Sometimes you might feel that there is a poor match between you and your supervisor, as Lisa does. Or you may feel poorly matched temperamentally. Research indicates that psychology interns who are matched with a theoretically compatible supervisor are often happier with how supervision goes (Putney, Worthington, & McCullough, 1992). However, differences can be an opportunity for mutual learning and growth. Try to be open to the different perspectives and new insights that the supervisor brings to your clinical work.

You may wish to talk to someone you trust to get feedback about working more effectively with your supervisor. Get advice from someone who is knowledgeable, discreet, and practical. If there is someone with your graduate program that you feel comfortable talking to, this would be a good choice since someone in your academic program will then know that you proactively addressed the issue. Discuss the situation with your consultant in a nonblaming, nonjudgmental manner. Ask for honest feedback and practical suggestions for working more effectively with your supervisor.

Try to consider all options. Perhaps your expectations were too unrealistic, and you need to refocus on learning what the supervisor has to teach. Perhaps you may have some emotional issues that need to be addressed in therapy. Perhaps a different supervisor would be more helpful to you.

COPING WITH THE DISENGAGED SUPERVISOR

Rebecca Goldberg is worried about her supervision. She talks to her supervisor on a weekly basis for an hour about her cases. Sometimes during supervision, he closes his eyes and appears to be napping. At times, he has even snored. She has no idea what to do during these times, so she just continues to talk about what she has done with the clients until he appears more alert.

Marcus White is worried about his supervision. He likes his supervisor and finds him helpful when they do meet. He has supervision scheduled on a weekly basis, but the supervisor is often late, cancels at the last minute, or just does not show up. Then on some weeks, the supervisor is out of the office on other business and makes no arrangements for backup supervision coverage.

These vignettes describe supervisors who are not meeting their responsibilities. As in these examples, the supervisor may be inattentive or unavailable. Or the supervisor may not be timely in assisting with paperwork or reports. The supervisor may not make arrangements for supervision coverage when absent.

If you have a supervisor who is not meeting responsibilities, you should address this as tactfully as possible with the supervisor first. Rebecca might ask if they could talk about the process of supervision, and then say, "I'm noticing that you seem a little sleepy during some of our supervision sessions. Would it be possible to move the supervision to another time that works better for you?" Marcus might state, "I really appreciate your insights about my work with my clients, but I'm realizing that you haven't been able to meet with me every week. I feel that I really need weekly supervision. Would it be possible for us to work out some way to meet more regularly on a weekly basis?" If your efforts are not successful, you should consider bringing this problem to the attention of your academic program and/or the staff member who is in charge of training at the facility.

COPING WITH THE INAPPROPRIATE SUPERVISOR

India Turner is worried about her supervisory relationship. She has moved from New York City to a southern state. Her supervisor tells her that she would look much more attractive if she didn't wear as much black and if she got rid of those "ugly glasses." He tells her that he wonders whether wearing black means she's depressed. India thinks that her wardrobe is chic, and she wonders why her supervisor thinks it is appropriate to tell her how to dress more attractively.

The example of India's supervisor illustrates inappropriately critical remarks on the part of the supervisor, coupled with poor boundaries. The supervisor should not be critiquing India's wardrobe unless she is dressing unprofessionally, nor should he be advising her on what would be most attractive. Depending on her assessment of the situation, India could consider waiting to see whether this was a one-time slip on the part of the supervisor. Depending on the quality of their relationship, she might consider discussing the remarks with the supervisor. Alternatively, she might prefer consulting with a trusted faculty member at her academic program and/or the training supervisor at the site. Depending on what happens subsequently in the supervisory relationship, she might consider asking for a different supervisor.

COPING WITH THE INCOMPETENT SUPERVISOR

Jessica Hill is worried about her supervision. She is working with a client who has presented with depression. The client has a history of closed head injury during a car accident a few years ago and has amnesia for the accident. The client has not been able to get her life back in order and seems unable to work. Jessica's supervisor insists on doing a structured relaxation protocol with the client. Jessica asks whether she should talk to the client about her depression. The supervisor replies, "Why would we want to open that can of worms?"

Brandon Adams is worried about his supervision. He is working with a gay high school teacher who has not come out to his colleagues or family. His supervisor is a strict Catholic. The supervisor's first question about the client is, "Is he sexually abusing any of the kids at his school?" Brandon is offended and sees that his supervisor holds uninformed and damaging misconceptions about gays. The supervisor goes on to insist that Brandon ask about guilt when Brandon feels that the client's primary issues revolve around coming out to his family.

In both vignettes, the supervisees are struggling with supervisors who have inadequate knowledge and/or skill to address the clients' issues. Jessica can see that the supervisor is fearful of addressing the client's depression. In addition, neither Jessica nor the supervisor has sufficient clinical knowledge to realize that the client's problems may be due in large part to brain injury. However, Jessica recognizes that the supervisor's clinical competence is very limited and not sufficient to assist her with this client. Brandon's supervisor is remarkably ignorant; he also is incompetent to address the particular case at hand.

When you are worried that the supervisor is not sufficiently competent, this problem is too large for you to address on your own with the supervisor. You may wish to discuss this issue first with a trusted older colleague or friend. However, it is essential that you bring this problem to the attention of faculty in your academic program. They should assist you in bringing it to the attention of the staff member who is in charge of training at the facility. These individuals should provide you with a different supervisor immediately, and they should take appropriate action to address the supervisor's deficits.

COPING WITH THE CULTURALLY INCOMPETENT SUPERVISOR

Joanie Stewart is worried about her supervision. She is working with an older lesbian woman who was a nurse in Vietnam during the war. Joanie is a lesbian as well. The client's presenting problem is panic disorder. Joanie asks the client whether she suffered discrimination or sexual harassment in the military. The client changes the subject. Joanie then asks about the client's relationships while in the military, and the client changes the subject again. When processing the session afterward, Joanie's supervisor (who is aware of Joanie's sexual orientation) criticizes her for bringing up these subjects, saying, "These lesbian issues aren't the point here. Why do you need to go there?" Joanie feels criticized and attacked.

Joanie's supervisor, unfortunately, is being both critical and culturally incompetent. Also, both of these issues are not "lesbian issues." A helpful supervisory intervention would have been to help Joanie explore why the client avoided discussing these issues in therapy. Joanie understands that a more detailed understanding of the client's history can help put the current anxiety symptoms in context, but she was unable to elicit this information.

Mental health trainees who belong to minority groups of all kinds can have negative experiences in supervision. In a recent qualitative study, *all* the supervisees of color in a small sample had experienced a culturally unresponsive event in supervision, while more than *half* of European American supervisees had as well (Burkard, Johnson et al., 2006). In another recent qualitative study, Constantine and Sue (2007) cataloged seven types of racial microaggressions that Black supervisees experienced from White supervisors. These included invalidating racial-cultural issues brought up by the supervisee, making stereotypical assumptions about Black clients, offering culturally insensitive treatment recommendations, and blaming clients of color for problems stemming from oppression. Difficulties between the supervisor and supervisee included making stereotypical assumptions about the Black supervisee, focusing primarily on the supervisee's clinical weaknesses (giving the impression they thought the supervisee was incompetent), or seeming reluctant to give sufficient constructive feedback (probably for fear of being seen as racist). Unfortunately, many supervisors have little training in multicultural issues, while many supervisees are much more knowledgeable.

Depending on her assessment of the supervisor's openness to feedback, Joanie might give the supervisor feedback on his handling of the supervision session. However, Joanie might prefer getting input from her academic program and/or the training supervisor at the site about how to address this supervision problem.

COPING WITH THE IMPAIRED SUPERVISOR

Michael Bell is worried about his supervision. His supervisor at the community mental health center is likable. But the supervisor talks so much about the helpfulness of Valium that Michael wonders whether she is addicted. The supervisor also has employed a former client who comes to her home and types up her psychological reports from her handwritten notes. Michael knows this former client and is aware that he has borderline traits.

M. V. Ellis (2001) suggests that supervisees be aware of their rights and responsibilities as well as the rights and wrongs of supervision so that they can seek help if they need it. In the case of Michael, the supervisor may be impaired through prescription drug abuse and clearly has impaired judgment as well. The supervisor clearly has violated appropriate boundaries with patients, used poor judgment, and violated patient confidentiality. This is an example of a supervisor who is engaging in professional misconduct. Michael should not address the issue directly with the supervisor. Instead, he should discuss his concerns with an appropriate authority and request a different supervisor.

THE PRODUCTIVE SUPERVISORY RELATIONSHIP

Rob Martinez, a mental health trainee, looks forward to his supervisory meetings with his supervisor, DeAngelo Williams. Rob feels supported by DeAngelo and appreciates hearing about the struggles that DeAngelo has had with his own clients. He feels that DeAngelo is interested in his ideas about how to work with his clients, and DeAngelo has a way of giving input that helps Rob enhance his own ideas and make them more workable. When Rob is confused, he finds that DeAngelo has a way of talking about clinical work that cuts through his confusion and clarifies the situation. Rob feels comfortable in the supervisory relationship and knows that he can count on DeAngelo to be there for him and his clients.

Vivian Medina, a mental health trainee, feels supported by her supervisor, Marianne Bishop. Vivian has had some struggles in her personal and professional life since starting graduate school. Marianne has been a mentor to Vivian and has provided her with invaluable professional advice, in addition to helpful supervision with Vivian's clients. Vivian and Marianne have had many discussions about challenging transference and countertransference issues. When Marianne suggests that Vivian seek therapy, Vivian knows that Marianne wants the best for her. While some of these discussions have been difficult, Vivian does not feel judged; instead she feels that Marianne has supported and mentored her.

As a beginning therapist, you will be anxious, and you need to be able to talk about these feelings with your supervisor. Some of the work you do with your clients may be "sensitive and challenging, and sometimes painful and difficult" (Walker & Jacobs, 2004, p. 13). Your relationship with your supervisor must be solid and supportive for you to be able to develop confidence in difficult clinical situations.

Give the supervisory relationship some time to grow and develop. Try to be appreciative of the strengths of your supervisor. Not every supervisor will be a good mentor, but he or she may still have helpful knowledge to impart to you that will help you grow as a professional. Even within an overall good supervisory relationship, counterproductive events can occur (L. A. Gray et al., 2001). It is hoped that some of the examples in this chapter will help you decide whether to address these directly at the time or try to let the mistake go—since we can all make mistakes.

RECOMMENDED READING

Berger, S. S., & Buchholz, E. S. (1993). On becoming a supervisee: Preparation for learning in a supervisory relationship. *Psychotherapy, 30*, 86–92.
   The authors talk about appropriate education for supervisees who are beginning the supervisory process. As the supervisee, this article will inform you about important yet more advanced supervision topics, such as stages of development and parallel process.

Constantine, M. G., & Sue, D. W. (2007). Perceptions of racial microaggressions among black supervisees in cross-racial dyads. *Journal of Counseling Psychology, 54*, 142–153.
   Constantine and Sue use qualitative research methods to study adverse supervisory events experienced by Black psychotherapy trainees.

EXERCISES AND DISCUSSION QUESTIONS

1. How could you work productively with a supervisor who is competent but is a mismatch with you in terms of temperament?
2. What if you and the supervisor are not matched in theoretical orientation?
3. What policies and procedures does your academic program have if you have supervisory difficulties? How could you address this kind of problem effectively and appropriately?

Chapter Three

The Therapeutic Frame

The *therapeutic frame* is a term drawn from psychodynamic literature, which likens the therapy to a painting (A. Gray, 1994). With a painting, the frame defines where the artwork begins and ends. With therapy, the *therapeutic frame* defines how, where, and when the therapy begins and ends. So the therapeutic frame refers to the structure of the session, including the location, frequency, duration, and charge for the sessions as well as what happens if the client misses or cancels any appointments. The therapeutic frame gives the client a stable structure for therapy.

When we consider the therapeutic frame, we also can think about when we are *not* doing therapy, for example, during routine phone calls, over e-mail, and so on. We do our utmost to keep therapy out of these instances where it does not belong (in chapter 6, client–therapist e-mail issues are covered). We never do therapy with adults in inappropriate locations, such as restaurants, bars, social events, and so on.

However, in rare instances, we might consider a home visit if the client has prolonged physical illness, or we might visit a client in the hospital if ill (Gutheil & Gabbard, 1993). In addition, behavioral treatment of phobias could appropriately involve meeting in an elevator, plane, or other phobic locations. Gutheil and Gabbard (1993) counsel that "the existence of a body of professional literature, a clinical rationale, and risk-benefit documentation will be useful in protecting the clinician in such a situation from misconstruction of the therapeutic efforts" (p. 192).

THERAPIST'S RESPONSIBILITIES TO
MAINTAIN THE THERAPEUTIC FRAME

To maintain the therapeutic frame, you have certain basic responsibilities. You must be on time for the scheduled therapy appointments, and you must not forget appointment times. Of course, none of us is perfect, so if you do forget a session, apologize, discuss the impact of this on the client as needed, and move on. However, if you find yourself forgetting more than one therapy appointment per year, you should talk to your supervisor to devise a better system to keep track of your responsibilities. Similarly, if you are running late, apologize, discuss the impact on the client as needed, and move on. If you find yourself running late for over 5% of your appointments, you should discuss this with your supervisor and address your lateness issue proactively.

Do not answer phone calls or pages during a psychotherapy session. The session belongs to the client, and you should not be distracted. However, in rare instances, you may be expecting an emergency call—in this case, inform the client at the outset of the session. If the emergency call comes though, allow additional time at the end of the client's session or reschedule another session the same week at no charge (paragraph informed by Gabbard, 2000a).

THE OFFICE ENVIRONMENT

Your office can tell a lot about you; "visual cues available in the therapist's office speak abundantly of the character of the occupant through the order or disorder of the office contents, the expression of taste—or lack of it—in the décor, and the comfort or discomfort of the furnishings" (Gutheil & Gabbard, 1998, p. 412). As a beginning therapist, you may have little control over the actual furnishings of the office. However, be aware that your clients may look at your office and draw conclusions about you from what they see.

In a review of the very limited research on the psychotherapist's office, Pressly and Heesacker (2001) recommend that the clinician personalize the office with artwork focusing in nature or animals (preferably not posters) and plants (if appropriate to the environment). Comfortable furniture, rugs, and nonfluorescent lighting are recommended. Soft surfaces help to reduce office noise. If the client is seated on an easily movable chair or a couch, she can moderate the interpersonal space between the two of you to a comfortable distance; these distances typically vary between individuals and cultures. Of course, the office should be handicapped accessible whenever possible. See chapter 20 for recommendations concerning safety issues and your office. Finally, I recommend avoiding potpourri, scented candles, and so on because of potential client allergies.

ATTENDANCE POLICIES

Cancellation and No-Show Policy
If you need to cancel, please call at least 24 hours ahead.
Cancellation fees are as follows:

- *24 hours or more: No fee*
- *Less than 24 hours: $100 fee*
- *If you do not show up for your appointment and do not call, there is a $100 fee as well.*

Special Circumstances or Emergencies: If you have a crisis or illness and can't attend your appointment, call me, and we will talk about it.
My signature below shows that I understand and agree to comply with the cancellation policy.

As a beginning therapist, you will probably be first working at an agency. The agency is likely to have a policy in place regarding clients canceling or not showing up for sessions. You need to know what that policy is and to be sure that the client has been informed of it in writing or verbally prior to or during the first session.

In a private practice setting, a policy, such as the one quoted previously, might be given to the client to sign as part of the intake materials filled out prior to the first session. As recommended by Gans and Counselman (1996), this policy sets clear guidelines that the session fee is to be paid in case of absence but that the psychotherapist is willing to have some flexibility as well.

CLIENT NO-SHOWS

Tom Johnson lives with his mother and has schizophrenia. Tom is low functioning, and he tends to be disorganized. He has again missed his regular appointment with his therapist this month. He is pleasant and engaged when he is in the office. Tom's therapist calls and talks with Tom about attending his next appointment. He asks Tom if it is okay to talk to Tom's mother and ask her to help him with his appointment time. Tom says yes and hands the phone to his mother. She agrees to help Tom remember to attend his next appointment.

Greg Campbell is a high-functioning client who has dropped out of therapy on two previous occasions per his self-report. He does not show up at his weekly psychotherapy appointment. Lately, he has been canceling more frequently. Greg's therapist knows that he is not a high-risk client and realizes he may be dropping out again. The therapist leaves a message about the missed appointment on Greg's cell phone and requests that Greg call. When he doesn't call within a week, the case is closed.

Do not take no-shows personally; they happen to every therapist with every population, at least occasionally. Give the client 15 minutes to be late for the session, then call. If the client does not pick up, you might leave a message like this:

> "Hi Tom, this is [therapist name], and I'm calling you at 2:15 Thursday afternoon. I'm calling because I had you down for an appointment at 2:00 today. Perhaps we had a miscommunication or you are running late. Can you give me a call about this soon? Thanks so much. Goodbye."

If you reach the client, just ask,

> "Hi Tom, this is [therapist name]. How are you? I'm calling because I had you down for an appointment at 2 this afternoon. Is that what you had?"

Of course, you must document the no-show in the client's chart along with whatever phone calls or other activities you did to address it. Note, however, that some supervisors will advise that you not call high-functioning clients who have no-showed; discuss this issue with your supervisor. If you have many no-shows with several of your clients, it may be helpful to discuss rapport building with your supervisor.

If the client does not show up or call, consult with your supervisor about what the next step should be. Depending on the clinic policies, the risk level of the client, and the functioning level of the client, you might close the case after waiting a week or so, you might make another outreach call, or you might send a letter—with or without another appointment time.

You should never let the client develop an expectation that you will be waiting at the next regularly scheduled appointment time after a no-show. If you have a hunch that the client might show up next week, even after this week's no-show, you might leave another phone message:

> "Hi Tom, this is [therapist name]. I need to let you know that I can't hold your appointment for next Thursday unless I hear from you by Monday. Please let me know what you would like to do."

CLIENT CANCELLATIONS

Juan Martinez is a mental health trainee. His client, Melinda Fox, has problems with chronic pain. He has been working with her on relaxation tech-

niques and coping skills that she can use to increase her functional ability and her activity level. The client keeps canceling her appointments. She often cancels at the last minute, stating that she has medical appointments—that she has probably known about for weeks. Or she leaves a vague message that she "isn't feeling well" today. Juan feels that she is not respectful of the time that he has dedicated to her therapy on a weekly basis. He is aggravated and resentful about these frequent cancellations. Clearly, he thinks, other matters are more important to the client than her psychotherapy or treating her therapist with respect. Juan discusses the issue with his supervisor, who suggests that he broach the issue with the client nonjudgmentally. At the next session, Juan states, "Melinda, I'm noticing that you've canceled your appointments several times over the past 2 months. It seems that you've been having a lot of health problems. I'm concerned about how this is affecting you. Can you tell me about that?"

Do not be concerned about an occasional cancellation. Clients vary. Some attend very regularly and never cancel except for extreme emergencies. However, others cancel at the last minute all too frequently. When you've gotten a cancellation message, return the call, let the client know that you got the message, and remind the client of the next appointment time. Gans and Counselman (1996) recommend that any symbolic or emotional issues about the canceled session be addressed in the next session prior to talking about any fees due.

Try not to be concerned if your client has canceled for the first time. However, make a note of the cancellation in the chart, along with the circumstances around it, specifically, what the excuse was and how much notice was given (e.g., 1 hour or 2 days). If canceling becomes a pattern, it will be helpful to have these notes to review later.

If you have a client like Juan's, you will need to address the frequent cancellations in therapy. It is likely that this will be a fruitful avenue of inquiry, informing you about some of the dysfunction in the client's life as well as giving you and the client an opportunity to address it and reduce the number of cancellations.

If the client is canceling frequently (at least one session in three), there is a good chance that the client is thinking of dropping out of therapy. When you suspect this, do not hesitate to comment on it:

"I'm worried that you are having some mixed feelings about therapy since I see you so irregularly. Can you talk to me about that?"

If several of your clients are canceling frequently, discuss this issue in supervision. Your supervisor may have some insight into any issues that you may have with building effective therapeutic relationships with the clients.

CLIENT SHOWS UP LATE

Kimberly Shaheen is a high-functioning client who has bipolar disorder. She tends to run off to her appointments after spending extra time winding up things at work. She speeds to the session in rush-hour traffic and always arrives distracted and late. After problem solving about when to leave work has not solved the problem, her therapist, Michelle Park, asks her about the lateness at the beginning of the session: "Kimberly, I'm noticing that you are still having problems with being late, even though we moved our appointment time back. I'm guessing you might have this problem in other areas of your life. How is that affecting you?" Later in the session, Michelle expresses concern that Kimberly has not been able to prioritize her health highly.

Lateness can be a rare event with a particular client, or it can be part of a pattern. In most cases, if the client is late, you should still end the session at the usual time. Extend the time only if you believe that the lateness is a fluke, you won't be late for the next client, and you aren't at all pressed for time. Be aware that if you extend the session, you may set up unrealistic expectations that you will extend the session every time the client shows up late. These unrealistic expectations can then lead to disappointment and conflict between you and the client later on. However, if the client is in crisis and you are concerned about risk, take whatever time is needed.

As with cancellations, lateness can be a pattern. Each time a client is late, document at the beginning of the progress note how late she was so that you can refer to it again later. Once this has become a regular pattern, it is time to address it, as Michelle did in the previous vignette.

If the client blames a logistical reason, consider problem solving with her:

> "So you get out of work at 5:00 and take the bus, which sometimes runs late, so you get here at 5:45 instead of 5:30. How about if we move your appointment to 6:30 on Wednesday instead? Then you won't be so rushed."

However, often problem solving will not resolve the client's lateness. After a couple more episodes of lateness, you may wish to ask about it again, as Michelle did in the previous vignette. Note that the question is not whether the lateness is occurring in other areas—it almost certainly is. Instead, Michelle asks how it is affecting the client since this is less likely to provoke defensiveness. By discussing the lateness, you are likely to elicit useful information about the client and her struggles in all areas of her life.

IRREGULAR ATTENDANCE

Angelina Ramirez is a new psychotherapy client for Jordan Ross, a mental health trainee. Angelina came in 15 minutes late for her appointment on the first session. Before the second session, she called stating that she had forgotten the time of the session. She came on time for her third session but came an hour late for the fourth session, insisting that Jordan had made an error in his calendar.

Martin Brooks is another one of Jordan's new psychotherapy clients. Martin attended his first session on time. The next week, he canceled at the last minute, stating he had to take his mother to a doctor's appointment. The third week, Martin came up 25 minutes late with a crisis to talk about. The fourth week, he had a doctor's appointment for himself that conflicted with the therapy session time, and he canceled again, leaving a message the morning of the appointment. The week after that, Martin comes in 15 minutes late, saying that all the buses are running late today. At that appointment, Jordan says, "Martin, I'm worried about you. I'm noticing that you're having a really hard time getting to your sessions regularly and on time. I see that you have a lot of responsibilities. I understand that, but I'm concerned because you aren't getting the treatment that you need. Realistically, we can't make much progress if I don't see you for the full session every week. Can we talk about this? I'd really like to help you with it, if I can."

Unless there is a life-threatening crisis, do not focus on any other therapeutic issues until the attendance issue is resolved. Irregular attendance needs to be addressed before any other progress can be made because you can't effectively treat a client who is not coming regularly to therapy. Next time you get the client in the office, bring up the subject gently, as Jordan does in the previous vignette.

When your client is disorganized about appointments, it is impossible to provide an effective treatment, so you need to determine the cause. There are many reasons why clients do not regularly attend their psychotherapy sessions. Here are some of them:

- Thought disorder
- Attention deficit disorder (ADD), with or without hyperactivity
- Client is characterologically disorganized
- Client is used to living a chaotic, disorganized lifestyle, going from one crisis to the next
- Client does not make own therapy a priority; others' needs come first
- Ambivalence about therapy
- Anxiety about therapy
- Client doesn't understand how weekly sessions can help more than crisis sessions as needed

If your client has a history of bipolar disorder, psychotic disorder, or major depression, evaluate for thought disorder and other psychotic symptoms (see chapter 9). If any of these appear to be present, communicate with the client's psychiatrist about it. The psychiatrist can prescribe medications that will almost certainly help.

Here is how an articulate client might talk about her continued difficulties with mild thought disorder:

> "I can't seem to get organized. At home, the house is a mess. I just stand there looking at it, and I can't decide what to do first, so I don't do any of it. I'm overwhelmed with e-mail at work and find myself spacing out at times. When I'm driving, other drivers honk at me because I can't seem to focus on the traffic lights all the time. I've had two accidents in the past 3 months."

Alternatively, your client may have ADHD, so screen for that as well (see chapter 9). Medications can help concentration. In addition, you can take a problem-solving approach with ADD clients.

If the client is habitually disorganized or her life has been chaotic, try a problem-solving approach. Ask if the client has a calendar, PDA, or phone with appointment capability with her. If so, remind her to put the appointments in it. If not, suggest that the client get one of these, keep it with her at all times, and use it regularly. She may have some resistance to doing this ("My dad has one of those, not me!"). You can explore it as needed in the session:

> "I'm concerned that your forgetfulness might be creating problems for you in other areas of your life. How is that affecting you?"

There is also a possibility that the client does not make his needs and health a priority. Discuss what the personal costs have been to the client of ignoring his mental health. Help the client problem solve about how to assertively address situations that might interfere with therapy.

If you suspect that the client is ambivalent about coming to therapy, this issue should be discussed immediately. Be aware that often the ambivalent client may make different excuses every week and may see your concern about attendance as criticism. Try to bring up the issue gently:

> "I've been very concerned about you, since I've noticed that you've been canceling a lot of appointments for medical reasons. It seems that these medical issues are having a negative impact on your ability to get things done that you want to do. Can we talk about this for a while? I want to know more about how this is affecting you."

You may find that exploring attendance in detail has not caused attendance to improve. Discuss this with your supervisor before implementing any further interventions. Keep in mind that it is not ethical to provide a treatment that you know is ineffective. Additionally, this puts you in a problematic situation with respect to professional liability. Perhaps you may wish to continue to schedule the client if he is high risk and seems to derive a modicum of increased stability from having a therapist. Document this decision and your reasoning thoroughly in the chart. Or you may decide to be a little more confrontational:

> "I see that you are still struggling with getting to your therapy appointments regularly and on time. I'm wondering if this is the right time in your life for you to be in therapy. Perhaps the other things in your life are more important right now. What do you think?"

Often clients will agree, and the case can be closed.

CLIENT WON'T LEAVE AT END OF SESSION

Certain clients want to linger at the end of the session time. Many therapists, consciously or unconsciously, develop behaviors that signal to the client that the session is over. Perhaps you might close your notepad, sit forward on the edge of your chair, or move to check the next appointment time in your calendar. Developing a cue such as this will help the client know that it is time to wind up. If you tend to run late with many of your clients' sessions, discuss this issue with your supervisor.

If there is a problem with ending a particular client's sessions on time, first try to problem solve. Try to figure out why the client is likely to linger. If he lingers to pay his bill, have him pay it at the beginning of the session. If he lingers to talk about schedules, coordinate schedules at the beginning of the session. Try to figure out how long the client is lingering. If he lingers for 5 minutes, make a gesture that you are done 5 minutes before the end of the session time. If he loses track of time, see if you can arrange the office so that he can see a clock.

If you find that despite your best efforts to end the session on time, the client still lingers, you will need to address that with him directly: "I'm noticing that our sessions always seem to run late. I'm hoping that you can help me with this by trying to help me end the session on time." If this is not effective, you will need to determine why the client feels a need to keep you late. Bring this up at the beginning of another session:

> "It seems that despite our best efforts, our sessions are still running late. I'm wondering if we could talk about this for a little bit. What are your thoughts about that? Is there any way in which you feel it is helpful if our sessions run late?"

CLIENT CHATS AT LENGTH ON PHONE

Sometimes you might need to call a client to reschedule an appointment or address another business matter. You know that the client is stable. However, the client wants to keep you on the phone and starts talking about recent personal events. What do you do?

Unless it is a crisis, it is best to confine therapeutic material to the psychotherapy session. You are a busy health care professional and cannot be expected to talk at length on the phone. When the client takes a breath, interrupt her and state kindly, "I'm so sorry. This sounds very important, but I only had a few minutes to call you about rescheduling. I really have to go. Can we talk about this when I see you on Monday?" Do not let the client develop an expectation that if she gets you on the phone, she gets a impromptu brief minisession.

CANCELLATIONS DUE TO THERAPIST'S MINOR ILLNESS

You will occasionally need to cancel appointments. In most cases, this will be due to a minor illness on your part. Do not try go to therapy sessions when you are preoccupied by how unwell you feel. Minor sniffles are okay, as are occasional aches and pains, but carefully consider any illness beyond that to determine whether it will distract you too much from your clients' needs.

When you are ill, you should cancel the appointments yourself if possible. Call your supervisor if you don't have the clients' contact information. If you feel that you may be getting sick while at work, take home the clients' phone numbers so that you can cancel your appointments over the next few days.

Call the clients and leave a brief message:

> "Hi, this is [therapist name], and I need to cancel your appointment today because I am not feeling well. Let's meet again at your appointment next Tuesday at 5:00."

Avoid providing too many details about your illness, and if the client asks at his next session, just briefly state, "I'm feeling much better, thanks for asking," and change the subject.

Certain dependent or highly attached clients can become upset when you are ill. You will need to be alert to the client's affect when asking about your illness, and if the client seems distressed, you will need to explore this issue in the next therapy session—but not over the phone when you are ill.

CANCELLATIONS DUE TO
THERAPIST'S FAMILY EMERGENCY

You may also need to cancel at times because of a family emergency. You might say,

> "Hi, this is [therapist name]. I'm afraid that I've had a family emergency, and I will need to cancel your appointment for this week. I'll see you next week as scheduled."

Always remind clients to come in next week since otherwise they may be uncertain about the length of the family difficulty. If the client expresses sympathy or concern, answer briefly as you feel comfortable, say thank you, and move on. However, again, in certain circumstances, the client will have an emotional reaction to your personal situation that will need to be explored in therapy.

Sometimes serious situations arise. A family member could be seriously ill. Or you might lose a close family member to death. In these cases, you need to accept that for at least a brief period of time, you will not be able to be emotionally available to your clients. As soon as you realize that you are in this type of situation, contact your supervisor and make arrangements for coverage and cancellations as needed. Change your professional voice-mail message and indicate who your clients should contact if a crisis should arise in your absence. The voice mail should also include when you expect to be back in the office.

Two types of errors can occur in these situations. One error is overestimating how much you can handle and not make appropriate clinical arrangements during the time when you do not have the physical or emotional resources to cope with your clients. The other error is underestimating your ability to be present with the client even though you are not feeling 100% back to normal. As Walker and Jacobs (2004) suggest, sometimes "competence can be good enough" (p. 101). Remember that even if you are not able to as attentive or engaged as you typically are, your clients may still benefit from your concerned presence. Discuss this issue with your supervisor if you are unsure whether to return to work yet.

THERAPIST VACATIONS

Clients need advance notice of your vacations. I recommend at least 3 to 4 weeks' notice. Choose a specific week in which to begin notifying all clients.

> "I wanted to let you know that I will be out of the office for 2 weeks starting on April 10, so I will have to cancel two of your weekly therapy sessions next month."

See what comments the clients have. Most clients will be fine. However, certain clients, especially those who feel very dependent or have abandonment issues (Kernberg, Selzer, Koenigsberg, Carr, & Appelbaum, 1989), may have strong reactions to your absence. Discuss how to handle these client concerns with your supervisor. Two weeks before the vacation, mention it again: "I just wanted to remind you that I will be out for two weeks, starting two weeks from now." One week before the vacation, remind the client once more and also remind the client of the next appointment date:

> "Since I'm going to be out starting next week, I just wanted to be sure that you have the date of our next meeting in your calendar. That will be on April 27 at 4:00 P.M. Should I write that down for you, or do you have your calendar with you?"

Before you go on vacation, you must obtain clinical coverage for your client caseload. Every active client needs to know who will be covering their case while you are gone and how to contact the covering clinician in your absence. Perhaps the covering clinician will be your clinical supervisor, the client's psychiatrist, another treatment team member, or perhaps another practitioner at the facility. If the client knows the person who will be covering, just tell the client who it is. If the covering clinician is not known to the client, write out the name and phone number of this person for the client. In all cases, you should document in the chart that the client has been informed of your absence and that the client is aware of who is covering while you are away.

You should change your voice-mail message during your absence. Specify on the message the exact dates that you are out and returning. Specify that you will not receive any messages during that time. Leave the name and number of the covering clinician and any additional information that might be helpful in case of emergency while you are gone. State that callers can leave nonurgent messages and that you will call them back on your return.

Work closely with your supervisor, the treating psychiatrist, and/or the treatment team to be sure that unstable clients have the treatment they need in your absence. Certain unstable clients may need to have a session or two while you are gone. Decide in consultation with your supervisor and the client whether sessions should be scheduled during your absence or whether sessions are optional and up to the client's discretion. Begin discussing these coverage plans 2 to 3 weeks in advance of your vacation.

FEE ISSUES

Holly Gibson is a mental health trainee working in a community mental health clinic affiliated with her training program. There are undergraduate assistants who work at the front desk. Clients are supposed to stop at the front desk before their psychotherapy sessions to pay their fees. The clinic director informs Holly that a client of hers has been giving excuses each time she is supposed to pay her fee and now has not paid for the past three sessions. Clinic policy is to refer clients out if they have more than three fees unpaid. The clinic director tells Holly to address this issue with the client at the next session. Holly feels confused about how to address this issue with the client. Holly, herself, gets no money from the fees that are paid to the clinic. She worries that she is not doing a good job with the client and, deep down, worries that the client may not be getting her money's worth anyway.

Women therapists particularly, socialized to prioritize others' needs, may be painfully mindful that we earn a living from the suffering of others. In the short step from empathizing with our clients to identifying with our clients, we find ourselves considering that we take a vacation or make an extravagant purchase that our clients could not afford, using money that represents the sacrifices they make to pay for therapy. Because the exchange of money in therapy takes place in an intimate context, therapists, especially those paid directly by their clients, are faced daily with questions about economic injustice in a way that those who work for a paycheck are not. (Hill, 1999, p. 1)

As Hill so eloquently states, even experienced psychotherapists can struggle with emotional and social justice issues with regard to the psychotherapy fee. Therapists with a strong impulse to nurture may feel an obligation to take care of their clients and may have some intrapsychic conflicts about taking a fee. Beginning therapists can be insulated from most fee issues, as in the previous vignette, so when the fee needs to be addressed, they can feel especially uncertain.

As in the previous vignette, beginning therapists may be insecure about how much they can help and not feel justified in collecting fees. In fact, in a study of clients at a mental health training clinic (Aubry, Hunsley, Josephson, & Vito, 2000), most clients indicated that they had gone to the clinic because they could get a reduced fee, but nearly 90% of clients were satisfied with paying the reduced fee they had been charged for their psychotherapy.

McWilliams (2004) wisely points out that when the therapist does not collect a fee, the client is being exploitative of the therapist. There are undoubtedly emotional issues that contribute to the client feeling entitled in this way, and these should be explored in therapy. However, you still need to collect the fee now. You might wish to call the client, then state the policy clearly and confidently:

"The clinic policy is that when a client owes three session fees, we need to get payment in full to continue therapy. So please bring payment with you at the time of your next appointment."

Two legal issues are important for therapists to know about fee payment. First, psychotherapists are sometimes tempted to accept the payment from the insurance company as payment in full; keep in mind that you should not do that since it is considered insurance fraud and may get you into legal trouble (Simon, 1995). The second issue is that if you stop psychotherapy abruptly for a client who is not paying the fee, this could be considered abandonment (R. F. Small, 1994). In the case of a high-functioning low-risk client who is fully capable of seeking treatment elsewhere, this is not a significant issue. However, if the client is low functioning or high risk, you may need to see the client again and during that session work with the client to contact an alternative low-cost or free alternative and set up an appointment. You should follow up by phone to ensure that the client attended the appointment (and therefore is not abandoned). Carefully document all your efforts in this regard in the chart.

RECOMMENDED READING

Gans, J. S., & Counselman, E. F. (1996). The missed session: A neglected aspect of psychodynamic psychotherapy. *Psychotherapy, 33,* 43–50.
The authors discuss many of the potential meanings behind clients' cancellations and make practical suggestions about managing policies about missed sessions.
Bender, S., & Messner, E. (2003). *Becoming a therapist: What do I say, and why?* New York: Guilford Press.
The authors have a chapter on setting fees and billing that will be helpful for any beginning therapist. They provide sample discussions with clients about fees so that you can see how experienced clinicians can address fees productively with clients and deal with related emotional issues. However, the billing practices and fee policies that they suggest are not the most effective. For better recommendations on billing and fee policies, see H. A. Hunt (2005).

EXERCISES AND DISCUSSION QUESTIONS

1. How would you like to personalize your office? What would these items say about you? What would you say if clients asked you questions about them?
2. What is the no-show and cancellation policy at the agency where you are working? What is the rationale behind this policy? If you were setting the policy, what policy would you set? Why?
3. When you are out of the office, who covers your clients? What are all the logistical steps to make that happen effectively and inform everyone who needs to know?
4. What difficulties do you expect to encounter in collecting fees from clients? How do you think Holly should collect the fee from her client? What client issues might contribute to nonpayment of fees?

Chapter Four

Boundaries

Like any relationship that the client has with a health care professional, the main focus of the psychotherapy relationship is the well-being of just one person: the client. Among the client's relationships with health care professionals, the psychotherapy relationship is unique because the focus is on the client's emotional well-being rather than physical well-being.

To keep the focus on the client, you need to refrain from talking too much about yourself. You need to maintain a *boundary* between the client and your personal activities, needs, emotional functioning, and so on. This boundary allows the client's difficulties to be addressed productively, without your personal issues intruding. This also allows your personal life to remain separate from that of the client, which is important in fostering your own emotional well-being.

This chapter is about therapeutic *boundaries*, defined by Gutheil (2005) as "the edge of appropriate professional conduct" (p. 89). *Boundaries* can also refer to what topics belong in the session and what do not.

BOUNDARY CROSSINGS

Rajiv Kumar is a psychotherapy trainee. A couple that he was treating for marital therapy canceled their termination session since their baby was born a little earlier than had been expected. He sent the couple a card congratulating them on the birth of the baby and indicating that he'd be happy to reschedule the appointment whenever they were ready to do so.

Alexandra Gutierrez, a psychotherapy trainee, goes outside after her last client and finds a blizzard. As she is exiting the parking lot, she sees her last client trudging through the snow. She knows that the client walks about 10 blocks to the train stop. She stops and offers him a ride to the train.

Gutheil (2005) defines *boundary crossings* as "transient, nonexploitative deviations from classical therapeutic or general clinical practice in which the treater steps out to a minor degree from strict verbal psychotherapy" (p. 89). Glass (2003) adds that "boundary crossings relate to the therapist's attempts to enhance the treatment, while boundary violations, which more grossly breach the patient's physical or psychological subjective space, often do so in the service of the therapist's interests" (p. 432). Gutheil (2005) defines *boundary violations* as "essentially harmful deviations from normal parameters of treatment—deviations that *do* harm the patient, usually through some sort of exploitation that breaks the rule 'first, do no harm'" (p. 89).

Examples of boundary crossings include offering a crying patient a tissue, helping a fallen patient up from the floor, helping an elderly patient on with a coat, writing cards to a patient during a long absence, home visits based on the patient's medical needs, calling a client who is apprehensive prior to a surgical procedure, suggesting a decreased fee for a client who has lost a job, or allowing sessions to run over the allotted time when the client is tearful, needy, or deeply upset (Glass, 2003; Gutheil, 2005). The previous two case vignettes are additional examples of boundary crossings. If limited and empathetic, occasional boundary crossings can be appropriate therapeutically. However, they should be discussed at the next psychotherapy session, and they should be carefully documented.

The context in which the boundary-related behavior occurs is of vital importance in assessing its significance (Gutheil, 2005; Gutheil & Gabbard, 1998). Gutheil (2005) goes on to clarify that "the definition is highly context-dependent. The relevant contexts might be the treater's ideology, the stage of therapy, the patient's condition or diagnosis, the geographical setting or the cultural milieu among others. . . . Context is a critical and determinative factor" (p. 89). For example, in certain circumstances, it may be appropriate for the therapist to engage in case management activities in addition to traditional therapy, which could entail securing services, financial assistance, or food for the client. It may be appropriate for a behavioral therapist to accompany a client in his car if they are doing a desensitization hierarchy regarding driving across bridges. Alternatively, a psychodynamic psychotherapist accompanying a client in the car would generally be considered a boundary violation.

BOUNDARY VIOLATIONS

Lauren Smith is a psychotherapy trainee. She is getting a divorce and needs to find a new condominium. One of her clients is a real estate agent who has some similar problems. She confides some of her concerns in him, including a brief description of her marital difficulties, and asks him for advice on real estate.

Jonathan Paul is a psychotherapist in private practice. He has a low-income client who recently lost her job. Jonathan decides to help her out by hiring her to do his filing, clean his office, and run personal and professional errands for him.

Al Chavez is a psychotherapy trainee. He is working with a client, Sally Ruiz. Sally suffers from depression and has a physically abusive boyfriend. Al is concerned about Sally, who often comes in highly distraught. He violates clinic rules by staying late to see her for 2-hour sessions during her more stressful periods (the clinic forbids trainees seeing clients after clinic hours are over). He gives Sally his cell phone number, and she calls him one or two times every week to discuss her difficulties. He doesn't tell his supervisor about this because he doesn't want to hear what his supervisor will say. He feels that he is doing the right thing for Sally and that his supervisor wouldn't understand. However, he is starting to feel overwhelmed by Sally's demands for his attention. After one particularly intense session, Sally becomes very angry at Al for refusing to schedule her again later that week. Al won't stay late that day because he has preexisting plans, and he feels that it is time to set some boundaries with Sally. Sally leaves in a rage. The next week, she files a complaint at the clinic alleging that Al exploited her sexually. Al feels that now he has to admit everything to his supervisor. However, his supervisor does not know what to believe since Al had been secretive about the other boundary violations in the past.

Examples of boundary violations include attending a social function with a client, eating out or going to a bar with a client, employing a client, getting a client to do errands for you, violating policies for a "special" client, and sexual contact with a client. A partial list of what does *not* belong in a session includes repeated detailed descriptions of client's sex life, any significant body contact, any detailed personal information about your personal life, or using the client as a resource. An example of the latter would be asking your client, a financial planner, for investment advice. The previously mentioned vignettes are also examples of boundary violations. Sexual contact between therapist and client is the most egregious example of a boundary violation. Note that sexual attraction alone, if not acted on, is not a boundary violation; this subject is discussed further in chapter 22.

Therapists may be especially vulnerable to boundary violations when they feel overwhelmed by a client, when they are having a life crisis, or when they feel lonely and want to confide in someone (Gabbard, 1996). They may also have a strong need to rescue others and enact this need through boundary violations (such as Al did in the previous example). If you are uncertain whether a behavior is a boundary crossing or a boundary violation, Gutheil (2005) suggests that you consider whether you would be comfortable discussing the behavior in question with a colleague. If not, it is probably a boundary violation.

Trainees should be aware that *"fact finders*—civil or criminal juries, judges, ethics committees of professional organizations, or state licensing boards—*often believe that the presence of boundary violations (or even crossings) is presumptive evidence of, or corroborates allegations of, sexual misconduct"* (Gutheil & Gabbard, 1993, p. 189). I have provided the example of Al and Sally to illustrate this point. Respecting and maintaining appropriate boundaries with clients must be a top priority of all psychotherapists. The remainder of this chapter details some common boundary issues in therapy and how to address them.

CLIENT ASKS PERSONAL QUESTIONS

Kyle Warunrit is a psychotherapy trainee who has a client who distrusts him. The client has borderline personality traits. She tells him that she can't tell him anything about her life until she knows more about him. She starts with asking appropriate questions about his training and qualifications. Every session, she asks slightly more intrusive questions, until Kyle finds that she is asking him about his sexual orientation, relationships, and so on.

Clients ask us personal questions for a variety of reasons. Your client might ask you questions simply because she is curious about you. Or your client might feel that he cannot share personal information of a sensitive nature with you unless he knows more about you. Or your client may fear that you will think negatively of her because of differences between the two of you. Or he might want to gain power over you by learning more about you. Or there could be many other reasons for asking.

If the client asks for some simple demographic information, for example, "Are you married?" "Do you have children?" or "How old are you?" you may wish to make an initial assumption that the client is just curious. In these cases, it is okay to answer these questions briefly and move on. However, it should be noted that even these simple questions could be fraught with personal meaning for the client (Wachtel, 1993).

Wachtel (1993) points out that your response to questions from the client should depend on your assessment of why the client is asking the question. He suggests making this remark to clarify the situation: "I'd be happy to tell you, but I don't feel clear about what it is that you are really interested in knowing (p. 227)."

If there are more than a couple questions or questioning occurs frequently, it is helpful to gently ask the client about the significance of this information:

> "I've noticed that you have asked me a number of personal questions and I'm wondering—how is it helpful to you to get this information?"

Never answer any question that feels too intrusive to you, even if on the surface it seems innocuous.

Even if you think that the client is asking just out of curiosity, you might not want to answer. For example, in certain instances, you might be in a treatment setting where personal information given to one client will quickly spread throughout much of the client population. In those cases, you can consider responding,

"I'm sorry, but I have a policy of not answering personal questions. But I'm curious, would you mind telling me how it would be helpful to you to know this?"

CLIENT ASKS ABOUT THERAPIST'S
MENTAL HEALTH HISTORY

Carrie Schmidt is a mental health trainee who has just started working in an outpatient alcohol treatment program. Carrie has a history of problem drinking in the past and a family history of alcoholism. For these reasons, Carrie has abstained from drinking alcohol for the past 4 years. Many of the other counselors are open about their substance abuse histories, but Carrie does not want to discuss her past drinking with clients. One of Carries clients asks her, "Are you a recovering alcoholic?" Carrie says, "I know that your group therapist talks a lot about his history as an alcoholic, but my approach is different. I would like to spend all of our time helping you focus on your personal problems, and it's my policy not to discuss my personal history."

Your client may blurt out personal questions about your mental health history such as these: "Have you ever been depressed?" "Have you ever been in therapy?" "Have you ever taken antidepressants?" or "Have you ever heard voices?" Your client might be asking because she is worried that you won't understand her. If you think that this is the case, you need not answer the question—instead, show that you understand by making an empathetic remark based on the material that preceded the question (e.g., "It seems that you've been suffering from this depression for a long time and you've had a hard time getting people to understand how difficult it is.").

You may or may not have a history of mental health treatment, but in almost all cases, you should not answer these questions. However, the fact that the client is asking the question is important, and you need to understand what her motivation is. Here are some possible responses to the question:

"I'm wondering how it would help you to know whether I've been depressed in the past."

"It seems that you may be concerned that if I haven't been depressed, I won't be able to relate to what you're going through."

Your client may also ask you about substances: "Are you an alcoholic?" "Have you ever been a problem drinker?" or "Have you ever used cocaine?" It is, in fact, common for many substance abuse counselors to talk openly about their own past substance abuse problems. If you would like to take this approach, discuss the implications thoroughly with your supervisor first. Alternatively, you can take the approach that Carrie does in the previous vignette.

Some clients have experienced a fairly rare event and worry that you won't understand their situation: "Have you ever been in combat?" "Have you ever heard voices?" or "Have you ever been manic?" Often in these cases, the client's underlying worry may be about your knowledge base and competence. In these cases, an alternative approach can be okay:

> "No, I've never been in combat, and I'm sure that I'll never understand it exactly the way that you do. However, I'm hoping that I can help you with your problems anyway."

Sometimes the client wants a therapist who has had the same problems he has. Explain that this can't always be the case ("If you had a heart attack, would you insist on having only other doctors and nurses who had had heart attacks themselves?") but that your training and knowledge can be helpful nonetheless. If this continues to be an issue, there may be underlying issues of distrust that will need further exploration over time.

If you do have a history of mental health treatment, think long and hard about revealing it to a client. Despite her questions, the client does not need to know about your emotional issues. Talk it over thoroughly with your supervisor first before revealing anything to a client. If you don't feel you can discuss the issue with your supervisor, you should not reveal it to your client.

CLIENT CRITICIZES OTHER HEALTH CARE PROFESSIONALS

Tim Browne, a new client, comes in for his first session. Immediately, he starts criticizing his primary care physician: "That guy's a quack. He only made me worse after seeing him." He then moved on to criticize his psychiatrist: "She's a bitch, and rude besides. She can't get my meds right. She's torturing me with all these blood tests she thinks she needs. Those people in the lab are vampires. I don't see why they need all that blood."

Keep in mind that the client may or may not accurately represent what happened with the previous health care professionals. Perhaps the client has borderline personality disorder and is now devaluing the past professional. Perhaps the client is paranoid and thinks that the professional was out to get him. Maybe the client takes minor complications like rescheduling as a personal insult. Maybe the client is suspicious of everyone because of a history of childhood trauma and neglect. Thus, you cannot know whether the previous professional is actually at fault, and it is inappropriate and unprofessional for you to join in with the criticism.

Maintain appropriate professional boundaries by empathizing with the client without necessarily agreeing with the client's perspective:

- "I'm sorry that didn't work out for you."
- "It sounds like you were disappointed in how things went with your previous therapist."
- "It sounds like you're feeling angry at your psychiatrist right now."

Be wary of these criticisms. If you take them at face value, this may result in a worst-case scenario, which is commonly called "splitting." Splitting occurs when the staff has split opinions and is arguing and in turmoil over a client. Splitting also occurs when one staff member believes that the client has to be protected from other staff who she thinks will victimize the client. If you recognize that splitting is happening, point this out to other staff so that it can be discussed at the staff level.

A CRISIS INTERFERES WITH THE NEXT APPOINTMENT

Armani Mosley is a mental health trainee. His client, Rose Washington, has come to her appointment feeling suicidal. Armani spent Rose's whole session talking with her about this and realizes that she needs to be hospitalized. He knows that he will need to spend at least the next hour working with his supervisor and Rose's psychiatrist to make this happen. Armani has a client scheduled for the next therapy session, and the client is now outside his office waiting. Rose has agreed to hospitalization and understands why it is necessary. Armani feels that it is safe to leave Rose alone for a few minutes. So Armani asks her to wait outside his office and asks the other client to come in briefly. Armani does not have a client scheduled for the following hour, so he says, "I'm really sorry, but I've had an emergency come up with another client. I estimate that I'll be available in about an hour, but I can't be sure of the exact time. Would it be possible for you to wait until then, or should I reschedule you?" The client states that he understands since he has been in crises himself in the past. The client says that he will just come back later in the week. Armani gives him another appointment and then proceeds to help Rose with her hospitalization.

In rare events, a client's crisis or a personal crisis will interfere with another client's appointment. As Armani did in this vignette, you must evaluate this and make a plan before you can end the session. In most cases, you will feel that it is safe to leave the crisis client briefly in your office or in another location, as Armani did, and spend a few minutes addressing the other client's appointment briefly.

You may feel that the crisis will be very time consuming, or you have a very tight schedule, so you can't run late all day. In that case, this would be more appropriate: "I'm sorry, but a crisis has come up with another client, and I have no idea how long this will take. I don't want to waste your time and keep you waiting. Is there any chance that you could come back later this week for your session?"

Most clients will be understanding, but when you see the client for the session that was postponed, it is wise to apologize again and ask about the client's feelings about the canceled session.

THERAPIST SEES CLIENT IN A PUBLIC PLACE

My private practice is in the relatively small suburb where I also live. I inevitably run into clients when I am with my spouse or with a friend, be it at the grocery store, at a street carnival, leaving a movie, etc. So, part of my orientation "spiel" to new therapy clients is to point out the likelihood/possibility of this happening eventually. I let the client know that my approach will be to not acknowledge in any way that I know them, unless they approach or acknowledge me first, and even then to keep it brief and casual. If/when I run into someone this way, I always bring it up (if feasible) in our next session. Of course, there is always that one client who not only has no qualms about being recognized or encountered but who will want to strike up a detailed conversation, ask my wife questions, etc. My wife and I have agreed that if we're out somewhere, and I spot one of these situations about to happen, I say a certain innocuous word or phrase that we've agreed will signal to her that I'm about to have an awkward clinical moment. She doesn't know if it's a current client, former client, referral source, or what, but she's prepared to handle it. She doesn't ask, "So where do you guys know each other from?" She doesn't encourage conversation. She'll "rescue" me by reminding me that we're late for something *and* she won't ask questions about it. Being with friends is trickier, but again my good friends know what I do, what the limitations are, and don't expect me to introduce them to everyone I meet. (Anonymous private practice psychotherapist, personal communication, January 24, 2007)

Sooner or later, you will probably run into one of your clients in a public place. Psychotherapists who practice in a university community or a rural area generally have this experience most frequently; in fact, 95% of therapists at college counseling centers had encountered clients in public (Sharkin & Birky, 1992). During these encounters, therapists need to be concerned about the risk for confidentiality violations and boundary violations.

If you are aware of any situations where you are likely to run into clients, it would be helpful to address this proactively at the beginning of therapy, as in the previous vignette. For example, my private practice, my home, and my gym are all within a couple miles of each other. Thus, I've learned that whenever clients mention going to a gym, I ask them where they go, and if they go to the same one, we have a brief conversation about that. One might simply say, "One thing I wanted to mention to you was that occasionally I will see a client in a public place. My policy is not to greet you to preserve your confidentiality. If you would like to say hi, please go ahead and do so. But to preserve your confidentiality, we cannot have any discussions outside of the office." See if the client has any reactions to this statement and explore them as necessary.

If I see a client in a public place and we have not discussed the issue, I will do my best to avoid any eye contact or any other signs that I have recognized the client. I will move in the other direction, away from the client, as soon as possible. However, the next time I see the client in therapy, if I think there was any chance that the client might have seen me, I may bring this issue up. I will explain to the client that I thought I saw him or her but that I did not approach or say hi to protect confidentiality. Sometimes you will need to address the issue further, but usually the client will be fine with what you have done and appreciate your concern for his or her well-being.

If the client sees you, approaches you, and greets you, you should not introduce any family member or friend who may be with you to the client (Woody, 1999) unless the client insists and there is no way to avoid it. It is better to keep moving, smile, and say, "It was good to see you—sorry, I've got to go."

There is always a risk that a client can observe you in any public place without you knowing about it. There is a chance that the client might observe behavior that is suitable to the venue but not particularly professional (e.g., holding hands with your partner, joking loudly with friends, or trying on clothes in a large group changing room at a discount store). This may provoke feelings in the client that will then need to be explored in therapy.

If you work in a rural setting, often you cannot avoid running into clients in a public place and even interacting with them regularly. For example, your client might work at the only gas station for 50 miles. It is unreasonable to assume that you can keep track of his work hours and get gas only when he is not there. If you are working in a rural setting, you should read about how to manage these situations effectively (C. D. Campbell & Gordon, 2003; Speigel, 1990).

Both you and the client may be members of a small subgroup within a larger area, increasing the likelihood for extratherapeutic encounters. The subgroup might encompass similarities in interests, ethnicity, religion, or sexual orientation. When this similarity is detected and you assess a moderate to high likelihood of encountering the client outside therapy, it would be wise to discuss the issue in advance. For a discussion of issues that arise when the therapist and client are members of the same lesbian, gay, and bisexual community, see L. E. Kessler and Waehler (2005).

THERAPIST–CLIENT TOUCHING

Jamie Thompson, a psychotherapist, has a long-standing therapeutic relationship with a high-functioning schizophrenic client. The client has always been pleasant and appropriate during their sessions, and they are clearly fond of one another. As she passes him in the waiting room, she touches him on the shoulder and tells him that she will be back to see him in about 5 minutes.

There is considerable debate about appropriate therapist–client touching, and full discussion of the issue is beyond the range of this volume. Until you have a chance to review the literature on this complex issue, I would suggest that you err on the side of minimal touch with clients.

If you or the client would like to shake hands at either the beginning or the end of the session, that's fine (Gutheil & Gabbard, 1993). These touches would be considered socially appropriate in almost any social setting. To be maximally safe and appropriate, I recommend that, as a trainee, you refrain from any other touches with clients. However, often experienced therapists do not hold themselves to this strict standard, as you can see in the case of Jamie in the previous vignette.

Prominent mental health practitioners have written about special situations of client touching. In one example, Koocher (2006) held the hand of a dying cystic fibrosis patient in a hospital. In another, Yalom (2002) ran his hands over the thin wisps of a cancer patient's remaining hair. I encourage you to read both of these examples to learn more about the specific situations and how these experienced therapists handled them.

As you can see, there is no single rule that every therapist adheres to about physical contact with clients. I recommend that you talk to peers and supervisors about the issue, asking questions about what they do and why they feel comfortable with their choices. You should also do some professional reading in this area. This will help you learn what feels right for you as well as what is safest from a risk management perspective.

CLIENT WANTS A HUG

Melissa Roberts, a psychotherapy trainee, has just had a very emotional session with her high-functioning female client. They both feel very close to each other during the session. Melissa's client impulsively grabs her for a hug at the end of the session. Melissa accepts the hug briefly.

Amy Zhang, a psychotherapy trainee, has been working for several months with a client who is low functioning and has schizoaffective disorder. The client is socially isolated and is difficult to tolerate because of his angry preoccupations with paranoid ideation. However, he is very grateful to Amy for her attention to him, and at their last session, he left saying, "I love you!" She has not addressed this in today's session since he is both emotionally fragile and not very cognitively intact. At the end of the session, he says he wants a hug and starts to reach for her. Amy sticks out her right hand and tells him, "Since we have a professional relationship, I prefer to shake hands. I'll look forward to seeing you in a couple weeks."

Tom Taylor, a psychotherapy trainee, has been working with a client, Glenn Vanderhook. Glenn has a relationship with a girlfriend. He has borderline traits. At the end of the emotional fourth session, Glenn indicates that he would like to hug Tom. Tom quickly realizes that since Glenn has borderline traits, maintaining appropriate boundaries may be a continuing issue, and he decides to decline the hug. Tom puts his hand out instead and says, "Since we have a professional relationship, I prefer to shake hands." At the 10th session, Glenn reveals that his girlfriend abruptly ended their relationship when she discovered that he has been having casual sexual relations with men.

Sometimes, the client will want to hug. This generally comes spontaneously at the end of the session, with little time to discuss the impulse, as in the previously mentioned cases. Be aware that refusing the hug, as Amy and Tom did, is the most conservative and safest approach from a risk management point of view. It can *sometimes* be okay to accept a hug, as Melissa did in the previous vignette, as long as there is a long-standing therapy relationship without any signs of erotic interest on the part of the client.

Never hug a client routinely; this is likely to be the start of a slide along the slippery slope of boundary violations (Gabbard, 2000a). Never hug a client if you don't think you can discuss it later with the client *and* your supervisor (Gabbard, 2000a). As Amy does, never hug a client if there have been signs that the client may have some erotic feelings toward you. If the client has issues that might lead to later misinterpretation of the hug (e.g., borderline traits), do not hug. As the third vignette illustrates, even a client's initial presentation of a sexual orientation that excludes the therapist (here the client, Glenn, has a girlfriend initially, and the therapist is male) is not necessarily a sign that accepting a hug is an appropriate therapeutic step.

As a beginning therapist, I recommend that you practice gently refusing to hug the first several clients who may want a hug, whoever they may be. As a mental health practitioner, you must develop the confidence and self-possession to refuse hugs from clients. Sooner or later, a client who should not be hugged under any circumstances will ask for a hug. You must be ready for that.

When you refuse to give a hug, or if you accept a hug that you later regret, address this in the next session. How to address the issue will need to be considered carefully. In Amy's case, because of the fragility of the client and his limited insight, the simple behavioral intervention of requesting a handshake instead is sufficient. In most other cases, you should ask the client about it if the client does not bring it up. Tom might say, "Glenn, I wanted to ask you something about your last session. At the end of the session, you asked for a hug, and I told you that since we have a professional relationship, I prefer to shake hands. I'm wondering if you have any reactions to that."

CLIENT GIVES YOU A GIFT

Before leaving his training site, Brian Nelson is having his last session with a client who has schizophrenia. The client is socially isolated and had become very attached to Brian during the year they worked together. The client's hobby is to collect trash and natural items, such as branches and pinecones, and put these together to make small sculptures. Brian had encouraged this artistic outlet. The client had talked about her art projects often during therapy and had brought in some of her artworks to show Brian. Brian expressed his genuine appreciation for them. At the last session, the client brings in a sculpture to give Brian. Brian thanks her graciously and accepts the gift, admiring its artistic qualities.

Tiffany Allen is seeing a successful businessman in therapy. The client is married and has two teenage boys. His second wife told him that she was going to divorce him unless he went to therapy and stopped cheating on her. Tiffany had noted that the client had narcissistic traits, and she had often felt that he was looking at her breasts, although his behavior had otherwise been appropriate. One of their sessions happens to fall on February 14. The client comes to the office and hands Tiffany a diamond tennis bracelet purchased from a famous jewelry store. Tiffany refuses to accept the gift, although the client insists that it cannot be returned. She insists that they explore the meaning of this gift and how this relates to his feelings and ideas about women.

Sooner or later, one of your clients will bring you a gift. This will almost always happen unexpectedly. It may be more likely to happen around holidays or when you are leaving a training site, but it could occur at other times as well.

Your first decision, when faced with a gift from a client, is whether to accept the gift. There is no definitive rule about gifts from a clinical perspective, but the facility where you are working may have some guidelines, and if they do, you should know them. However, here are some general guidelines. First, you should never accept an expensive gift. I would be reluctant to accept any gift that I thought cost more than $25 (or possibly $5, if it was from a low-income client), although I might consider accepting a somewhat more expensive gift if the client's income level was high and I was reasonably certain that no complex therapeutic issues were involved. Personally handcrafted items and small gifts of food are generally acceptable. Second, do not accept more than one gift from a client in a calendar year—or if you do accept the second gift, you must talk about it and dissuade the client from further gifts. Third, do not accept any inappropriate (e.g., romantic) gift, like the one that had been offered to Tiffany in the previous vignette.

If you are thinking of accepting a gift, consider carefully what you know about the client's issues so far. The gift may simply be an expression of appreciation and gratitude, or it may have a secondary, more complex meaning (Hahn, 1998). By accepting the gift, you are giving a message that giving the gift is okay; this is why you would never want to accept an inappropriate gift. If you reject the gift, the client may feel rejected, and it may be more difficult to explore the meaning behind the gift; however, sometimes this is unavoidable. In practice, therapists do sometimes accept gifts they consider somewhat problematic in order not to unduly disrupt the therapeutic relationship (S. Knox, Hess, Williams, & Hill, 2003).

Here are some more considerations for whether to accept the gift (adapted from S. Knox et al., 2003). Is it an appropriate gift-giving occasion, such as a holiday or termination of therapy, or not, such as early in therapy? Does the gift seem to blur the therapist–client boundaries in an uncomfortable way? Does the gift somehow feel manipulative or aggressive?

Your second decision, when faced with a gift, is whether to explore its meaning further in therapy. You might not want to explore the meaning when this might be seen as a sign of rejection to a fragile client (Hahn, 1998). In addition, you might not explore the meaning if the client is low functioning and the gift seems to have a clear meaning, as in the case of Tom's client in the previous vignette. Finally, you may not wish to explore the meaning if you do not see the gift as problematic (S. Knox et al., 2003).

Gifts may have varied and complex meanings (Hahn, 1998; S. Knox et al., 2003). A gift could mean appreciation, gratitude, thanks, or good-bye. It could be symbolic of some aspect of therapy, such as a plant symbolizing the nurturing of the therapeutic relationship. It could also have a more complex meaning, such as garnering special treatment, equalizing power, or being "a good client."

If you explore the meaning of the gift, your goal is to understand "the emotional meaning of the gift within the patient's subjective perspective" as it relates to the therapy relationship (Hahn, 1998, p. 79). This exploration must be empathetic and gentle. In response to an appropriate gift of an inexpensive outdoor thermometer, Hahn suggests the following comments and questions:

> "Oh, what a beautiful thermometer. It's the kind I can use outside [pause for patient to comment]. . . . This is such a nice gift. What made you pick it?" (p. 81)

Later, after exploring the meaning further, the therapist remarked, "No matter how you feel when you come to therapy, I am always here for you. And by taking this gift home, I will be reminded of how important our therapy has been for you."

Exploring the meaning of a gift you have refused to accept is more difficult. In that situation, your client is likely to be feeling rejected or defensive. If you personally have always had problems accepting gifts, you need to address this issue before you are faced with any client who attempts to give you a gift. Your difficulty will probably be seen as rejection by the client, who will probably be feeling vulnerable at that point anyway. Talk this over with your supervisor and/or your therapist to avoid disrupting your clients with your own issues.

Accept gifts that do not match your taste in a heartfelt but strategic manner:

> "I can see a lot of skill and care went into this needlepoint pillow. Thank you so much. I will take it home with me tonight."

This ensures that the client will not be expecting to see the needlepoint pillow in your office, and, if you like, you can safely give it away to someone else who would like it more than you do.

Finally, always document in the chart any gift that the client has given you, along with its likely cost. Explain briefly in the chart why you accepted the gift. Summarize any discussion that you had with the client about gift giving.

INVITATIONS TO CLIENT PERSONAL EVENTS

I have attended a client's wedding. I did so for many reasons—though only after having a thorough discussion with the client about her interest in me being there, how I would introduce myself to others, and my decision not to attend the reception. This was a client I had worked with for quite a long time and had a good working relationship with. My attendance was important to her, as her family had rejected her because of her sexual identity and my attendance was in lieu of "family." It was only after we talked about this quite a bit that I decided to go. I sat separately from others but not so distant as to call attention to myself.

I do not have a policy against this, as I think that because of cultural scripts of clients, attending a personal event can enhance the therapeutic alliance. For me it is a case-by-case basis and always understanding the intent behind the request. If confidentiality can be preserved and if it makes therapeutic sense for me to attend, I would consider it. Since I see clients from the gay/lesbian community, running into them at various events is common, and so attending something of importance for clients is something I now consider within the client's cultural frame. (Anonymous psychotherapist, personal communication, July 2, 2007)

I have attended events for patients. Working with kids, I am often invited to bar/bat mitzvahs, plays, recitals, and funerals. I don't attend them all and generally make it policy not to accept those invitations. But there are some circumstances which compel me to attend. I work with many special needs kids, and completing the effort needed for a bar/bat mitzvah or recital is very much a part of our work together. So I attend those events. I do not attend any party or reception that follows. Another part of my work is with parents who have had children die and families who have had a parent die. When my work with these people begins before the death occurs, I usually attend those funerals. For others, if there is a memorial planned at the anniversary, I attend those also. This type of work exceeds the bounds of traditional psychotherapy. In those treatment relationships, I typically do not attend events. (L. Weiss, personal communication, July 3, 2007)

I do attend those events, usually. In general, I attend the main event but not the receptions. In part, this is because I hate receptions, but on a more therapeutic level, it can be quite awkward to be asked how you know the bride, bar mitzvah boy, birthday girl, etc. I always discuss this with the client so that we have a plan and I know what they are granting me permission to say. I have no problem being an old friend of the family or some other appropriate but vague designation, but I want the client to be comfortable with how I introduce myself. Nevertheless, despite that difficulty, I consider it an honor to be invited, and if my schedule permits, I attend.

I have never been asked to any event that felt inappropriate for me to attend. I know two colleagues, however, who have been asked to attend the birth (and I mean invited to be in the delivery room) of a child. They did decline! And of course, I think these decisions must be explored therapeutically, both the invitation and the declining.

I could imagine a situation in which, knowing a client, an invitation should be explored and probably declined on therapeutic grounds. Perhaps issues of boundaries or a covert agenda. The point is if we know our clients well, then we will have a sense of other issues entwined with the invitation which might make it problematic. Whether or not these issues are discussed at that time depends on our evaluation of the client's readiness to explore them. It's possible that declining with regret may be the best path to take for the moment. (V. Seglin, personal communication, July 5, 2007)

These examples from psychotherapists provide carefully thought-out rationales for attending select client events. However, a large number of therapists, perhaps the majority, make it a policy to *never* attend any client events. Either choice can be valid, depending on the circumstances.

If you decide to *never* attend client events — an equally valid choice — be prepared to explain your policy to your clients:

"Thank you so much for inviting me to your wedding. That is very thoughtful of you. However, I must explain that I have a policy of not attending any client events. This is because of my concern about preserving your confidentiality. If I am there, people may start conversations with me and ask me about my connection to you. I certainly wouldn't want to violate your confidentiality by talking about you being in therapy, and I wouldn't feel comfortable lying either. There's also a chance that we might know someone in common and that person will figure out why I am there without my saying anything. So I'd feel most comfortable that your confidentiality was best preserved if I did not attend. I'd like to see the pictures, though, so if you'd like to bring some in, e-mail me a few, or send me a link to your photo album, that would be great. And of course, I'd like to hear all about it."

Here the therapist is expressing interest in the event and gratitude for being invited, yet shares his policy and the rationale for the policy: his concerns about violating confidentiality by attending. If the client continues to insist, the therapist might ask, "How do you feel that it would be helpful to you if I attended the wedding?" and then explore these feelings as a therapeutic issue.

If you do not attend the client's important event, you can mark the event in other ways. You might express your interest in hearing about the event and seeing pictures. In certain special circumstances, you might even mark the event with a card or a very small gift, such as a picture frame.

If you are willing to consider attending the client's event, it should carefully be considered on an individual basis. The experienced therapists quoted previously provide some useful guidelines. If the event is in some way a culmination of the work you have done with the client (e.g., graduation or a recital), it may be relevant to the therapeutic process to attend. There also may be some cultural reasons to attend, as the therapists quoted previously have noted. However, think carefully about what your comfort level would be attending the event. Consider the following issues:

- Is the event large enough that you can remain relatively anonymous?
- What would you say if someone decided to make conversation with you? Discuss this with your client proactively. If you are uncertain whether you could cope with that kind of inquiry effectively, it might be better not to go.
- Can you get there as it is starting, sit by yourself, and leave quickly? Discuss with your client what you intend to do at the event and what to expect of your presence ("I need to leave quickly after the service to minimize any chances of inadvertently violating your confidentiality, so I'll have to provide my congratulations to you in advance.").
- Can you figure out how to gracefully avoid staying around for any reception or social interactions afterward?

As a trainee, you should never agree to attend a client event without the approval of your supervisor. If you have a policy not to attend any client events or your supervisor does not want you to attend any client events, be prepared to address this appropriately with your client. If, after considering the previously mentioned issues, you would like to attend the client's event and you think your supervisor might approve, tell the client that you will consider it and that you will inform the client of your decision next week. Then discuss the issue thoroughly with your supervisor and arrive at an agreement about the appropriate course of action.

THERAPIST SELF-DISCLOSURE

Therapist *self-disclosure* is "verbal statements that reveal something personal about the therapist" (S. Knox & Hill, 2003, p. 530). Additionally, Knox and Hill talk about different types of self-disclosures. You may disclose facts. Or you may disclose your feelings, insights, challenges, or coping strategies when faced with a situation similar to the client's. Or you may reassure the client that the client's feelings about a situation are common by citing your own experience. Finally, you may talk about your emotional reactions to how the client is presenting in therapy.

If used properly, research suggests that clients find self-disclosure helpful (S. Knox & Hill, 2003). They see the therapist as more real and human, and they feel reassured and that their experiences are more normal (S. Knox,

Hess, Peterson, & Hill, 1997). Self-disclosure can be especially helpful in cross-cultural therapist–client dyads (Burkard, Knox, Groen, Perez, & Hess, 2006), especially those where the therapist is White and the client is of color. In a qualitative research study, they found that therapists' self-disclosure of their feelings and reactions to clients' experiences of racism and oppression helped to facilitate therapy.

An appropriate self-disclosure is brief, generally no more than one or two sentences long. Do not be too intimate in your self-disclosures; rather, give an example of your own human behavior that normalizes the client.

Never self-disclose about current personal problems (Gabbard, 2000a), unless totally unavoidable (e.g., you have cancer, have to take time off for treatment, and will be looking different afterward). If you still have intense feelings about the topic, you should not self-disclose; disclose only about resolved issues. Be certain that you do not disclose in a way that meets your needs more than the client's, that overburdens the client with your personal issues, or that blurs boundaries.

> Wrong: "When my husband divorced me, I hated men. It took years for me to get over the pain and bitterness."
> Even more wrong: "I'm getting divorced now too. It's a terrible experience. My husband has more money than I do and is fighting for full custody. I don't know how I'm going to get through this. Sometimes I feel that I can't bear it [more details about divorce process]."
> Right: "I can sympathize. I know from personal experience that going through a divorce is an emotionally difficult period and that it takes a while to reorient your life."

In day-to-day interactions, we are not used to the kind of self-editing that needs to transpire as part of the therapeutic interaction. Therefore, generally, for beginning therapists, it is wise to err on the side of volunteering little personal information. Experts indicated that self-disclosure is a potent intervention and recommend that therapists self-disclose infrequently (S. Knox & Hill, 2003); otherwise, it might be indicative of poor boundaries.

If you are tempted to share a personal experience with the client, it may be wise to refrain and discuss this issue with your supervisor after the session. If you can't see yourself discussing the personal experience with your supervisor, this is a sign that you should not discuss it with your client, either. You can be sure that if the client's issue is important, another opportunity to share the experience will arise later if you and your supervisor agree that it would be therapeutic to do so. An experienced therapist may very occasionally tell about personal experiences, but these have been carefully chosen and edited for therapeutic effect.

SEXUAL BOUNDARY VIOLATIONS

Next to suicide, boundary problems and sexual misconduct rank highest as causes of malpractice actions against mental health providers. (Norris, Gutheil, & Strasburger, 2003, p. 517)

Having occasional sexual feelings toward clients is normal (Bernsen, Tabachnick, & Pope, 1994) and is further addressed in chapter 22. However, having sexual relations with clients or former clients is never acceptable. In his intensive study and treatment of therapists who have committed sexual boundary violations, Gabbard (1996) has unearthed some important cautions that all therapists should be aware of. He reports that the transgressing psychotherapists are not "bad apples" or "psychopathic" but instead therapists who have started down a "slippery slope" through unexamined, seemingly minor boundary crossings with clients. These continue unexamined, leading to greater inappropriate personal involvement between the therapist and client.

Norris et al. (2003) characterize some personal situations that may put a therapist at risk of greater boundary crossings. A life crisis or transition, such as aging, illness, career change, marital conflict, or other personal difficulty, may put a therapist at risk. The therapist may feel lonely and want someone to confide in. The therapist may see a particular client as "special" and particularly appealing in some way. Maintaining appropriate boundaries in small towns or in some subcultures can be a continual negotiation and challenge. Gabbard (1996) emphasizes that many therapists who commit sexual boundary violations were emotionally vulnerable because of an impoverished social life, divorce, or loss.

Jackson and Nuttall (2001) did an anonymous survey of various mental health practitioners. They found that while only one of 200 female therapists had ever had a sexual encounter with a client, one of 12 male therapists had. The therapists who were especially at risk were those who were male *and* under emotional stress *and* who had a history of having been intrusively sexually abused (these therapists had a 60% chance of having had a sexual encounter with a client, but note that there were a very small number of therapists with these characteristics in the sample, so it is unclear whether the same risk would be seen in a larger sample). All three of these risk factors alone and in combination also increased the risk of inappropriate sexual boundary crossing. Jackson and Nuttall (2001) recommend that therapists with these risk factors avoid the isolation of private practice, seek regular supervision/consultation regarding boundary issues, and get personal therapy to address trauma-related concerns.

Gabbard (1994, 1996) reports that in most cases, sexual transgression started with a nonsexual hug between the therapist and client. Or the therapist might have become informal, friendly, and self-revealing, perhaps to the extent of talking about the therapist's own personal difficulties at length. Other boundaries may weaken, such as staying later than the 50-minute therapy hour or talking to the client at night. The therapist was in denial that there are significant boundary crossings taking place. The therapist had difficulty setting limits and feels that he or she is being aggressive when doing so. Some therapists feel that they are falling in love with the client and that this justifies the sexual boundary violation (Gabbard, 1994).

To prevent starting on this slippery slope, Gabbard (1996) emphasizes that "specifically, those aspects of their [the supervisee's or consultee's] thoughts, feelings, or actions that they would most like to keep secret from the supervisor are precisely the issues that should be openly discussed in supervision" (p. 317).

THERAPIST PREGNANCY

During the course of my pregnancy, preoccupation with the well-being of my self and baby, anxieties related to changing body boundaries, and heightened conflicts around issues of control and achievement, affected my willingness, at times, to actively explore transference material that was related to my pregnancy as well as to facilitate the expression of patients' aggressive or envious feelings toward me. In certain instances, these dynamics contributed to a tendency to distance myself from highly charged affects in the treatment and to a collusion with patients' denial and avoidance of these affects. . . . I was retrospectively aware of my wish to withdraw from threatening aspects of patients' feelings and associations and enacted this wish by sharpening the boundaries between us. This dynamic was most apparent with patients who were either intrusive or demanding, or whose crises resonated with some personal anxiety about my pregnancy. . . . Trying to listen to patients' ostensible concerns about my pregnancy and to hear the layered transferential meanings presented an ongoing challenge throughout my pregnancy. (Bienen, 1990, p. 611)

A brief discussion of therapist pregnancy is included in this chapter on boundaries, as this is an example of a very personal event in the therapist's life that makes itself obvious to clients. Pregnancy involves some crossing of boundaries between the therapist's personal life and her professional life and forces some therapist self-disclosure. Bienen (1990), quoted previously, clearly a psychodynamic therapist, describes her interpretations of how her pregnancy had an impact on her clients and on her emotional responsiveness to them.

As soon as you feel comfortable doing so, tell your colleagues and supervisor about your pregnancy so that everyone can work as a team to support you and your clients during this period. Keep them informed of any limitations that your obstetrician places on your activities (Tinsley, 2000).

Prior to announcing your pregnancy to your clients, you should read up on the literature in the area so that you will be prepared for some of the emotional reactions that clients may have. Would you prefer to tell your clients about your pregnancy or wait for them to ask about it? The literature is unclear about which would be the most therapeutic course of action (Tinsley, 2000), so discuss this issue carefully with your supervisor and colleagues so that you can decide what would be best for your clients. However, if the client does not bring up your pregnancy, you should do it several weeks (at least) before you start making plans for coverage in your absence. Clients who have abandonment issues are most likely to have difficult reactions to the pregnancy (Tinsley, 2000).

So that your clients feel more comfortable with your impending absence, work carefully with your supervisor and colleagues to transfer clients or to provide coverage for them in your absence (Stockman & Green-Emrich, 1994). Be sure that all your clients have a plan tailored to their needs and that they know what to do if you need to stop work unexpectedly early (Tinsley, 2000). Allow yourself flexibility concerning when you will again provide clinical coverage since many aspects of pregnancy, delivery, and infant behavior are unpredictable. Before you return to work, think about how you will handle clients' questions about the baby, baby gifts, or requests to see photos of the baby (Tinsley, 2000).

THERAPIST'S SERIOUS ILLNESS

During the month following the discovery of a lump in my breast, it felt urgent to me to schedule immediate medical consultations and procedures. The regularity of my schedule with patients was disrupted by my need to consult with physicians. This appeared to me to be inescapable. I typically telephoned these patients whose appointments conflicted with my doctors' appointments with a statement such as, "I need to cancel and hopefully reschedule our appointment next Wednesday." I had to reschedule some patients' appointments two to three times over the course of a few weeks. My patients had come to depend on me for my consistency; in my mind, they were no longer able to do so. . . . It was at this point that self-disclosure appeared inescapable to me. (Kahn, 2003, p. 54)

Illness that is serious enough to disrupt client care or personal appearance, such as Dr. Kahn's breast cancer in the previous quote, is also an example of unavoidable therapist self-disclosure. Since these types of illnesses have a profound emotional impact on the therapist, continuing regular consultation is recommended to ensure that the therapist is coping realistically and effectively with her clients' needs during her illness (Philip, 1993). It is essential that the therapist consider whether treatment can be continued effectively and that clients be prepared for any disruptions that might occur.

RECOMMENDED READING

Gabbard, G. O. (1996). Lessons to be learned from the study of sexual boundary violations. *American Journal of Psychotherapy, 50*, 311–322.
   Dr. Gabbard talks about the slippery slope leading to sexual boundary violations.
Gutheil, T. G., & Gabbard, G. O. (1993). The concept of boundaries in clinical practice: Theoretical and risk-management dimensions. *American Journal of Psychiatry, 150*, 188–196.
   A helpful article in understanding boundary crossings versus boundary violations with regard to sexual misconduct. The article is available on the Web in the Boundaries section of Ken Pope's website: http://kspope.com/ethics/boundaries.php.
Gutheil, T. G., & Gabbard, G. O. (1998). Misuses and misunderstandings of boundary theory in clinical and regulatory settings. *American Journal of Psychiatry, 155*, 409–414.
   This classic article provides a sophisticated discussion of the role of context in deciding whether a therapist's behavior is a boundary crossing or a boundary violation. The article is available on the Web in the Boundaries section of Ken Pope's website: http://kspope.com/payton/gutheil-gabbard.php.
Knox, S., Hess, S. A., Williams, E. N., & Hill, C. E. (2003). "Here's a little something for you": How therapists respond to client gifts. *Journal of Consulting Psychology, 50*, 199–210.
   Knox and colleagues examine 12 therapists' descriptions of gifts received.
Knox, S., & Hill, C. E. (2003). Therapist self-disclosure: Research-based suggestions for practitioners. *Journal of Clinical Psychology, 59*, 529–539.
   Knox and Hill provide a thorough discussion of therapist self-disclosure with recommendations to maximize therapeutic effectiveness.
Tinsley, J. A. (2000). Pregnancy of the early-career psychiatrist. *Psychiatric Services, 51*, 105–110.
   Even though targeted at psychiatrists, Tinsley's article provides a useful review of the literature on the pregnant therapist and helpful suggestions for coping.

WEB RESOURCE

http://www.kspope.com/dual/index.php
   Dr. Kenneth Pope is a psychologist and author. This page from Ken Pope's extensive website provides immediate access to many useful articles by a variety of authors on the subjects of dual relationships and boundaries.

EXERCISES AND DISCUSSION QUESTIONS

1. What personal questions from a client would you be willing to answer?
2. What if the client asked about your sexual orientation? Would your response depend on the interaction of the client's issues (e.g., homophobic or struggling with coming out) and your orientation?
3. How would you address running into a client in a public place? Would you discuss this issue with all clients ahead of time or just the ones you think you'd be more likely to see? If you do see a client in a public place and you are not sure the client has seen you, would you try to avoid her?
4. Are you willing to touch clients (other than shaking hands)? If so, when would you feel comfortable and uncomfortable with this?
5. Would you ever be willing to attend a client event? If so, what kind of event?

Chapter Five

Therapist–Client Differences and Coping with Prejudice

Twenty-first century mental health trainees are usually well educated about individual differences. However, applying this knowledge to clinical practice is a complex task. It is impossible to address all the clinical issues that might arise from therapist–client differences, but in this chapter my aim is to discuss some complex clinical issues that can arise.

RELIGIOUS DIFFERENCES

Aaron Schwartz is a Jewish mental health trainee working with a predominantly African American population. He is a Reform Jew and does not wear a yarmulke. He lives and works in New York City, which has a large Jewish population. One of his clients, a Muslim, notices that he is out of the office for Yom Kippur (in areas with high Jewish populations, many people are aware of the occurrence of Jewish holidays from grocery store displays, newspaper articles, and so on). There is a lot of conflict in the Middle East, and the client has been talking to Aaron about how upset he is regarding Muslims' treatment by the international community. When Aaron returns from the holiday, the client asks him, "Why didn't you tell me that you're Jewish?"

Crystal Cooper is a Christian mental health trainee who grew up in the rural South. She is now working at a clinic in a major metropolitan area. She has a few items of personal significance in her office to make herself feel more at home. One of them is a picture frame that her mother gave her when she moved away. It has writing about Jesus and the importance of family on the frame and a picture of her family inside. She also wears a small gold cross necklace that her parents gave her for her college graduation, which has

great sentimental value to her. She is assigned a new client who is having dif-
ficulty accepting his attractions for men. She notices that the client keeps fo-
cusing in the sessions on how his family's religion does not accept gays.

Religious symbols and behavior vary from those that are religiously required
(e.g., a yarmulke for an Orthodox Jewish male therapist or observing certain religious holidays) to those that are voluntary (e.g., a cross necklace worn by a
Christian therapist). While mental health practitioners tend to be less religious
than the general population (Hage, 2006), still many do actively practice within
a spiritual tradition. Knowledge of the therapist's religion will inevitably elicit
reactions in some clients—positive and negative—including the following:

* Being happy that the therapist has the same religious background
* Assuming that client and therapist religious values are the same if client and
  therapist have the same religion, which well could be in error (Gabbard,
  2000a)
* Not being pleased at being treated by a religious therapist or a therapist of
  a different religion (possibly the case for Aaron, described previously)
* Altering behavior to seek approval of the therapist (e.g., Crystal, described
  previously)
* Having concerns but being unwilling to talk about them (probably also applicable to Crystal's client)
* Being concerned about differing religious values and, hence, whether the
  therapist will be respectful of the client's religious values (also possibly the
  case for Aaron's client)

Because of the likelihood of getting negative reactions and hence imped-
ing the therapy, whenever possible many therapists prefer to confine their display of religious symbols to their homes and areas of their offices that are not
readily observable by clients. As Gabbard (2000a) states, "Revealing one's
religion is rarely productive in psychotherapy" (p. 47).

However, another equally valid perspective emphasizes communication,
acceptance, and mutual respect. In these cases, directly addressing any questions in a very matter-of-fact manner and assuring clients that you are respectful of their differences can sometimes be sufficient. In other cases, a
more detailed exploration of the client's reaction is necessary.

If you suspect that the client may be concerned about known or suspected
religious issues but hasn't brought up the topic, consider asking the following:

"I'm wondering, do you have any concerns about our religious differences?"

"I'm thinking you've probably noticed [religious item or clothing]—I'm wondering if you have any reactions to that."

Be proactive and discuss any of these types of issues with a supervisor as soon as you recognize that they might be relevant in any of your current (or future) cases.

A related issue is how the nonreligious therapist might address religious issues with a religious client. There is a growing literature on the importance of cultural competence regarding religious differences (as cited by Hage, 2006). Addressing these issues of cultural competency is well beyond the scope of this volume, but trainees should be aware of the importance of cultural knowledge of the client's religion and seek information out as needed (a good source to start with is Schultz-Ross & Gutheil, 1997).

DIFFERENCES IN AGE AND LIFE EXPERIENCES

During our first year as psychiatric residents at a veterans' hospital, any patient could reliably stump my colleagues and me by asking one simple question: "If you weren't in Vietnam, how can you possibly help me?"

We hadn't been to Vietnam. We were in high school during the worst years of the war. And no, we had never been ambushed, cradled a dying buddy in our arms or dodged land mines. It was a mocking question, really—"Were you in Vietnam?"—and it left us tongue-tied and apologetic.

What were the patients really saying to us? Nancy's patient, we determined, was testing her perseverance: would she really try to know him? The veteran John was seeing, it soon became clear, was keeping him at arm's length to conceal a heroin habit. Matt's patient—the one who told him haughtily at the start of every session, "Really, now, college boy, this will be pointless"—was so ashamed of his tattered life that he had to demean his therapist.

My patient, Rich B., was a former tunnel rat, a wiry soldier who could navigate the Vietcong underground networks. His diagnosis was "anxiety." Mr. B. was in the habit of quizzing me disdainfully. "What were the dates of the Tet offensive? What happened at My Lai? Do you have any idea what it's like to go down in a tunnel?"

At first I was defensive. But then I said: "Of course I don't know these things, Mr. B. You do. Tell me everything." That seemed to break the ice. Our therapy became a bit like a tutorial, and the patient realized I valued his knowledge. . . .

I now hear the question "Have you been there, done that?" for the proxy it often is. In his practice, the psychotherapist Saul Raw finds it a common query. "I find it can reflect more profound difficulties in forming collaborative relationships based on trust," he told me, "and, at the same time, recognizing that all empathy has imperfections."

For other patients, though, the "Have you ever . . ." question is less a therapeutic riddle to be solved—as it was in the case of Mr. B—than an expression of genuine skepticism that they can indeed be helped.

It is the kind of question asked by a person who believes his very soul has been warped by calamity. "Sometimes a patient expresses frustration that I can't possibly help him because I never experienced the trauma that he did," said Dr. Walter Reich, a professor of psychiatry at George Washington University and a former director of the United States Holocaust Memorial Museum, whose patients have included Holocaust survivors. . . .

Addiction, too, can be an intense and defining experience. "I have heard patients say that if you haven't been there you can't help me," said Keith Humphreys, a Stanford psychologist. "So I tell them, 'I can help you live a sober life because it's all I have ever lived.'" (S. Patel, M.D., writing in the *New York Times*, June 12, 2007)

Adam Robinson is a 25-year-old mental health trainee who looks somewhat younger than his age. He is working with a 55-year-old client who repeatedly asks his age and asks Adam if he's experienced enough. Since this is Adam's first clinical training experience, he has some doubts as well. He is uncertain what to say to the client.

At times, clients with different life experiences from ours will doubt that we can be effective with them. Clients wonder whether you can understand them because your personal experiences have been different (e.g., you are not a survivor of trauma, you are of different ethnicities, and so on).

Age difference is one difference that comes up commonly with beginning therapists. Your insecurity about your experience level may make you feel tongue-tied if you are asked about this unexpectedly. Older clients' concerns will usually decrease naturally over time as you demonstrate your empathy, interest, and competence.

When the client has concerns about differing life experiences, I recommend that you try something like this:

> "I realize that you have many experiences that I have not had. However, I hope that you will be willing to give me a chance to learn about what you have experienced in your life and learn how this has affected you. I can assure you that I will do the very best I can to help you. I think that the things I have learned as a therapist may be helpful to you as well. I hope you will be willing to give me a chance to work with you."

If the client still seems reluctant, suggest a trial period of four to eight sessions, at which point you can reevaluate and see if the client still feels the same way.

You might be working with an adult client on his child's behavior issues. Often clients will ask you at this time whether you are a parent. Depending on your theoretical orientation, you might prefer to answer this question directly, or you might prefer to inquire about the client's feelings regarding the question first. In any event, you can take a similar approach of confirming differences while suggesting that your knowledge might be helpful and asking that the client give you a chance to help.

Be aware that sometimes this concern about differences might reflect some underlying interpersonal issues. The client may be fearful of opening up to others, may have had some negative experiences with others who are demographically similar to you, may have narcissistic issues ("I want only the best, most experienced therapist"), or may have a multitude of other concerns.

RACIAL AND CULTURAL DIFFERENCES

Justin Lee is a White mental health trainee preparing to work with a predominantly Native American population for the first time. He is concerned that he will make inadvertently tactless remarks. He is trying to learn about Native American culture but is aware that there are significant differences between various Native American cultural groups that may be insufficiently described in the literature. He worries that his clients will not like him because he is White and still has a lot to learn about their cultural background. He wonders when and how best to address these differences.

Michelle Kim is a Korean American mental health trainee working with a substance abuse recovery program that is in a predominantly African American neighborhood. She asks a new client whether experiences of racism have any relationship to her substance abuse and recovery. She is surprised that the client changes the subject.

Carefully consider the clinical needs of the client when thinking about client–therapist cultural/racial or other differences. When the client is new to therapy, these issues might be too sensitive to bring up until a level of trust has been developed. If a client is dealing with a crisis situation, you may wish to establish your concern and credibility by working to stabilize the client as soon as possible. If a client is beginning work on substance abuse recovery, after a "hitting bottom," his top priority must be his abstinence and recovery; all else is secondary for now. So while Michelle's question in the previous vignette might be a fruitful course of inquiry for an advanced recovery client, her new client may be more focused on basic needs, such as maintaining jobs, reestablishing trust with family, financial stability, and so on.

Consider the difference between *content* and *process* when thinking about differences between the client and yourself. If you address these differences through the *process* of therapy, you show through your behavior and your verbalizations that you understand, are knowledgeable about, and are respectful of the client. Through the *process* of therapy, right from the beginning, you make certain points to the client through how you treat him or her rather than by overtly discussing the interpersonal differences. If you address differences in the *content* of therapy, this means you will be asking the client directly to talk about the therapist–client differences. Once trust is established, it can sometimes be helpful to overtly discuss individual differences in psychotherapy. There is a growing literature on this subject (much is referenced by Maxie, Arnold, & Stephenson, 2006) that you may wish to explore.

When working with racial/cultural or sexual minority groups, the majority-group psychotherapist can take three effective steps to maximize effectiveness and the therapeutic alliance. First, the psychotherapist must be sufficiently knowledgeable about cultural, societal, familial, developmental, assimilation, and spiritual issues within the minority group (Baker & Bell, 1999) and balance this knowledge with an accurate understanding of the uniqueness of the client. Second, the psychotherapist must have done personal work on her own attitudes toward the minority group and on her own identity formation (Burkard, Ponterotto, Reynolds, & Alfonso, 1999, show that White therapists' identity formations are related to their effectiveness with Black clients; Gelso, Fassinger, Gomez, & Latts, 1995, found that therapists' homophobia was related to ineffectiveness with a lesbian client's relationship issues). Third, Sue and Zane (1987), in a classic article, stress the importance of being *credible* and *giving* to the ethnic minority client. Being *credible* consists of being able to collaboratively form a conceptualization of the problem, means for problem resolution, and goals for treatment that are culturally relevant to your unique client. By *giving*, Sue and Zane (1987) refer to the importance of using interventions that help the client achieve significant gains early in treatment.

Research on client–therapist ethnic matching has had mixed results. Some studies have found that ethnic matching can result in improved outcomes, while others found that if the client returns after the first session, there is little effect (Zane et al., 2005). Perhaps a more important consideration is agreement between the therapist and client about the perception of the problem, coping orientation, and goals for treatment, referred to as *cognitive matching* (Zane et al., 2005).

SEXUAL ORIENTATION DIFFERENCES

David Bailey is a mental health trainee who is working with young adults in a mental health training site. David has been assigned a new psychotherapy client by the intake coordinator. The client is a 19-year-old male who is struggling with his attraction toward other men, especially with respect to his Christian background. While David is heterosexual, he has had some struggles with his own Christian background as well. David attended a Christian university and has recently started a graduate program at a university unaffiliated with any religion. At his undergraduate university, he was aware that the gay and lesbian students were deeply closeted. As a consequence, he has never been personally acquainted with anyone who has been open about a gay, lesbian, or bisexual orientation. David is eager to learn, but he has doubts about his level of knowledge and whether he can help the client. He also feels unsure about how well he will relate to the client, and he has some religious concerns as well.

Multiple studies have confirmed that lesbian, gay, and bisexual (LGB) clients see psychotherapists at a higher rate than heterosexuals (Burckell & Goldfried, 2006). So every psychotherapist must be prepared as a part of basic cultural competency training to see LGB clients. LGB individuals are likely to seek psychotherapy at a higher rate because they commonly experience significant life stressors that heterosexuals do not. It is essential to understand such basic topics as the coming out process, family adaptation to learning about the client's sexual orientation, dealing with heterosexism, and internalized homophobia (Baron, 1996). In addition, it is important to realize that gay and lesbian versus bisexual clients have some similar and different issues. For example, bisexual individuals may be less open about their sexual orientation and may be less connected with a community (Balsam & Mohr, 2007).

Psychotherapists of all sexual orientations may need to look deeply into their own personal attitudes about LGB clients and make an effort to address any internalized homophobia through psychotherapy, supervision, and education. In an analogue study, Gelso et al. (1995) found that psychotherapists with greater homophobia tended to avoid helping a lesbian client with her relationship issues. If you have some religious concerns about working with LGB clients, consider seeking out a religious leader of an LGB-affirmative religious group for dialogue. It is essential that psychotherapists recognize that there is no scientific evidence that sexual orientation can be changed through psychotherapy and that efforts to do so will almost certainly result in lasting psychological harm to the client (Burckell & Goldfried, 2006).

Beginning psychotherapists may wonder when it is helpful to disclose their sexual orientation to clients. If the LGB client asks you what your sexual orientation is, in most cases you should go ahead and openly answer that question. The client is likely asking you because she wants to know if she can feel safe and accepted with you and/or she might be thinking about looking for an LGB therapist. She may also ask you whether you feel comfortable working with LGB clients. Be prepared to answer that question:

"Yes, I have a lot of experience with people who are lesbian and gay." (Note that it is okay if some of this experience is in your personal life).

"Yes, I very much hope that I can help you with your difficulties."

Research has shown that knowledgeable heterosexual therapists can be seen as effective and helpful by their LGB clients (Burckell & Goldfried, 2006). If LGB clients have a strong preference for an LGB therapist, they usually will look for one to begin with. Another common scenario is the LGB psychotherapist with the heterosexual client. In general, if it isn't relevant to the client's psychotherapeutic issues, there is no reason to disclose your sexual orientation to the client. If you are LGB and feel that it would be helpful for your LGB client to know this, discuss how you might self-disclose to the client with your supervisor. In addition, you may wish to read about some of the issues that may arise when you are a member of the same LGB community as your client (L. E. Kessler & Waehler, 2005).

A more complex situation is when a client who is confused or conflicted about his sexual identity asks a therapist about his sexual orientation. Depending on the client's tolerance of ambiguity and the strength of the therapeutic relationship, you might want to explore the implications of your response before you self-disclose: "I don't mind answering that question, but before I do, would you mind telling me a little bit about how it would be helpful to you to know the answer?" The therapist might follow up with the following:

> "How do you think you would feel if you learned that I was gay? How would you feel if you learned I was heterosexual?"

Balance these two considerations: first, telling the client about your own orientation (especially if you are not LGB) may inhibit the client's self-exploration process; however, alternatively, not telling the client while asking questions might raise his anxiety level higher than he may be able to tolerate well. Decide what is best for your particular client's situation.

Note that I have not addressed any of the treatment issues of *intersex* and *transgendered* individuals in this section; fewer individuals identify as intersex or transgendered than lesbian, gay, or bisexual. *Intersex* individuals' sex chromosomes, genitalia, and/or secondary sexual characteristics are not exclusively male or female (in the past, the outdated term *hermaphrodite* was often used). *Transgendered* is a difficult term to define and often relates to individuals who are in the process of transitioning between genders but may also describe others who do not identify as strictly male or female in other ways. These clients have specific treatment issues that are beyond the scope of this book. Suffice it to say that the psychotherapist should not treat an intersex or transgendered client without, at a minimum, an intensive effort to learn the professional literature about these groups and, preferably, knowledgeable supervision or consultation as well.

OTHER NONOBVIOUS DIFFERENCES

Vanessa Morgan is a mental health trainee. She has been working for a year and a half with Mark Phillips, and Mark's depression and social isolation have improved significantly. In today's session, Mark tells Vanessa that he went hunting with his brother and his two nephews. He volunteers to bring her some venison next time he comes. Ordinarily, Vanessa would be willing to accept a small gift from a client, and she knows that Mark simply wants to show his appreciation. However, Vanessa is a vegetarian and thus really does not want a large slab of deer meat in her office. She fears that if she does not tell him that she is a vegetarian, she will be presented with a gift of meat sooner or later. On the other hand, she fears that if she tells him that she is a vegetarian, he will see this as an implicit criticism of his hunting. After weighing her options, she decides that the relationship is strong enough to handle this. She states, "Thank you so much for thinking of giving me some of the meat, but since I'm a vegetarian, I'm afraid that I have to decline."

A therapist who adheres to strict Jewish or Muslim dietary standards would not eat the deer meat, either, because it was not killed according to the appropriate religiously specified protocol. Another example of nonobvious differences would be a client asking whether a therapist likes barbecued ribs — and the therapist keeps kosher or is Muslim or is a vegetarian.

If the relationship is more tenuous, the therapist may gently indicate that the therapist doesn't care for the particular food being mentioned and steer the session in another direction. Other examples of nonobvious differences would be parenting status, family-of-origin differences, and so on. At times, ethnic and cultural differences can be nonobvious differences as well.

Generally, letting our clients know about some of our personal differences yet still being able to maintain a close therapeutic relationship helps all of us learn to respect and accept these differences. However, you must weigh the risks and benefits of sharing nonobvious personal differences in a particular situation individually. Too much information about you can become a boundary violation over time. After the client asks several questions about your personal matters, it must usually be explored as a therapeutic issue. (See chapter 4 for further discussion of personal questions from clients.)

COMPLEXLY DIVERSE CLIENTS

Angelica Lopez is a mental health trainee who is being assigned a new client. Her client is a second-generation Syrian American, Jason Al-Khani, who is just realizing that he is gay. The client's parents are university professors at a major university in Texas, and he grew up there. She cannot even begin to speculate how these varying cultural influences will interact in the client.

Modern 21st-century nations are tremendously culturally diverse. Clearly, we must have exposure and understanding of individual differences, acculturation, biculturalism, and other diversity topics. However, no textbook or article can cover all the possible interactions between different cultural, societal, and family influences in a particular client. Like Angelica, we might see clients whose multiple influences confuse us. Or we might see emigrants from nations whose cultural backgrounds we know little about and cannot learn much about from the psychological literature (e.g., Greeks or Egyptians). In these situations, we must be open to getting information from our clients about their cultural influence to arrive at a complete conceptualization.

COPING WITH CLINICAL ERRORS RELATING TO CULTURAL DIFFERENCES

Ebony Jackson is a mental health trainee working with a middle-aged female client of Puerto Rican background living in a major urban area. They have had several sessions and have developed a good rapport. Ebony has demonstrated her understanding of the client's bicultural struggles as they affect her role in the family (traditional mother versus cobreadwinner). Her client is having problems with her adult stepdaughter, who the family refers to as "Baby." The client feels that her husband is overly protective of "Baby." Ebony blurts out, "Well if everyone calls her Baby, no wonder she behaves that way! What is her real name?" The client tells her the name, then gently informs her that all the Puerto Rican families she knows call the youngest child in the family "Baby," even as an adult. Ebony apologized to the client, who was amused by the error.

Heather Parker is a White mental health trainee with an African American young adult client. The client is very close with her sister, and they raid each other's closets all the time. The sister stays over at the client's apartment even though they live in the same city. They are often loaning each other small amounts of money back and forth. Heather conceptualizes this behavior as "enmeshed" and encourages her client to have more separation from her sister. Later Heather's supervisor reminds her that resource sharing and family closeness is common in the client's cultural group, and so the client's behavior is totally normal. At the next session, Heather apologized to the client for her misunderstanding.

None of us has any desire to make the types of clinical errors that Ebony and Heather have made. But it is almost inevitable that all of us will, sooner or later. As the case of Ebony demonstrates, we might understand basic cultural issues but still be surprised by unexpected traditions that mean something very different from our initial interpretation. As the case of Heather demonstrates, we might have an intellectual understanding of cultural differences, but applying this knowledge takes time and experience.

If you do make this kind of clinical error, as you can see from the previous examples, it is unlikely to cause a permanent rift in the therapeutic relationship. However, it is important to apologize to the client as soon as you realize that you have made an error. Then, as necessary, explore how your error has impacted the client.

COPING WITH PREJUDICED CLIENTS

Pablo Sanchez is a mental health trainee working with a lower-functioning population. The group members do not know that Pablo is gay. He is coleading group therapy when a group member starts to use offensive language when talking about a supposedly gay person. Pablo and his cotherapists (who know that Pablo is gay) are shocked and don't know what to say, and the moment passes.

On occasion, one's clients in therapy will make discriminatory remarks toward a group. Commonly, this is done toward a group that the client does not belong to and thinks that the therapist does not belong to. Often, when first encountering this behavior from clients, therapists may be shocked and uncertain about what to do.

The therapist in this situation often has at least two concerns about these remarks. First, these remarks are not socially appropriate. Persons making these types of remarks are unlikely to have positive relationships with individuals of other groups, which is dysfunctional, given the increasing diversity of 21st-century nations. Even more important, the therapist does not want to give the client the impression that he or she agrees with the discriminatory remarks by not commenting on them. This leaves the therapist with the challenge of how to address the remarks appropriately in therapy.

Laszloffy and Hardy (2000) suggest that the therapist should first validate some aspect of the feelings that the client has in the situation: "It sounds as though you were very frustrated with how that other passenger treated you on the train." Note that in this reflection, you do not use the discriminatory language that the client used. This provides the client with an implicit message that you will not engage in using this language during their interactions.

At this point, you should consider the client's functioning level. If the client is low functioning, you might simply request that discriminatory language not be used during the individual or group therapy session: "I'd appreciate it if you did not use those words during our meeting."

If you believe that the client has the capacity to tolerate it, you might ask some of these questions:

"How do other people respond when you use that kind of language?"

"What kinds of feelings do you have about [group]? How did you develop those? Do you know anyone who is [group]? Do you use that term around her? Why not?"

If questions about the client's experiences and language are asked gently, this will minimize defensiveness, and the client is more likely to see this behavior as inappropriate as well. In addition, consider that Hamer (2006) suggests that racist remarks of a client can often be indicative of underlying issues, often regarding transference and anger, which can be productively explored in therapy.

COPING WITH CLIENTS WHO ARE PREJUDICED AGAINST YOU OR YOUR DEMOGRAPHIC GROUP

Ryan Yamamoto is a Japanese American mental health trainee doing a rotation at the Veterans Affairs Medical Center. He is interested in working with Vietnam veterans and has been assigned to work with a staff psychologist leading a psychotherapy group. The psychologist will be Ryan's supervisor for this training experience. Before going to the group, the psychologist warns Ryan that the group may react negatively to his ethnicity. During the first group session that Ryan attends, one group member refers to him by an ethnic slur and insists that he cannot work with Ryan.

Dominique King is an African American mental health trainee working with a rural southern population. She has a new White female client who has been treating her in a strange way that she can't exactly describe. She asks the client if she has any concerns about working with an African American therapist. The client says, "No, of course not. I'm used to having Blacks take care of me."

The appearance of each therapist, including gender, age, ethnicity, and any other obvious attributes, is a stimulus that will cause emotional reactions in some clients. These stimulus issues are unavoidable and intrinsic to who we are. Ethnic minority therapists may be especially plagued with insensitive remarks and prejudicial attitudes, as noted in the previous vignettes. It is beyond the scope of this volume to thoroughly address each possible example of demographic difference since each situation will have unique elements that need to be thoroughly explored in supervision as well as with demographically similar peers and mentors (M. Harris, 2005).

Therapists often have very legitimate concerns about the client's negative reactions toward the therapist. If the negative reactions are trauma based and the client is willing to continue to work with the therapist (as with the example of Ryan), the relationship may be difficult at first but has the potential to be especially therapeutic for the client. The client will have an opportunity to face and resolve fears about a particular demographic group, which can foster much-improved functioning.

Clients' prejudices can present themselves overly or covertly. Unfortunately, the literature on therapist–client racial differences focuses almost entirely on the White therapist–Black client dyad (Laszloffy & Hardy, 2000) and ignores the concerns of the racial minority therapist.

After one very overt remark or several subtly prejudicial remarks, the therapist may wish to ask the client,

> "I'm wondering if you may have any discomfort or concerns about working with a [fill in the blank] therapist?"

In the case of an overtly prejudicial client, it can sometimes be best for the case to be transferred to a therapist more demographically similar to the client who can address dysfunctional aspects of the client's prejudicial attitudes more comfortably over time. On the other hand, if the therapist is able to tolerate the client and continues to gently question the client when these issues come up, the client may be able to develop a greater maturity as well as tolerance and understanding for others. However, if the client insists on a transfer at any time, it is wise to accommodate that request.

As a supervisor and/or fellow group coleader, I would offer different feedback and assistance to the previously mentioned trainees, depending on the situation. Specifically, for Ryan and Pablo, who are dealing with prejudiced group members, we would work together to establish a group rule that no prejudicial comments are allowed. Given that Pablo's clients are low functioning, the simple goal of encouraging socially appropriate behavior, such as avoiding prejudicial remarks, might be sufficient. However, the issues that Ryan's client has are likely related to hypervigilance and post-traumatic stress disorder. These symptoms should be addressed directly, even while asking that the client talk to Ryan and the group appropriately. When the client gets used to Ryan and sees him as a helping professional, this will be a huge step in his recovery.

Dominique, on the other hand, is in a more difficult situation. The client is overtly cooperative with treatment but has an underlying prejudicial attitude toward the therapist. Dominique should discuss this situation carefully with her supervisor. On the one hand, a White therapist might be more accepted by the client. On the other hand, if Dominique can stick it out and gets help coping with the inevitable countertransference (since working with a client who is prejudiced against the therapist is an especially emotionally taxing situation), perhaps Dominique's assistance will help this client gain respect for African Americans as professionals and individuals over time. Later, when they develop a stronger bond, it may be possible to address this comment directly.

UNDERSTANDING UNCONSCIOUS CULTURAL PREJUDICES

I mean, you got the first mainstream African-American [Senator Barack Obama] who is articulate and bright and clean and a nice-looking guy. (Senator Joseph Biden, as quoted in the *New York Observer*, by J. Horowitz, February 4, 2007)

When whites use the word [*articulate*] in reference to blacks, it often carries a subtext of amazement, even bewilderment. It is similar to praising a female executive or politician by calling her "tough" or "a rational decision-maker." "When people say it, what they are really saying is that someone is articulate . . . for a black person," Ms. Perez said. Such a subtext is inherently offensive because it suggests that the recipient of the "compliment" is notably different from other black people. "Historically, it was meant to signal the exceptional Negro," Mr. Dyson said. "The implication is that most black people do not have the capacity to engage in articulate speech, when white people are automatically assumed to be articulate." (L. Clementson, *New York Times*, February 4, 2007)

Boding poorly for the start of his presidential campaign, Senator Biden apparently meant to compliment Senator Obama in the previous quote. Instead, he ended up revealing his (probably unconscious) racial prejudices by oddly describing him as "clean." And as the second quote reveals, even the seemingly positive adjective "articulate" can carry a loaded subtext.

It is easy for the rest of us to be appalled at Biden's obvious prejudices. However, cognitive psychologists have learned much about prejudices in the past 20 years, and what they've learned is that everyone within the culture is well aware of negative cultural stereotypes and that, unfortunately, these stereotypes are automatically elicited (Devine, 1989). However, just because one is aware of stereotypes does not mean that one has any desire to implement them.

Research has shown that low-prejudice individuals establish a personal belief structure that allows them to consciously counteract the known, automatically elicited cultural stereotype. In addition, research has shown that education (Rudman, Ashmore, & Gary, 2001) is effective in reducing prejudice and stereotypes.

As therapists, we must acknowledge that, like everyone else in the culture, we have ingested unhealthy racial and cultural stereotypes and prejudices. This issue is further discussed in the context of the therapist's emotional reactions to the client in chapter 22. Modern psychotherapy training programs emphasize multicultural education and training, an essential step in helping us to cope effectively with these cultural influences.

RECOMMENDED READING

Bieschke, K. J., Perez, R. M., & DeBord, K. A. (Eds.). (2006). *Handbook of counseling and psychotherapy with lesbian, gay, bisexual, and transgender clients* (2nd ed.). Washington, DC: American Psychological Association.
Many contributors to this edited volume provide enhanced expertise and assist the psychotherapist in learning about cultural contexts and affirmative counseling with lesbian, gay, bisexual, and transgender clients.

Devine, P. G. (1989). Stereotypes and prejudice: Their automatic and controlled components. *Journal of Personality and Social Psychology, 56*, 5–18.
In this now classic article, Devine describes the process of automatic racial stereotype activation.

Hamer, F. M. (2006). Racism as a transference state: Episodes of racial hostility in the psychoanalytic context. *Psychoanalytic Quarterly, 75*, 197–214.
Hamer's discussion of how he, an African American therapist, addressed clients' racist remarks in therapy is well worth reading for therapists of all racial backgrounds and provides invaluable insights into the psychodynamics of racism.

Larson, D. B., & Larson, S. S. (2003). Spirituality's potential relevance to physical and emotional health: A brief review of quantitative research. *Journal of Psychology and Theology, 31*, 37–51.
Larson and Larson provide an informative and evenhanded review of the literature on spirituality and health; this is a good introduction to the topic.

Nesbit, R. E. (2003). *The geography of thought: How Asians and Westerners think differently . . . and why.* New York: Free Press.
This fascinating work summarizes research describing cultural and cognitive differences, showing how people from different cultures actually see the world differently.

EXERCISES AND DISCUSSION QUESTIONS

1. Given your age, ethnicity, sexual orientation, and other factors, what challenges do you anticipate having with clients who are different from you? Which of these challenges are more likely to be related to prejudice and

which to a lack of understanding? How will you or the client know the difference?

2. What thoughts do you have about addressing a client's prejudicial remarks toward you? Would it matter if the client did or did not know that you belong to the group he is prejudiced against?

3. How would you address a client's prejudicial remarks toward others?

Chapter Six

Professional Electronic Communications

Electronic communications are fraught with potential for therapeutic problems, including misunderstandings, inappropriate remarks, legal liability, and breaches of confidentiality. However, although electronic communications are an essential part of modern life, the mental health literature provides limited guidance. Yet I understand that you, as a beginning therapist, still need input on these matters. I will draw on the literature that does exist and my personal experiences and those of other mental health practitioners I know.

CHOOSING YOUR E-MAIL ADDRESS

A training site supervisor is reviewing vitas of mental health trainees that might be matched to the site. He sees that one student's personal e-mail address is foxyshrink12345@aprovider.com. He thinks that the student has poor taste, poor judgment, or both. The student is not offered an interview for that site.

If you can choose an e-mail ID at work, choose something simple and recognizable. For example, you might choose kellyreed@thisclinic.org or kreed@thatclinic.com. If you enter a tagline on your work e-mail, enter your job title. This will help people learn who you are. Never choose anything religious, irrelevant, distracting, personal, or (supposedly) humorous.

Your personal e-mail address should be one that you can keep indefinitely (e.g., Hotmail or Yahoo!). For example, you don't want your university to terminate your e-mail address when you are applying for your first job. That would impede your professional networking at a crucial point. However, some universities do let alumni keep their e-mail addresses indefinitely.

PROFESSIONAL E-MAIL

Two mental health trainees at a training site are good friends. They send each other e-mail about how things are going. They are using the training site's e-mail system for these messages when they are at work. One sends the other an e-mail criticizing his supervisor. When the other trainee is reading it, she is thinking about how she needs to forward a different e-mail to that supervisor; then she absentmindedly forwards the negative e-mail to the very supervisor the first student is criticizing. Professional embarrassment and interpersonal difficulties ensue.

Professional e-mail has a very different tone than personal e-mail. Many clinics and medical centers have a secure internal e-mail system where you can safely discuss patient care issues with other professionals. Remember, you should consider that all e-mail might be retrievable by a superior at any time. Here are some don'ts:

- Don't ever send any e-mail that you would not want everyone in the clinic to read. E-mails can get mistakenly forwarded or, worse, maliciously forwarded.
- Don't talk negatively about anyone, clients or staff, on e-mail.
- Don't ever write an e-mail when you are angry. Cool off and later handle the situation tactfully, in person.
- Don't ever write anything in an e-mail that would humiliate or endanger you or anyone else if you had to talk about it in a court of law. E-mail is discoverable.
- Don't use e-mail abbreviations (e.g., BTW [by the way] or LOL [laugh out loud]). Many of your colleagues will be old enough that they don't understand what you're saying. Besides, it looks unprofessional.
- Avoid or use very few "emoticons." These often come across as juvenile or overly silly to your older colleagues.
- Don't use professional e-mail systems for personal chitchat. Use your personal e-mail address and the recipient's personal e-mail address for this instead. Again, if it is ever discovered or forwarded, you will regret it.

SENDING E-MAIL ABOUT CLIENTS TO OTHER PRACTITIONERS

E-mail can help tremendously in coordinating care between different professionals, but use it carefully. If sensitive information must be conveyed, a voice mail is preferable, as voice mail is generally more secure.

If you do send e-mail, you should first consider the type of e-mail system that you are sending the e-mail on. If you are sending it from one e-mail address to another within the same clinic or hospital, it is possible that the e-mail system has been protected with sufficient firewalls that you can send identifying information safely by e-mail. Never send identifying information unless you have first asked your supervisor and/or the computer network administrator about the internal security of the system.

Even on a secure e-mail system, confine your discussion of client issues to bare facts as much as possible. Especially if they are electronic and readily accessible, let your progress notes speak for themselves and just send an e-mail pointing out that there is important information in them.

> Wrong: "Hi Lori: Bob was at his session today and talked about killing himself again. I'm sick and tired of all his manipulation. Anyway, can you fit him in sooner for meds?
> Right: "Hi Lori: Please see my note for today on Bob. Can you fit him in sooner for meds?

The first note makes unkind negative statements about Bob, which should never be done in an e-mail (if you feel that way about Bob, you need to discuss your countertransference about him in supervision instead). The second e-mail refers to the note instead.

Never, ever, send any unsecured e-mail that mentions a client by name or that gives any identifying information about the client. Unsecured e-mail would be any e-mail account that you have personally or through your school, but other e-mail accounts can be unsecured as well. Here are two examples of unsecured e-mails that you might consider sending:

> Wrong: "Hi Lori: I'm referring you a 27-year-old Filipino American male client, Roberto P. He's a graduate student at Xavier University and has been struggling with depression for years. I'm worried about suicidality and want to talk to you about it before his first appointment. Call me."
> Right: "Hi Lori: I'm referring you a new client, R.P. I'm faxing you a release today. There are some urgent issues, so please call me about this client before the first appointment. Wednesday morning is a good time to reach me."

Even though the first example does not include the last name, too much identifying information has been included in the e-mail. The second example includes only initials—and not even the gender—which is enough information that Lori can identify the client when he calls, especially when Lori finds out that you referred him. Often one or two initials are sufficient for the recipient to figure out what client you are referring to, so using any names at all should be avoided. In addition, never post too much identifying information to a listserv.

COMMUNICATING BY E-MAIL WITH CLIENTS

Many therapists communicate with clients by e-mail. I do as well. However, before I even see new clients, they must fill out a form indicating their understanding of my e-mail policy. I indicate that they should not use e-mail to contact me in an emergency and that they need to be aware that e-mail is not a confidential medium, so any sensitive information should be brought up during the session instead.

You should never give an e-mail address that you share with a family member to a client. If you give an e-mail address to a client, it must be one that is used by you alone (Woody, 1999).

Most therapists prefer to confine e-mail exchanges to minor issues such as appointment scheduling. Here is a sample of this kind of e-mail:

> Hi Connie: I'm realizing that I have schedule problems next week. Can we move our appointment to 5:00 instead of 3:00? Thanks, [your name]

Never give out your e-mail address without discussing it with a supervisor. There may be some relevant clinical issues that should be discussed when you are tempted to share your e-mail address. Why can't the client just call? Case reports in the literature suggest that e-mail may be more subject to misinterpretation and boundary crossing than other types of communication (Gutheil & Simon, 2005).

Keep in mind that clients might be able to get your e-mail address through your university's website—so a client may decide to send you e-mail without discussing it with you first. If you think this is likely, discuss e-mail issues with the client proactively. At times, despite your requests, a client may send clinically relevant information to you by e-mail. In these cases, they often just want to give you an update but don't need much of a response from you. Here is an appropriate response:

> Hi Connie: Thanks for sending me this information. I can see that this is very important, and I look forward to hearing more about it when I see you on Wednesday. Sincerely, [your name]

Note that the response is respectful of the importance of the e-mail without commenting on its contents. Don't comment on the information by e-mail since you will be more effective dealing with it during the therapy session. Too much detail and emotion is lost through e-mail communications to address the issue effectively (Gutheil & Simon, 2005). When you see the client next, you might suggest that the client write in her journal about the issue instead, then bring her writings to the therapy sessions to read to you there. Emphasize your concerns about her privacy and confidentiality as you make this suggestion.

Another reason to avoid most e-mail communications with clients is that research indicates that e-mail communication is especially vulnerable to expectancies and stereotypes (Epley & Kruger, 2005). From this, it is not a large leap to conclude that there is a risk that transference issues could become overly intense and problematic through e-mail.

People have been found to overestimate their ability to convey emotion and tone over e-mail. This overconfidence is related to our innate egocentrism (Kruger, Epley, Parker, & Ng, 2005). The obvious implication is that we must all assume that our e-mails will be occasionally misinterpreted by others in ways that we are unable to predict.

You should save a copy of any e-mail that you have sent or received from a client that has clinically relevant information in it. E-mail can be printed out and placed physically into the chart, or you can copy it into an electronic medical record instead. Some might advise that you save every e-mail from a client, whereas other clinicians would not bother saving e-mails that solely deal with routine scheduling or billing issues, so opinions differ. Discuss this issue with your supervisor and do as she suggests.

ONLINE CONSULTATION AND TREATMENT

Online treatment is a rapidly developing area, with evolving norms and protocols. Having any type of online relationship with a prospective client may legally create a doctor–patient relationship (Simon, 2004), which would mean that you would have a responsibility to do appropriate assessments in case of a crisis, suicidality, and so on, which is nearly impossible to do online. However, be aware that online treatment is not advised for any client who has any suicide or violence risk. Too little information is available compared to an in-person meeting. Be aware that practicing online consultation is a dangerous clinical activity from a risk management perspective.

TEXT MESSAGING AND INSTANT MESSAGING

You should never text-message with a client. Because of their brevity, text messages are highly prone to misinterpretation, projection, and so on. In the unlikely event that a client somehow figures how to send a text message to you, reply with a request that the client call you instead about the matter. Instant messages are too intimate and are likely to veer into chat. They are intrusive on the time outside the session and should also be avoided.

YOUR PERSONAL INFORMATION ON THE WEB

Many people have a prominent Web presence. They may have a page on a social networking site or a personal Web page. They may post vacation pictures online or have a blog. Maybe they do online dating. These are normal everyday activities, but as psychotherapists we need to think carefully about what we have online about ourselves.

Preserve your privacy carefully. If you ever decide to do online dating, consider not posting a picture and instead send it by e-mail to a select few who you are interested in meeting. If you post snapshots online, do not use any ID that can link your snapshots to you through search engines. Delete your online information *now* since search engine caches will keep it available to searches for a while after it is deleted.

Carefully review everything you have put online. Potential employers or supervisors may look you up online and judge you negatively. This has now become common (Finder, 2006). Even more upsetting is the likelihood that sooner or later an intrusive and disturbed client will find this material. At best, it will be awkward or disruptive to the therapeutic process. ("Hey, I see on your MySpace page that you're not single anymore—what's up with that?" or the client sends you an invitation to be "friends.") At worst, it may aid in stalking and otherwise harassing you.

As a professional, I advise removing *all* personal information from open access on the Web. If you insist on having personal information available on the Web, do this only if there is a way to make it privately available only to your friends, family, and others you specify. For example, networking site entries should be not be available to the general public because they include too much personal information (e.g., relationship status, sexual orientation, religion, income, and zodiac sign).

Blogs also contain too much personal information. I recommend avoiding writing blogs altogether, although in certain cases you might want to blog a special event, such as a vacation, limiting access to friends and family. Therapists should *never* have blogs about their personal or professional lives freely available to anyone on the Internet. And never, ever, mention anything about a client in a blog.

RECOMMENDED READING

Gutheil, T. G., & Simon, R. I. (2005). E-mails, extra-therapeutic contact, and early boundary problems: The internet as a "slippery slope." *Psychiatric Annals, 35,* 952–960.
Some of the true but disguised case examples in this article will make you think very carefully about exchanging e-mail with clients.

EXERCISES AND DISCUSSION QUESTIONS

1. Some people feel that some of my advice regarding keeping your phone number unlisted and minimizing your Web presence in this chapter is too risk averse. What do you think? Are you going to make the recommended changes?
2. Is it too limiting of your personal life to avoid blogging or public Web pages?

Section II

GETTING STARTED
WITH PSYCHOTHERAPY

Chapter Seven

Informed Consent, Confidentiality, and HIPAA

This chapter discusses some important factors to consider regarding the client's understanding of the therapy process and confidentiality. Health Insurance Portability and Accountability Act (HIPAA) regulations are included in this chapter as well. All these issues are presented to the client in written or verbal form at or before the first therapy session. If done in writing, the client reviews written information about these subjects and signs to indicate understanding and agreement. Then you provide an opportunity to ask questions as needed. Resources are provided at the end of this chapter if you need assistance in developing client information materials.

INFORMED CONSENT FOR PSYCHOTHERAPY

Informed consent requires a mentally competent person who has a good knowledge of what will occur in treatment, freely chooses to be treated, and is documented in the record as such. If any of these is lacking, its absence must be documented, explained, and responded to. (Zuckerman, 2003, p. 172)

The basic elements of informed consent are competence, information and voluntariness. (Simon, 1992, p. 123)

What is meant by *informed consent*? These two quotes cover the significant points; the informed consent process involves the following:

• A mentally competent client
• Education about the treatment process and treatment options, including risks and benefits
• Voluntary consent to treatment
• Documentation of the above

Clearly, not all the possible risks of treatment can be predicted since you do not know how the client's social and professional circles will react to the changes made in therapy (Beahrs & Gutheil, 2001). To ascertain whether a client is mentally competent to provide fully informed consent, a client must be able to comprehend relevant information, appreciate the relevance of the information provided to the situation, be able to weigh the risks and benefits against alternatives, and make a clear choice to participate (Eyler & Jeste, 2006). If the client is cognitively limited or has severe mental illness, the client may not be able to provide fully informed consent. Read more about this issue if you are working in a setting where this is a concern.

Our professional ethics codes require that we, as mental health professionals, obtain informed consent (American Counseling Association, 2005; American Psychiatric Association, 2006; American Psychological Association, 2002; National Association of Social Workers, 1999). Across mental health professions, differing standards are written into ethics codes about whether informed consent should be oral, written, or both. One code explicitly requires that informed consent be documented as well (American Psychological Association, 2002), although we can safely assume that other professions would also endorse documentation. Additionally, informed consent requirements encoded in law can vary by state (Braaten, Otto, & Handelsman, 1993).

However, fully informed consent is often not obtained by psychotherapists (Somberg, Stone, & Claiborn, 1993). This is a professional danger since large sums have been awarded in certain legal cases where informed consent was not obtained (Beahrs & Gutheil, 2001). Research suggests that professionals who engage in informed consent procedures may be seen by their clients as having more trustworthiness and expertise (T. Sullivan, Martin, & Handelsman, 1993). All these considerations make it a necessity that psychotherapists obtain and document informed consent from their therapy clients.

Braaten et al. (1993) summarize areas that various authors have suggested should be covered in the informed consent process: (a) the nature of treatment; (b) benefits and risks of treatment; (c) likely alternative treatments and their benefits and risks; (d) the probability of reaching successful outcomes; (e) limits of confidentiality; (f) financial costs and arrangements; (g) time, place, setting, and duration of treatment; (h) therapist training, qualifications, and theoretical orientation; (i) the procedure for handling grievances; (j) a statement that any questions about procedures will be answered at any time; and (k) a statement that therapy can be discontinued at any time. Clearly, this is an extensive list, and a detailed verbal examination of all these points with every client would be a waste of time and an unnecessary burden to many clients. For this reason, written informed consent procedures have been developed so that clients can learn about their treatment. Then you provide an opportunity for the client to ask questions during the initial session and subsequent ones as needed.

Your first option in obtaining informed consent is to use a written format; see Zuckerman (2003) for a complete and detailed description of five different ways in which informed consent can be obtained in a written format. When informed consent is obtained in writing, a copy of that form is kept in the client's permanent chart, and you may not have to also document informed consent in the progress notes as well. However, you may wish to give the client an opportunity to ask questions and document this interaction in the chart.

Your second option to obtain informed consent is to use a verbal rather than a written format. In fact, some experts prefer this option as being better tailored to the needs of the client (Beahrs & Gutheil, 2001). For your reference, I have outlined in appendix 2 the process of obtaining verbal informed consent with a mentally competent adult.

An interesting third option, with the aim of engaging the client more actively in the informed consent process, is to provide the client with a list of potential questions to ask about therapy that is supplemented by oral and written information (Handelsman & Galvin, 1988; Pomerantz & Handelsman, 2004). See these references if you are interesting in learning more about this option.

As a beginning therapist, you will probably be entering into clinical situations where policies about how to obtain informed consent have already been established on a facility-wide basis. Your supervisor can orient you to how informed consent is obtained in your facility. If no written informed consent process is in place, I recommend that you carefully obtain verbal informed consent instead and document in the chart that you have done so. Be sure that the informed consent policy involves either written or verbal discussion of fee payment policies at the clinic so that future difficulties about fees are minimized.

Informed consent is a complex issue, and the process of obtaining it varies depending on population characteristics and circumstances. For example, the informed consent process differs significantly with children and adolescents (Beeman & Scott, 1991); detailing these differences is beyond the scope of this book. Sometimes informed consent cannot be obtained because of an emergency or other practical reasons (Zuckerman, 2003). Informed consent when the client is treated with psychotropic medications involves additional considerations (Schachter & Kleinman, 2004) that are also beyond the scope of this volume. Growing use of technology, including use of videoconferencing equipment for therapy or doing therapy over the Internet, may require special informed consent considerations (Recupero & Rainey, 2005). Finally, there are special considerations for the informed consent process when doing research (Davies, 2001; Wendler & Rackoff, 2001); read further about this issue as needed.

DISCUSSING SUPERVISION WITH CLIENTS

As part of the informed consent process, you will need to alert your clients that you will be supervised. I recommend something like the following script, which is modified from Walker and Jacobs (2004):

> Since I am a [insert type of psychotherapy student], I am regularly supervised on my clinical work. Part of getting supervision includes listening to audiotapes. I will be asking you to sign a form indicating that you consent to being audiotaped, and we will routinely tape our sessions. [pause for client comment] Do you have any questions or concerns?

You should tape every session, whether you expect your supervisor to listen to it or not, so that the client becomes less self-conscious about being taped (Walker & Jacobs, 2004). In some settings, verbal rather than written agreement is sufficient. In that case, be sure to document the client's agreement in your progress note.

Often clients will have a few brief factual questions. They may want to know who your supervisor is (tell them), why you need supervision ("It's part of my professional training and development"), and other questions. Answer the questions completely yet succinctly. Clients may also have some unique worries or fears about the supervisor or the supervision process. For example, some are fearful about their confidentiality, while others may fear being judged by the supervisor. These fears will often be useful clues about the client's interpersonal problems. These fears may be allayed somewhat by describing the supervision process in slightly more detail:

> "Yes, we will talk about your issues to some extent, but the main focus of supervision is to help me learn how to understand you and help you better."

CONFIDENTIALITY

Professional ethics codes (e.g., American Psychological Association, 2002) require that we discuss *confidentiality* at the outset of therapy with our clients. It is essential to know what the legal limits to confidentiality are in the state where you are practicing, and you must alert your clients to these limits either verbally or in writing as part of the informed consent process when beginning therapy.

Research has indicated that people can erroneously believe that everything said in therapy is confidential and that therapists often do not educate their psychotherapy clients about legal limits to confidentiality (Braaten et al., 1993). Legal limits to confidentiality would include state-mandated reporting of child and elder abuse and perhaps intimate partner violence. Specifically, certain identifying information must be released when the clinician makes a report of abuse. Another legal limitation to confidentiality may be reporting plans of violence against another person.

The client needs to understand that you will be discussing her with your supervisor and perhaps also others on the treatment team. In addition, if the client is involved in legal proceedings where a determination of the client's mental health is of importance, there are circumstances in which the therapy record can be subpoenaed. Although unlikely, you can release information that is needed to secure emergency medical care for the client, and you can release information to a coroner examining a client's death (Moline, Williams, & Austin, 1998).

Legal limits to confidentiality should be covered at the beginning of therapy. Many therapists prefer to do this in writing. They provide written material about the limits to confidentiality (for some examples, see Zuckerman, 2003) and ask the client to sign to indicate understanding. As needed, you should provide opportunities to discuss confidentiality in the first and subsequent sessions. Alternatively, many therapists prefer to discuss these issues verbally during the first session. A suggested verbal script for addressing confidentiality is provided for you in appendix 3. If you choose this option, you should carefully document what you discussed in the client's chart.

Be mindful about where you are discussing clinical issues. Treatment planning should not occur in restaurants, elevators, or other public places. Discussions about mutual clients should not occur in agency hallways. Find a private place to talk instead. However, you can discuss general (not specific) clinical issues (carefully) in public locations that are not connected to the work setting, such as having lunch with a colleague at a restaurant:

Right: "Tell me how you manage clients who aren't coming to their sessions regularly and always seem to have a good excuse."
Wrong: "I have this 50-year-old client who lives with his mother and always cancels at the last minute because he says he has to take his mother to the hospital again for treatment. What should I do?"

So you can discuss principles of treatment in public but avoid discussing the specifics of any particular client.

Special issues regarding confidentiality include children and adolescents, confidentiality after client death, and confidentiality when the client is at risk of spreading HIV, among others. If any of these issues (or any others I have not covered) are likely to arise in your client population, you may wish to review the literature on confidentiality in those circumstances. While those issues are beyond the scope of this volume, articles on these subjects and others are readily available through databases.

USING CASE MATERIAL IN COURSE WORK, LECTURES, WRITINGS, AND OTHER MEDIA

Ethical considerations (American Psychological Association, 2002) require that when case material is used in communications, "(1) they [psychologists] take reasonable steps to disguise the person or organization, (2) the person or organization has consented in writing, or (3) there is legal authorization for doing so." The American Psychiatric Association (2006) has similar standards: "Clinical and other materials used in teaching and writing must be adequately disguised in order to preserve the anonymity of the individuals involved. . . . It is ethical to present a patient or former patient to a public gathering or to the news media only if the patient is fully informed of enduring loss of confidentiality, is competent, and consents in writing without coercion (pp. 6–7)."

Your first consideration with using case material is how far the material is distributed. Case material that is discussed within a clinical treatment team or with a supervisor should not have any masking of the client's identity. Often students may need to write up or present case material as part of their course work. These training presentations are generally with one or two supervisors and a small group of peers. As long as you believe that there is almost no likelihood that your colleagues will know the client, a *mild disguise* will do. Mild disguise would include leaving off or changing the client's name, making the age vague (mid-20s versus 24 years old), and omitting any extraneous identifying details that are not important to the case presentation. Note that this type of case material should never be posted anywhere on the Internet, used in a larger professional format, or published since it is not well disguised and you may not have obtained informed consent to use the material.

As you advance in your work, you may have the opportunity to make presentations to a larger professional group or prepare professional articles or books. Case material can be helpful in illustrating your points to the audience. However, you must take great care in preserving the privacy of your clients in those instances. Any case material that is written in a book or journal article *must* be considered to be readily accessible by clients. Thus, in all these cases, more intensive disguising techniques should be used. You should also consider whether to get informed consent from the client as well.

Gabbard (2000a, 2001b) suggests a number of effective strategies for *thick disguise*. In all cases, you should falsify (rather than obscure) certain external features that are not pertinent to the clinical issues at hand. For example, changing the client's profession, ethnicity, or other identifying features will make the client more difficult to identify than if you are just vague about these. He also emphasizes that brief vignettes can be as illustrative of the clinical issues as longer case descriptions are and will be more protective of the client's privacy. You can make further efforts to maintain confidentiality by using composite cases, by writing joint papers (so that it is unclear who the treating psychotherapist was), and by using case materials from other psychotherapists in your presentations or writings.

As you may have noticed, all the case material in this book is presented in the form of vignettes. All the vignettes that are based on real events are heavily disguised and/or composite; however, many others are complete fiction, invented to illustrate a point. As a practical matter, you may decide not to use case material in a book or presentation until many years after you have seen the client. You may not have any practical way of contacting the client because of the passage of time and other barriers (e.g., you have different employment, you forgot names, and so on). In those cases, if you use the material, you must use thick disguise.

When presenting longer case material in a professional presentation or publication, the psychotherapist should consider obtaining informed consent from the client (Gabbard, 2000a). This is particularly pertinent if the case material is difficult to disguise. This consent can be written, or it can be verbal and then be documented in the progress notes. In this case, the client may be given a copy of the presentation or article for review before it is presented to the profession. Be aware that this request might inspire numerous and varied emotional reactions, including feeling honored, insulted, exploited, and many more (for an insightful discussion of possible clinical ramifications, see Gabbard, 2000a).

Finally, I agree with the American Psychiatric Association (2006) guidelines that require a careful informed consent process if clinical information about a particular client is to be presented in any forum for the general public, such as on the news or in a general interest publication. Probably a better alternative in that case would be to use composite cases with details carefully changed and combined so that no one could ever be identified.

SOME IMPLICATIONS OF HIPAA FOR THE TRAINEE

When health care practitioners are talking about HIPAA, they are usually talking about two separate rules that apply to all health care practitioners. These rules are the HIPAA Security Rule and the HIPAA Privacy Rule. Exploring all the implications of HIPAA rules is far beyond the scope of this volume. However, I will briefly discuss the focus of each rule and some implications for mental health trainees. Every institution or organization where you work should have a designated HIPAA security officer and a designated HIPAA privacy officer, who may be the same individual. These individuals are responsible for ensuring HIPAA compliance throughout the organization. Ask your supervisor who these officers are and ask them questions about HIPAA as needed.

Before discussing what the rules are, you need to know that *protected health information* (PHI) is "information, including demographic data, that relates to: the individual's past, present or future physical or mental health or condition, the provision of health care to the individual, or the past, present, or future payment for the provision of health care to the individual, and that identifies the individual or for which there is a reasonable basis to believe can be used to identify the individual. Individually identifiable health information includes many common identifiers (e.g., name, address, birth date, Social Security Number)" (U.S. Department of Health and Human Services, 2003 p. 4). Thus, PHI is any information that can identify the client or that describes the client's health care.

The HIPAA Privacy Rule controls when, under what circumstances, and to whom the health care practitioner intentionally releases PHI. Note that the Privacy Rule focuses on intentional releases of protected health information, while the HIPAA Security Rule focuses on safeguarding against unintentional disclosures (American Psychological Association Practice Organization, 2007). To comply with the HIPAA Privacy Rule, health care organizations develop a Notice of Privacy Practices form, among other activities. The HIPAA Privacy Rule has implications for mental health progress notes, which will be discussed in chapter 13. Your supervisor can guide you regarding when and how information about your clients is released. You may be responsible for having new clients sign a Notice of Privacy Practices form and answering any questions that the clients may have about privacy. Ensure that appropriate releases are obtained from the client at any time that information about the client is sent out of the health care facility.

As noted previously, the HIPAA Security Rule is about protecting electronic health information from unintended disclosure through breaches of security and from unintended loss, such as through fire or flood (American Psychological

Association Practice Organization, 2007). This rule is implemented primarily through appropriate electronic security measures and backup procedures.

HIPAA AND DATA SECURITY ISSUES

The HIPAA Security Rule is most applicable to mental health trainees with regard to computer security. Any computer, personal digital assistant (PDA), flash drive, CD, or other device or storage media must be properly secured if it contains any protected health information. Thus, for example, if you keep your clients' phone numbers on your PDA, in case you become ill and may need to cancel their appointments, the PDA—and the computer it syncs with—must be password protected.

If you share a computer that has PHI on it with anyone else, even your partner, you must set up a separate log-on for them so that they cannot have access to the PHI. Before disposal or donation, any device that has ever had PHI on it must have the memory completely wiped by a program designed to do so. Just deleting the files is not sufficient and is a security violation. And you should have appropriate firewalls, perform regular backups, and run updated antivirus and antispyware programs on your personal computer that contains PHI (Kibbe, 2005).

You may need to move from office to office if space is tight at your practicum site. If you use a flash drive to move clinical documents that you are working on (e.g., psychological reports), you must password protect the flash drive as well. You can purchase a secure flash drive that can be accessed only with a password you specify (for options, just run an Internet search for "secure flash drive" or ask for help at an office supply store).

Researchers have studied attempts to hack into computers and have seen what hackers try (M. Cukier, cited in personal communication from K. S. Pope, February 16, 2007). They have found that any computer connected to the Internet has about two attempts to hack it per *minute*. Given their research, here are some user names *not* to set up on any computer: root, admin, test, guest, info, adm, mysql, user, administrator, and oracle. For the password, do not use your user name, serial digits such as "1234," "password," "passwd," or "test."

As a general rule, any document that contains information about a client must not be available in a public place, even on top of your desk when other clients are in the room. Secure this information in a locked drawer or filing cabinet. Do not let clients see the names of other clients on your computer screen. Any client materials or contact information you have in your home (perhaps a case conceptualization you are preparing for class) should be under a password or kept in a locked drawer or cabinet.

CONFIDENTIALITY AND THE THERAPIST'S PARTNER

Sometimes I find myself talking briefly about challenging clinical issues that have come up [with my partner], without giving any names or identifying material. I'm very careful not to give identifying info [to my partner]. I also often find myself being asked to talk about, or wanting to talk about, mental health issues that are of interest to the broader population (like PTSD in the returning soldiers, the recovered memory debate, etc.), and it's often useful to use anecdotes from cases with which I've been involved. Again, I keep it pretty non-specific, and I've even changed pertinent personal details (age, sex). I guess, in the end, the people with whom I would ever have these conversations to begin with are also going to be people who will be respectful of my boundaries, however I feel I need to draw them. (Anonymous psychotherapist, personal communication, January 21, 2007)

I tend to share experiences [with my partner] that are "out of the ordinary" or that somehow impact me personally (for example, things that hit close to home, a strong emotional reaction). I am cautious never to share any identifying information and usually focus on my reaction. (Anonymous psychotherapist, personal communication, February 3, 2007)

I think carefully about revealing the all-too-human side of the work to a spouse who has been or is currently in therapy. It's a feeling of wanting to protect without impingement the sacredness of the partner's connection w/their own therapist without the burden of, "Hey, if my wife says that a client is frustrating, does my therapist ever find me frustrating? (boring? difficult?)." It's this need to uphold the illusion that their therapist would never have these mere-mortal reactions (and the protection that illusion affords the work). I'm especially careful to avoid at all costs being overtly critical of a client, with the possible exception of those few who have left while still owing me money. For some reason in these instances I'll have no trouble talking to my husband about the client's history of character pathology and their decision to not pay me (of course again, never jeopardizing confidentiality). I don't tend to talk to him about the nuts and bolts of the work. He's not interested on that level and I don't have the need to do it. Like the rest of us, I rely on consultation for that, have a few colleagues that I check in with whenever needed. (Anonymous psychotherapist, personal communication, January 24, 2007)

My partner is a psychotherapist as well, so we sometimes discuss clinical issues and consult with each other. When doing this in the past, we often included what we thought were benign bits of personal identifying information (profession, involvement in a community organization, etc.). On a couple of occasions, however, it seemed easy to "connect the dots" and make a pretty good guess as to who he was discussing or who I was discussing. When we realized this, we were both quite troubled to realize our lapses—we had simply said too much that wasn't essential to the peer consultation we were seeking from one another. We have since been extremely careful about this. There are definite advantages to being partnered with another therapist, but it is also easy to slip into less-than-rigorous standards of privacy when discussing our work. We have to be pretty vigilant about this, and it is not always easy. (Anonymous psychotherapist, personal communication, February 23, 2007)

As a practical matter, it is not possible to fully withhold all information about one's clients from one's significant other. At times, you may need to isolate yourself in a room at home and close the door to call a client in crisis; your partner is undoubtedly savvy enough to understand what is going on. You may need to stay late at work because of a client's crisis; you will probably need to tell your partner that you were delayed because of a client crisis.

Woody (1999) counseled against being lax about patient confidentiality. Clients should be able to leave a message for you on a secure voice-mail system, and you should listen to your messages from clients where no one else can hear them. Do not have confidential information faxed to a fax machine that is not in a secure clinical area. Consider computer safety carefully. Woody (1999) also advises against discussing case material with significant others, family members, or other persons who are not mental health practitioners.

Given the emotional intimacy of one's relationship with one's partner, it is difficult to withhold all information about one's day-to-day emotional reactions to doing psychotherapy, as the previously quoted psychotherapists describe. If you do talk to your partner, focus on your emotional reaction rather than the clinical situation as much as possible. Never share any client's identifying information with a partner, relative, or friend. Educate them about why you need to be circumspect. Further research and inquiry is clearly needed in this area.

RECOMMENDED READING

Gabbard, G. O. (2000). Disguise or consent: Problems and recommendations concerning the publication and presentation of clinical material. *International Journal of Psychoanalysis, 81,* 1071–1086.
   This article provides a detailed discussion of the issues involved in presenting clinical material to colleagues while maintaining client confidentiality.
Woody, R. H. (1999). Domestic violations of confidentiality. *Professional Psychology: Research and Practice, 30,* 607–610.
   Woody describes a number of unfortunately common scenarios where confidentiality is violated by mental health practitioners.
Zuckerman, E. (2003). *The paper office* (3rd ed.). New York: Guilford Press.

This helpful and essential resource provides forms and helpful practice guidelines for many important clinical situations, including those discussed in this chapter.

WEB RESOURCES

http://www.hhs.gov/ocr/hipaa
The Department of Health and Human Services has extensive information available on its website about HIPAA.
http://kspope.com/consent/index.php
Dr. Kenneth Pope is a prominent psychologist and author. This page from his extensive website provides immediate access to a variety of informed consent forms as well as standards for informed consent from many prominent mental health professional organizations.

EXERCISES AND DISCUSSION QUESTIONS

1. What are the procedures for informed consent, HIPAA, and informing clients about confidentiality at your site? Do you feel that these procedures are adequate? If not, how would you address this?
2. What information about clients is okay to talk about to your partner, a close friend, or family member? What should you avoid? Does it matter if the partner, friend, or relative is a mental health professional or trainee as well?

Chapter Eight

Making Clinical Observations

Well-trained mental health clinicians look at people with a trained eye. They know that careful observations help them zero in on the clients' problems more quickly and accurately. They learn to make a holistic evaluation of the client using how the client looks, talks, and behaves in addition to what the client says. This chapter will guide you in understanding the types of observations that trained clinicians make so that you can start doing this too.

APPEARANCE, CLOTHING, AND HYGIENE

Toni comes to the intake appointment today and meets with a mental health student. As Toni enters the office, the trainee notes that she is a white female of average height and weight with blonde hair. Toni's casual clothes are a bit rumpled, stained, and mismatched but apparently clean. Her hair is somewhat messy and maybe a little dirty. When asked about her ethnic background, she states that she is Polish and that both of her parents immigrated to the United States from Poland, although she was born here.

Alberto comes to the intake appointment today and meets with a mental health trainee. As Alberto enters the office, the trainee notes that he is neatly dressed in an immaculate dress shirt and tie. Alberto has a very dark complexion and is tall with an athletic build. His hair is carefully groomed and styled. When asked about his ethnic background, he indicates that he is a Latino of mixed black and mestizo heritage.

Ophelia comes to the intake appointment today at the college counseling center and meets with a mental health trainee. As Ophelia enters the office, the trainee can't help noticing that she is wearing a bright red dress with shiny

black patent leather high-heeled pumps. Her dress is very low cut. She has an
olive complexion and thick black, wavy hair. All the other students in the wait-
ing room were wearing sneakers and jeans. When asked, she indicates that
her mother is Mexican and that her father is Greek.

You can see that even though we know nothing of these clients' backgrounds, we already can generate some hypotheses and/or questions we need to ask them from their personal appearances. Depending on the circumstances, sometimes it can be helpful to describe the client's appearance in the chart. It can also be helpful to note any unusual ways in which the client chooses to appear, for example, sporting a dozen earrings on the left ear or having a prominent tattoo on the neck. You should also note any obvious physical disabilities, such as a missing limb or finger or a prominent burn scar on the face.

It is often unwise to guess at a client's ethnic background, as you can often be wrong. For example, the therapist might have guessed that Alberto identified as African American from his appearance. Asking a client, "What is the ethnic background of your family?" can be very informative, even for apparently White clients.

The client's way of dressing can give us clues about their mental state and their ethnic and socioeconomic background. What hypotheses might you generate about the previously mentioned clients with just the information you have now?

BEHAVIOR, MOTOR ACTIVITY, AND EYE CONTACT

During the interview, Toni sits calmly in the chair and appears to be attend-
ing to the trainee's questions. Occasionally, she looks around the room into
the corners of the ceiling, but the trainee knows that there is nothing interest-
ing there. She has poor eye contact.

As Alberto moves toward his chair, he places his takeaway coffee cup pre-
cisely in the corner of the student's desk and carefully folds his jacket and
drapes it over the back of the chair. During the interview, Alberto sits quietly.
He tends to look down instead of at the trainee when talking.

As Ophelia enters the room, she is visibly bubbly. She sits down in the chair
but often gestures dramatically to illustrate her points during the interview.
She has good eye contact, and she appears full of energy.

Observing any unusual behavior in your clients can be a useful clue as well. What might it mean that Toni is looking around the room? What might it mean about Alberto that he is so precise with his coffee cup and his jacket?

What might Ophelia's dramatic gestures mean? Given her ethnic background, you might wonder whether these gestures are normative or clinically significant. Be alert to any unusual physical symptoms, such as tics, tremors, or an unusual gait (*gait* means how the client walks). Ask your client about them to see if there has been a diagnosis or any treatment of the underlying condition.

Observe the client's eye contact. Poor eye contact can be indicative of a wide variety of different problems, from Asperger's syndrome (a milder disorder on the autism spectrum) to schizophrenia to depression to shyness. It can be a sign that, for whatever reason, the client cannot adhere to all appropriate social nonverbal behavior, at least right now. However, note that if the client is from a different cultural background than yours, it may be difficult to know what eye contact is considered appropriate in the client's cultural group since eye contact does vary from one cultural group to another (Mc-Carthy, Lee, Itakura, & Muir, 2006). Also note that less acculturated Asian Americans may tend to gaze downward in the presence of authority figures (Ling, 1997). This may also be the case for Native Americans.

Observe the amount of general *motor* (or physical) activity of the client. A low level of motor activity can be suggestive of depression. A high level of motor activity can be suggestive of mania or agitation. Agitation can be a sign of anxiety, anger, or even certain kinds of depression. Some clients with psychotic disorders can have a low level of activity, while others can be agitated.

There are a number of special motor issues with clients who are taking antipsychotic medications. First, clients may have a side effect to antipsychotic medication called *akathesia*, which causes them to jiggle their legs and have a profound feeling of restlessness. If you observe this, discuss the issue with the client and the psychiatrist; this side effect is often so intolerable that clients will stop taking their medications to get rid of it. Second, clients may also exhibit *tardive dyskinesia*, which is a mostly irreversible movement disorder that can occur in people who take antipsychotic medications for many years. Symptoms of tardive dyskinesia may include involuntary wriggling of the fingers, tongue thrusting, and/or facial grimacing. Discuss this issue with the psychiatrist to see how it is being managed. Third, if the client seems particularly stiff around the head or neck area or complains of muscle pain, cramping, or stiffness, this could be a side effect of antipsychotic medications. Have the client talk to a psychiatrist right away.

SPEECH AND THOUGHT PROCESSES

During the interview, Toni attends to the trainee's questions. Occasionally, she seems to "zone out," and questions need to be repeated. Her answers tend to be brief and uninformative, necessitating many follow-up questions. She uses a simple basic vocabulary and nonstandard English words such as "ain't." Her voice is not very expressive, and the trainee cannot tell how she is feeling.

Alberto listens carefully to the trainee's questions and responds completely and precisely. When he describes his job in the financial sector, he uses financial jargon that the student does not fully understand. His speech flows smoothly, and he uses complex vocabulary words occasionally. However, he tends to speak quietly and mumbles a bit.

Ophelia often interrupts before the trainee is done phrasing a question. She then talks at length and with great excitement about topics that are only peripherally related to the question at hand. Her voice is expressive of her emotions, and she talks overly loudly and at a fast pace. When the trainee asks her to slow down, she tries but then speeds up again.

Certain aspects of how a client speaks can be informative. Is the client's speech fluent or impoverished? *Impoverished speech* is speech that is especially uninformative and brief. Impoverished speech might be suggestive of mental retardation, other developmental disabilities, profound depression, or, in some cases, schizophrenia.

Be aware of how the client is processing what you are asking and telling her. Does she seem to understand your questions, or is she confused? Confusion can be a sign of thought disorder, dementia, or various other cognitive difficulties. Can the client remember the question that was asked? If not, she may be having some difficulties with attention and concentration. What does the client's vocabulary say about the client's likely *verbal intelligence*? (Note that it is impossible to estimate *general intelligence* from a verbal interview since *nonverbal* abilities—spatial, numerical, and others—are not observed.)

Can the client stay on the subject at hand? Repeated difficulties staying on the subject might be suggestive of mania, schizophrenia, or attention-deficit/hyperactivity disorder. Some clients have what is called *tangential* or *circumstantial* speech: they talk about several topics sequentially but idiosyncratically so that others find it difficult or impossible to follow their thought processes.

The qualities of the client's voice can be informative as well. Is the voice fast or slow? Is it quiet or loud? Is it expressive or monotone? Does the client speak clearly or mumble? What is the emotional tone of the voice? Different vocal qualities are suggestive of different problems. What do the different vocal qualities of the previously mentioned clients suggest about their problems?

Whenever you have any concerns about the client's ability to think clearly, it can help to determine whether the client is *oriented* to person, place, and date, that is, whether the client can answer these three questions:

"What is your name?"
"Where are we right now?"
"What is today's date?"

If the client can answer all these questions accurately, we say that the client is *oriented in all spheres* or *oriented times three* (usually denoted "OX3" in charts). Be a little flexible if the client is a little wrong about the date. However, if the client is not oriented (e.g., he says that he is in a different location than where he is or says that the date is 1990), there is a strong likelihood of medical illness affecting cognition. Get the client medically evaluated immediately.

AFFECT AND MOOD

The trainee watches Toni's face carefully but cannot detect any significant mood changes. Even when Toni talks about her mother's recent death and states how sad she was about the loss, she does not appear emotional.

Alberto's face looks drawn and sad during the interview. When talking about his daughter's recent cancer scare, his eyes become red and appear tearful, although he does not actually cry. When asked how he has been feeling, he readily states that he has been sad.

Ophelia is excited and even somewhat agitated throughout the interview. Her mood is very positive throughout, except she appears a bit irritable when talking about her roommate making her come to the college counseling center. She talks about her many plans for successful Web businesses that she will run out of her home and that will make a fortune for her.

It is important to ask clients about their mood and compare that to your observations. Generally, *mood* refers to what the client says about how she is feeling, whereas *affect* refers to your observations of how the client appears to be feeling from her facial expressions, voice, eye contact, and so on (Morrison, 1995). *Flat affect*, like Toni's, means that few facial indications of emotion are present.

Comparison of mood and affect can be very informative. Toni's verbally expressed sadness coupled with her flat affect (sometimes also called *blunted affect*) suggests that she has a psychotic disorder (although flat affect can also be found in depression, Parkinson's disease, and other neurological conditions;

Morrison, 1995). Alberto, on the other hand, expresses sadness in both his mood and his affect. Ophelia claims that her mood is fine, but the clinician observes excessively positive mood and grandiosity. *Grandiosity* means that she has an inflated view of herself, her abilities, and her importance. This suggests that she has no insight into the likelihood that she may be getting manic.

Labile affect describes a client whose mood varies widely and quickly during a session from one extreme to another. For example, she could be angry one moment, then making a joke and laughing the next. When you see it, make a note of emotional lability since it is of diagnostic importance. Most often, it is seen in clients with borderline personality disorder but also could be indicative of mania or histrionic personality disorder.

Inappropriate affect is also of concern. Odd emotional expressions (e.g., giggling at something profoundly sad) can be seen sometimes in individuals with schizophrenia (and sometimes neurological disorders; Morrison, 1995).

Sometimes people with post-traumatic stress disorder may talk in a strangely calm and collected manner about extremely traumatic material; unless this material has been thoroughly processed with a therapist, this is probably indicative of emotional numbing. *Emotional numbing* is a psychological defense mechanism in which the client is able to talk and function seemingly normally yet emotionlessly about experiences that would normally be considered to be extremely distressing.

In more extreme cases, a client may dissociate in a session. *Dissociation* is a more extreme psychological defense mechanism in which the client's thought processes are detached from emotions or bodily sensations when faced with highly distressing material. Dissociation can sometimes involve memory repression. The dissociating client will often look vague, break eye contact, or become nonverbal. Clients will often describe this as "shutting down." If a client responds this way, gently call the client's name, ask the client what was happening, and move on with the interview, changing the subject and avoiding the topic that triggered this response. Note this behavior and the topic that triggered it carefully in the chart. Discuss this thoroughly with your supervisor for guidance.

Be aware of how connected you feel toward the client during the interview and how the client appears to be feeling about your efforts to be of assistance. If you feel unconnected to the client, this generally indicates that the client has some kind of temporary (e.g., certain individuals with acute depression) or permanent (e.g., schizophrenia or Asperger's syndrome) difficulty with social interactions.

Be aware that some affects are expressed only fleetingly. These brief facial expressions of emotion are called *microexpressions* and last for only a split second (Ekman & O'Sullivan, 1991). These microexpressions have typically been studied in the context of detecting deception. However, clients may also exhibit microexpressions during psychotherapy. Asking your client about the feeling that you observed momentarily ("For a moment there, you looked a bit disgusted when talking about your brother") can yield further insights.

JUDGMENT AND INSIGHT

When asked why she came in for treatment today, Toni states that her father told her that she needed to come. She lives with him. She says that they have been arguing about the neighbors. Toni states that she feels that her father should confront the neighbors since they have been spying on her with tiny video cameras.

Alberto states that he had decided to come for treatment since he knows that he is getting more depressed. He says that he decided that he needed to get help before his work performance suffered.

Ophelia states that her roommates insisted that she come to the counseling center. She states that she feels so good that she knows she doesn't really need to be there.

Toni and Ophelia have very little insight into the fact that they are mentally ill. Toni is not exhibiting good judgment since she wants to feud with the neighbors over her belief that they are spying on her—which is a symptom of her mental illness. Ophelia's judgment appears impaired as well. Alberto, on the other hand, has good insight and is using good judgment to seek help before his functioning level at work deteriorates.

DOCUMENTING YOUR OBSERVATIONS

Now that we have reviewed the topic of making clinical observations, you've learned that observations can be helpful in making a diagnosis. You need not write down every single behavior that you observe. Some of these behaviors will only suggest to you that you should ask further questions (e.g., might Alberto's exactness in setting down his coffee cup and coat be indicative of some obsessive compulsive symptoms? Ask him.) Others are clinically significant (e.g., flat affect or euphoria). Share your observations with your supervisor and together figure out which ones are of clinical significance and how to document these in the progress notes.

OBSERVATIONS SUGGESTIVE OF LYING

Clients may lie about certain aspects of their current or historical situation. This is not uncommon, as research has indicated that lying is a frequent interpersonal behavior. Here are some indicators of possible lying (adapted from DePaulo et al., 2003):

- Liars provide fewer details in a more uncertain manner.
- Liars have more silent pauses and longer response latency to questions.
- Liars seem more tense and inhibited.
- Truth tellers are more likely to spontaneously correct themselves and admit that they can't remember everything.

However, DePaulo et al. (2003) conclude, "Behavioral cues that are discernible by human perceivers are associated with deceit only probabilistically. To establish definitively that someone is lying, further evidence is needed" (p. 108).

I suggest that you avoid any direct accusations of lying in the chart. However, be aware that there are certain established ways of phrasing comments in the chart that indicate that the client may be lying without outright stating it: "Since Mr. R's report of his past hospitalizations differed significantly from one session to the next, I consider him to be an unreliable informant." An *unreliable informant* is a client who cannot be relied on to provide an accurate history. You can also imply that the client may be lying by contrasting the client's statement with other information:

> "Ms. A stated that she had not used substances over the weekend; however, her urine toxicology screen was positive for cocaine."

Discuss with your supervisor whether you should just keep in mind that the client may be untruthful or whether you should attempt to verify the suspect information. You might consider interviewing family members to gather more reliable historical information.

OBSERVATIONS SUGGESTIVE OF MALINGERING

Most of your clients will have genuine problems. However, certain clients are motivated to present themselves as more ill than they actually are. Malingerers may fake mental illness, cognitive impairment, pain, and physical disability. Although it is notoriously difficult to study malingerers, my clinical experience is that while malingers do not have the mental illness that they present, they can have some serious problems—often emotional but maybe also coping deficits—that lead them to believe that malingering is a reasonable way to address their life problems. Often, the client's motivation to ma-linger is connected to financial benefits, such as collecting a settlement or disability payments due to illness. Malingering is more common in specific situations, such as in prisons or disability evaluations.

Sometimes the reason for malingering is emotional, and it may not be wholly conscious. The client may feel a desperate need to be taken care of. One way for the client to get this need met is to be mentally ill and have mental health practitioners concerned about her well-being. The client's supposed illness may entitle the client to extra caring and caretaking from family and friends.

There is a large and complex literature about assessing malingering. It is far beyond the scope of this volume to fully address this topic. Rogers (1997) provides helpful guidance in discovering whether a client might be malingering. Here are just a few indicators of possible malingering:

- The client describes obvious symptoms (e.g., crying, sadness, or hallucinations) but does not describe, demonstrate, or endorse commonly co-occurring subtle symptoms (e.g., appetite changes or thought disorder).
- Contradictions in the account of the illness become clear over time (but remember that memory does deteriorate normally).
- The client answers "I don't know" when an actual client would know (e.g., when asked about a hallucination: "Was that the voice of a male or female?").
- The client exhibits overly bizarre self-presentation, perhaps combining obvious symptoms of several different disorders.
- The client accuses the interviewer of thinking that he is faking.
- Symptoms that don't typically arise suddenly have a sudden onset ("I felt great on Wednesday, but on Thursday I couldn't concentrate on anything and felt incredibly anxious").
- The client describes pain or physical dysfunction that is not possible neurologically (consult a physician to be sure).
- The client exhibits disparities between reported and observed symptoms, such as an inability to sustain the symptom presentation over time when on an inpatient unit.

In conclusion, you must be very cautious about making a diagnosis of malingering because, unless you are a specially trained forensic psychologist, you probably do not have sufficient evidence to be absolutely sure. Document your observations carefully in the chart and try to be factual in a way that informs a knowledgeable reader about your suspicions without making explicit accusations (e.g., "Ms. T. reported that she had suddenly recovered from her depression last Thursday. No signs of mania were present.") Finally, do not make any accusations to the client without thoroughly discussing the issue with your supervisor first.

When you think a client may be malingering, discuss your concerns about the client's honesty with the treatment team or a trusted colleague. Carefully document factual information that would be of assistance later. For example,

> "Client stated that he was hearing voices, but when asked if they were male or female, he stated he did not know."

> "Client repeatedly asked whether I thought she was faking her symptoms."

Refer the client for a psychological assessment, preferably with a psychologist who is knowledgeable about detecting deception. However, any psychologist can be helpful, as the psychologist should be able to administer the Minnesota Multiphasic Personality Inventory-2 (MMPI-2), which would probably give useful information about the reliability of the client's self-report (for more information in using the MMPI-2 in this manner, see Rogers, Sewell, Martin, & Vitacco, 2003).

RECOMMENDED READING

DePaulo, B. M., Lindsay, J. J., Malone, B. E., Muhlenbruck, L., Charlton, K., & Cooper, H. (2003). Cues to deception. *Psychological Bulletin, 129*, 74–118.
DePaulo and colleagues provide an interesting review of psychological research on interpersonal detection of lying.
Rogers, R. (Ed.). (1997). *Clinical assessment of malingering and deception* (2nd ed.). New York: Guilford Press.
Although this volume is no longer fully current, it provides a helpful guide to the assessment of malingering.

EXERCISES AND DISCUSSION QUESTIONS

1. What are your diagnostic hypotheses about each of the three clients discussed in this chapter? Why?
2. List the symptoms that you have observed for each of the three clients. Have your observations confirmed enough symptoms to make a diagnosis in any of these cases?
3. How would you use your diagnostic hypotheses and what you know about the clients' symptoms so far to focus the rest of the intake interview?

Chapter Nine

Making a Diagnosis

Knowing your client's diagnosis allows you to access the large body of clinical and research knowledge. This will help you tailor the treatment to the client's needs more effectively. Many settings require that a diagnosis be made. Thus, I provide reference material for diagnostic screening in the appendices of this volume, which are referenced throughout this chapter. I recommend that you keep a copy of this book handy any time you will be doing an intake interview in case you need to reference or copy any of the materials. I have not provided any flowcharts or hierarchies; my feeling is that these would be more confusing than helpful. Your best resource in making a diagnosis quickly is your detailed knowledge of the behaviors and symptoms of mental illnesses.

To make a diagnosis, there are several steps:

- Understand the format for the diagnostic interview that your site requires or choose a format if you have that latitude. Several considerations on format are discussed later in this chapter.
- Gather information.
- Consider alternative causes of the apparent psychological symptoms: medical illness or substance abuse.
- Diagnose if you have enough information to be confident.

This chapter and the related appendices only begin to educate you about the complex process of making a diagnosis. I hope that you will look up the recommended readings as well, especially Morrison (2007). Your supervisor can also help guide you to consider appropriate diagnoses for your clients.

CHALLENGES IN MAKING A DIAGNOSIS

Making a full and accurate diagnosis is a time-consuming process. In an ideal world, the clinician might do a structured interview and an extensive diagnostic interview and then refer the client to psychological testing as needed to clarify any remaining questions, all this culminating in making a *disposition*, which means to arrange for appropriate treatment for the client. As you might imagine, this ideal assessment could take up to 3 hours, possibly considerably more.

In real life, agencies are often pressed for money, often resulting in clinicians being pressed for time. Thus, clients are usually allocated a 1-hour intake slot. As you can see from the ideal-world example, a 1-hour intake (or even a 90-minute one) ensures that the clinician will need to make some shortcuts and will sometimes miss important information. We have no choice but to accept this reality. This chapter will educate you in the processes that experienced clinicians use to work effectively under these real-world constraints.

INTERVIEW FORMAT: SITE SPECIFIC

The format for your initial diagnostic interview with a new client may vary by site. When starting in a new practice setting, discuss any requirements for the initial session with your supervisor. In many settings, the clinician is given a paper form (or a template in the electronic medical record) regarding the client that must be filled out; the form provides an outline for the initial session.

In other settings, no formal structure is provided. Beginning therapists often benefit from using a structured list of questions or topics to address during the first session. In appendix 4, I provide an outline of some topics to address in the initial session . If you use this list, ask your supervisor if there are additional subjects that you should explore with your particular client population. Look at any of the sources that I cited for the list to get a more detailed understanding of how to address these interview topics with the client.

INTERVIEW FORMAT: STRUCTURED INTERVIEWS

The most accurate way to make a diagnosis is to administer a well-validated structured diagnostic interview, such as the Structured Clinical Interview for the DSM-IV-TR (SCID; First, Spitzer, Gibbon, & Williams, 2002), which takes 2 to 3 hours to complete. After completing the SCID, the clinician is as confident as possible that an accurate and complete psychiatric diagnosis has been made. A valuable alternative is the Mini-International Neuropsychiatric Interview, a structured interview that was developed to take about 15 minutes (Sheehan et al., 1998). See the website referenced at the end of the chapter for more information.

MENTAL STATUS EXAM

Sometimes a formal Mental Status Exam (MSE) is required. The MSE is a semistructured way to ensure that you ask certain questions and make certain observations. Many of the observations that are part of doing an MSE are covered in chapter 8. There are standardized versions (Mini Mental State Exam; see http://www.minimental.com) and nonstandardized versions of the MSE (for instructions, see Morrison, 2007). Training you how to do a full MSE is beyond the scope of this book, but if your site requires it, your supervisor can quickly train you.

KNOW ABOUT COMMON DIAGNOSES

Certain mental illnesses are very common in the general population. One way to measure how common mental illnesses are is to determine the *lifetime prevalence*, which means the proportion of the population that has met the criteria for the illness sometime during the individual's lifetime. The following mental illnesses have at least a 4% lifetime prevalence in U.S. adults; the ones in italics have at least an 8% lifetime prevalence (R. C. Kessler, Adler, Ames et al., 2005; O'Leary & Norcross, 1998):

- *Adjustment disorder*
- Adult attention-deficit/hyperactivity disorder (ADHD)
- Agoraphobia without panic (panic disorder has a 2% to 3% lifetime prevalence)
- *Alcohol abuse/dependence*
- Bipolar II (also known as cyclothymic disorder)
- *Drug abuse/dependence*
- Dysthymia
- Generalized anxiety disorder
- *Major depression*
- Post-traumatic stress disorder (PTSD)
- *Simple/specific phobia (despite the high lifetime prevalence, many individuals with simple phobias are not particularly bothered with them on a daily basis)*
- *Social phobia*

You should be familiar with the symptoms of each of these diagnoses, as you will see clients with these problems in any setting. Learn as much as you can about how clients with specific mental illnesses look: how they talk, characteristic nonverbal behavior, what their eye contact is like, and so on (how clinicians systematically observe behavior is addressed in chapter 8).

KNOW ABOUT HIGH-RISK SYMPTOMS

All mental health practitioners should be familiar with symptoms of psychosis and mania. These symptoms are very disabling and indicative of a need for psychotropic medication. In addition, clients with these symptoms are at higher risk for suicide (see chapter 19 for more information).

KNOW COMMON DIAGNOSES WITHIN YOUR CLIENT POPULATION

Different client populations have higher rates of specific mental illnesses. For example, if you work in a prison, you may see more individuals with trauma or antisocial personality disorder. If you work at a college counseling center, prevalences of eating disorders may be high. Ask your supervisor about the population you are working with and be familiar with diagnoses that are common within that group.

ASK ABOUT SLEEP

Sleep patterns vary depending on the client's emotional problems. Thus, asking about sleep can provide a quick clue about the client's diagnosis. Appendix 5 outlines some important questions to ask about sleep and how specific sleep problems correspond to various emotional and sleep disorders.

BE ATTUNED TO CLUES

The client's presenting problem, your clinical observations of the client, and any sleep problems the client is having give you helpful clues about possible diagnoses. Let these clues guide your interview. Given the clues you have gathered, ask about the most likely diagnoses first. You can use the screening questions that I have gathered for you in the appendixes if you like. I hope that the sample questions that I have furnished will give you an idea about how to ask about various symptoms. To make the diagnosis, you need to remember enough of the symptoms, or you will need to have the *Diagnostic and Statistical Manual of Mental Disorders* (4th ed., text revision) (*DSM-IV-TR*, American Psychiatric Association, 2000) handy. Be sure to use the *DSM* criteria to make a more reliable and valid diagnosis.

BE PREPARED WITH SCREENING QUESTIONS

Screening questions are a shortcut to help us make a diagnosis efficiently. We may use one or several screening questions to help us determine whether we should ask further questions about a certain diagnosis or move on to other subjects. Realize that there is potential error with all screening questions. We might have a *false positive*; in other words, our client may answer the screening question in a way that leads us to believe that the client has the diagnosis, but on further questioning, it will turn out that the client does not. Or we might have a *false negative*; in other words, we erroneously skip asking more about a particular problem because the answer to the screening question suggests that the client does not have the problem.

Why are screening questions important? Many emotional problems and psychiatric diagnoses may not be immediately obvious even to a trained professional. Here are some examples from the literature:

- *Half the cases of PTSD were missed by clinicians* in a study comparing diagnoses made by unstructured interview versus structured interview (Zimmerman & Mattia, 1999). *Three-fourths of PTSD was missed* in a sample of substance-abusing veterans (Kimerling, Trafton, & Nguyen, 2006). Multiple studies have found that most clients with a history of trauma history will *not* volunteer this information to a therapist without being asked (Agar, Read, & Bush, 2002). These clients with undetected PTSD are not getting the correct treatment. Appendix 6 provides information about screening for PTSD.
- *One-third to one-half of clients presenting with a major depressive episode will have undetected bipolar I or II disorder instead*, as indicated in multiple studies cited by Bowden (2005). Since bipolar individuals are more likely to seek treatment when depressed, their histories of mania can be easily missed. This is a terrifying figure because many of these clients will get inappropriate and even harmful treatment. Antidepressants alone will often send bipolar clients into mania, worsening their mental illness (Angst & Cassano, 2005). Unfortunately, mania usually feels good, so the clients may not understand that they are *not* doing better. Appendix 7 provides information

about screening for bipolar disorder. Appendix 8 provides the Mood Disorder Questionnaire, which the clients can take to help the screening process for bipolar disorder.

• *About 10% of major depression is seasonal*, otherwise known as *seasonal affective disorder* (SAD, Levitt & Boyle, 2002). SAD is a specific type of major depression that occurs in conjunction with a specific season, usually winter. It is crucial to distinguish seasonal from nonseasonal depression because the recommended first-line treatments are different. A treatment that you should try first that has the highest likelihood of being effective is called a *first-line treatment*. Bright-light treatment is the first-line treatment for SAD (Lam & Levitan, 2000) and can be supplemented by psychotherapy and medications; in nonseasonal depression, bright-light treatment is not typically used as a first-line treatment. Thus, whenever you have a client presenting with depression in the winter, screen for SAD. Appendix 9 provides information about screening for major depression, and appendix 10 provides information on SAD.

• *Adults with ADHD present twice as often for treatment for emotional problems than for the ADHD itself*, so adult ADHD is easily missed by clinicians. This is probably because attention deficit disorder is so often comorbid with other psychiatric disorders (R. C. Kessler, Adler, Ames et al., 2005; R. C. Kessler, Adler, Barkley et al., 2005). In addition, the diagnostic criteria were developed for children and offer little guidance to the clinician in assessing ADHD in adults (R. C. Kessler, Adler, Barkley et al.). Appendix 11 provides information about screening for adult ADHD.

Beginning therapists also have difficulty knowing how to ask clients about their psychotic symptoms, so I have outlined a method of screening for psychosis in appendix 12. For completeness, I have addressed screening anxiety disorders in appendix 13, screening for substance abuse in appendices 14 and 15, and screening for eating disorders in appendix 16.

I recommend that you review all these appendices. You may wish to construct your own list of screening questions to keep handy, drawing on the ones that are most relevant to your client population or most difficult to remember. Or you may wish to keep this volume handy for reference.

ASK ABOUT FAMILY HISTORY OF MENTAL ILLNESS

Most types of mental illness can run in families. However, usually it is the class of diagnoses (e.g., anxiety or psychotic disorders) that runs in the family, and the relative might have a different specific diagnosis than the client. The mental illnesses of first-degree relatives, who share half the client's genes (parents, siblings, and children), are most predictive, followed by second-degree relatives, who share one-quarter of the client's genes (grandparents, aunts, uncles, nephews, nieces, and half siblings). If the client is unsure what the mental illness of the family member was, you can ask some of these questions:

"What did the relative do that was unusual?"

"Do you know what kind of medication your relative is taking?"

Of course, you can't diagnose this relative, whom you've never seen, but this information may provide some useful clues about genetic influences in the client's family. Be aware, however, that many people with mental illness don't have any relatives with a similar disorder.

Different mental illnesses vary in how much a predisposition to them is inherited. The following numbers provide a rough comparison of the relative heritability of different types of mental illnesses. These numbers are *odds ratios* (the proportion of first-degree relatives of the person with mental illness who have the mental illness themselves versus the proportion of first-degree relatives of a control—without mental illness—who have the mental illness themselves). All the odds ratios that follow are aggregates from literature reviews. A higher odds ratio indicates that the mental illness is more highly inherited:

- 3: Major depression (P. F. Sullivan, Neale, & Kendler, 2000)
- 4–6: Panic disorder, obsessive-compulsive disorder, generalized anxiety disorder, and simple phobia (Hettema, Neale, & Kendler, 2001)
- 9: Bipolar disorder (Merikangas & Yu, 2002)
- 10: Schizophrenia (P. F. Sullivan, 2005)

Since these numbers are from different studies, with undoubtedly different methodologies, realize that any direct comparisons of heritability will necessarily be inexact. But this gives you an idea of the relative influences of genetics on these mental illnesses.

GATHER INFORMATION FROM ALL SOURCES, WHEN POSSIBLE

When you see a client to make a diagnosis, you are seeing the client in *cross section*; that is, you are seeing the client at just one point in time. However, to make many diagnoses, information and observations about the client's functioning over time, or *longitudinally*, is especially helpful.

Clients may or may not be *reliable informants*, that is, a useful and reliable source of honest and accurate information about themselves. They may have cognitive difficulties that impair their abilities to report their histories. They may be too mentally ill to be able to provide a coherent narrative about the past. They may be confused about what happened. They may have limited insight into their illnesses. Clients may want to minimize their mental health histories and current symptoms to convince you or themselves that they are not mentally ill. Alternatively, clients may overexaggerate their mental health histories and current symptoms because they are motivated to appear mentally ill.

For all these reasons, other sources of information can be invaluable in making a more accurate diagnosis. These sources include the following:

- Old chart material at your site
- Old charts from other sites
- A description of the client's current and past functioning from partner, family, roommate, or close friend

You may not have time to gather sufficient historical information from these collateral sources during the first session. You may not even have time to gather all the pertinent social history from the client during the first session. Therefore, sometimes the client will have to remain undiagnosed until you can be more sure.

ASSESS FREQUENCY, DURATION, AND SEVERITY OF SYMPTOMS

When the client talks to you about symptoms, you should then assess and document the extent of these symptoms (Morrison, 1995). The follow-up questions that you will ask will depend on the nature of the symptoms. A symptom can be *discrete*, which means that the symptom has distinct occurrences, such as nightmares, hallucinations, or panic attacks. Or a symptom can be *continuous*, which means that it seems to be occurring much of the time, such as depression or anxiety.

For discrete symptoms, ask about frequency: "Out of 7 nights in a week, on how many of these do you have nightmares?" "During a day, how often do you typically hear the voices?" Phrase the questions in such a way that the client can tell what kind of answer would be helpful (e.g., knowing that nightmares occur three or four times per week is more helpful than "a lot"). For example, if you client has obsessive-compulsive disorder, you might want to know how often the client checks the stove daily or how much time is spent checking every day. If the client has panic attacks, you would want to know when the last one was and about how frequently the client has been having them.

If the client has difficulty providing this information, ask more specific questions:

"Did you have a nightmare last night?"
"Have you heard the voices so far today? How many times?"

Panic attacks are also discrete symptoms but are often less frequent and thus would require different questions:

"How often do you typically have panic attacks?"
"When was the last time you had a panic attack?"

Note that you would not want to ask these questions about panic attacks until you had determined that the client's anxiety episodes did indeed fulfill the criteria for panic attacks and you were sure that the client understood what you meant by the term "panic attack."

For symptoms that are more continuous, you will want to ask about duration and severity:

"How long have you been feeling depressed?"
"Has it gotten worse over time?"
"Tell me what you've noticed that lets you know you're feeling worse."

How much the mental illness impacts on adaptive functioning (e.g., whether the client is going to work or school, taking care of routine tasks, or seeing friends and family) is another indicator of severity.

Symptoms tend to gradually decrease or increase over time. Thus, documenting the frequency of symptoms in the first session sets a benchmark that will help you and the client compare current to past functioning after some progress in therapy has been made.

MEDICAL ILLNESS CAN CAUSE
PSYCHOLOGICAL SYMPTOMS

Possible medical reasons for the symptoms must be thoroughly evaluated before you can make a definitive diagnosis (Morrison, 1995). Many medical issues mimic mental illness. Here are just a few examples:

• Undiagnosed brain dysfunction from a closed head injury can look like depression with motivation problems.

- Hypothyroidism can look like depression because of the client's low energy level.
- Temporal lobe epilepsy can have many unusual symptoms that resemble psychosis or other mental illnesses.
- Sleep apnea can look like depression because of poor sleep quality, which results in daytime tiredness and low motivation.

Here are some situations in which you should refer the client for a medical evaluation to clarify the diagnostic picture (informed by Morrison, 2007):

- Client is having a first episode of mental illness, especially if client is 40 or older.
- Client has recently given birth.
- Client has a current major medical illness (such as diabetes or seizure disorder), past major medical illness, or family history of major inheritable medical illness.
- Client has a current or past endocrine disorder.
- Client has experienced a head injury, including sharp blows to the head without the skull being pierced.
- Client has neurological symptoms (such as weakness, tingling, numbing, trouble walking, tremor, involuntary movements, dizziness, or blurred or double vision).
- Client does not seem fully alert, has trouble with speech or memory, or cannot follow simple commands.
- Client is not oriented to person, place, and date (see chapter 8).
- Client has any behaviors that could cause vitamin deficiency (limited diet, large weight loss, or self-neglect).

I would also add that if your client has not seen a physician for more than a year, it would be wise to send the client for a routine visit, especially if the client is 40 or older.

SUBSTANCE USE CAN CAUSE PSYCHOLOGICAL SYMPTOMS

Alcohol and drug use, along with intoxication and withdrawal, can cause a plethora of symptoms mimicking mental illnesses. These include the following (American Psychiatric Association, 2000):

- Anger
- Anxiety

- Dysphoria
- Euphoria
- Hallucinations
- Impairment in attention
- Insomnia
- Paranoia
- Psychomotor agitation
- Psychomotor retardation

In addition, there is evidence (Liappas, Paparrigopoulos, Tzavellas, & Christodoulou, 2002) that alcohol abusers who are detoxing feel quite anxious and depressed at first but feel much less so after 4 to 5 weeks of detox. Therefore, other diagnoses sometimes need to be deferred in the presence of substance abuse until the client is abstinent and can be evaluated again.

BE ALERT FOR DIAGNOSTIC COMORBIDITIES

Diagnostic comorbidities are common but can be often missed. Of the 26% of the population who have had a mental illness in the past 12 months, about half have had two or more diagnoses (R. C. Kessler, Chiu, Demler, & Walters, 2005). Since these individuals with comorbidity are more likely to have greater distress, they may be more likely to present for treatment. So be alert to the potential for multiple mental health diagnoses in all your clients.

DON'T DIAGNOSE PREMATURELY

Tomas Figuerro, a licensed psychologist, has been working with a new client, Laurie Norris for several weeks. He knows that she has had some problems with depression, but some things continue to confuse him. He finds her charming, but at times she is disconcertingly blunt. She has an avid interest in literature. She talks about reading frequently and comes to each session carrying at least three different books that she is working on. She often talks about going to websites to read book reviews. Yet she seems satisfied with a job that is less than challenging to her high verbal intelligence. She is friendly and smiles often, yet her affect still seems somewhat blunted at times, even though she used to act in the theater semiprofessionally. She would often feel confused in social situations. After a while, even though she did not seem to fit the picture he knew, he started to wonder whether she had Asperger's. He found a questionnaire in an article and gave it to the client. Her answers were

consistent with that diagnosis and revealed some symptoms (such as a preoc-
cupation with numbers) that he had not been aware of. Laurie started to look
up information on the Internet, and they both discussed how this syndrome
had affected her life. Both of them learned about the differences between men
and women with Asperger's. Laurie soon felt much better about herself, and
they terminated therapy.

Sometimes, as in the previous vignette, you will need to patiently observe the
client longitudinally to gather enough data to make a diagnosis. At other
times, you will need another session or two to finish gathering pertinent data
and make a diagnosis. As long as the client is not in a crisis, it is okay for the
client to remain undiagnosed for a while. If the client is in a crisis, gather
whatever diagnostic information you need to cope with the immediate crisis,
then go back and finish gathering information when the crisis is over.

As you become more experienced, you will learn to recognize common
mental illnesses more easily. You will also become better at realizing when
you need to persist to get more information. As you can see from the previous vignette, even advanced clinicians can struggle to diagnose a client.

SELECTED DIAGNOSTIC CONSIDERATIONS
REGARDING ETHNICITY AND CULTURE

Diagnostic errors are common and some are specifically tied to ethnicity. One
error that has been commonly researched and cited is misdiagnosing African
Americans with schizophrenia when major depression with psychotic features
would be more accurate (Garb, 1997, reviews the literature). Studies have indicated that this error could be due in part to the greater prevalence of psychotic symptomatology (e.g., more psychotic depression versus nonpsychotic
depression) in African Americans relative to Whites (Strakowski, 2003).

You can reduce the likelihood of misdiagnosis of schizophrenia by ensuring that you ask psychotic clients about mood as well (Strakowski, 2003) and
ascertain the time lines of both affective and psychotic symptoms. In clients
who have major depression with psychotic features, depression will occur
first, followed by psychotic symptoms during the most acute period of depression. While clients with schizophrenia often become depressed, the schizophrenia occurs first, and the depression typically occurs in response to the
ensuing negative life events.

Most clinicians are savvy to this issue now, and there is some evidence that
this type of misdiagnosis may be disappearing (e.g., Neighbors, Trierweiler,
Ford, & Muroff, 2003); however, these researchers do cite another diagnostic

difference of possible concern: higher diagnosis of schizophrenia in African Americans versus higher diagnosis of bipolar disorder in Whites.

Another ethnic difference of concern is that Asians may express their level of distress primarily through volunteering information about somatic symptoms (K. Lin & Cheung, 1999). Possible reasons for these cultural differences in symptom expression include regarding body and mind as one (as opposed to Western dualism) and reticence about discussing one's private life. Direct questioning about psychological symptoms can elicit the needed information (K. Lin & Cheung, 1999).

A final diagnostic concern relates to culture rather than ethnicity per se. The *Canadian Journal of Psychiatry* (Lalonde, Hudson, Gigante, & Pope, 2001; Piper & Merskey, 2004) has published skeptical articles regarding the diagnosis of dissociative identity disorder (previously known as multiple personality disorder). The authors indicate that many Canadian mental health practitioners feel that dissociative identity disorder is culture bound (primarily to the United States) and can be *iatragenic*, which means that it is (unwittingly) caused by the practitioner. Clearly, further research is much needed in this area.

RECOMMENDED READING

Bowden, C. (2001). Strategies to reduce misdiagnosis of bipolar depression. *Psychiatric Services, 52,* 51–55.
Bowden's helpful and succinct article will aid you in more accurately diagnosing bipolar disorder when clients present with a depressive episode.

Lin, K., & Cheung, F. (1999). Mental health issues for Asian Americans. *Psychiatric Services, 50,* 774–780.
This article provides helpful cultural insights into culture and mental health for Asian Americans.

Morrison, J. (2007). *Diagnosis made easier: Principles and techniques for mental health clinicians.* New York: Guilford Press.
This helpful and well-written volume clearly describes almost everything you will ever need to know about the process of making diagnoses. Highly recommended for all mental health trainees and professionals.

Ramsay, J. R., & Rostain, A. L. (2005). Adapting psychotherapy to meet the needs of adults with attention-deficit/hyperactivity disorder. *Psychotherapy: Theory, Research, Practice, Training, 42,* 72–84.
The authors provide some helpful guidance for the clinician who treats adults with ADHD in psychotherapy.

Rosenthal, N. E. (1998). *Winter blues: Seasonal affective disorder, what it is and how to overcome it.* New York: Guilford Press.
The definitive book about seasonal affective disorder—it is helpful for clinicians and clients alike.

WEB RESOURCES

https://www.medical-outcomes.com/HTMLFiles/MINI/MINI.htm
   *This website requires you to register but then allows you to download the MINI
   (Mini International Neuropsychiatric Interview) for free, under certain conditions.
   This structured interview takes about 15 to 20 minutes, and it may significantly improve your diagnostic reliability and accuracy.*
http://www.med.nyu.edu/psych/assets/adhdscreen18.pdf
   *The National Comorbidity Survey at Harvard University has posted self-report
   screening questionnaires for adult ADHD that were developed in conjunction with
   a World Health Organization work group. This symptom checklist is in the public
   domain. There is a 6-item and an 18-item version, and it is in many different languages. This checklist operationalizes ADHD symptoms in terms of adult behaviors, assisting the clinician in making a diagnosis.*

EXERCISES AND DISCUSSION QUESTIONS

1. Annesha Banks is a new client of yours. You observe that she has difficulty maintaining eye contact with you during the interview and that her
   affect is flat. When asked what brought her to therapy, she indicates that
   she has been crying every day. When asked about her sleep, she says that
   she has been having vivid and disturbing dreams that disrupt her sleep.
   What else would you want to ask Annesha? What diagnoses would you
   consider for Annesha?
2. Theodore Packer is a new client. When asked what brought him to therapy, he says that he's been very anxious lately and that he can't concentrate at work and worries about losing his job. He says that his wife always
   complains that he doesn't listen to her, and their marriage is in trouble. His
   eye contact is good, and his affect is *euthymic* (normal, not depressed or
   manic). When asked about sleep, he says that it takes him a long time to
   get to sleep. What else would you want to ask Theodore? What diagnoses
   would you consider for Theodore?
3. Rodrigo Gutierrez is a new client. He is an Iraq War veteran. When asked
   why he decided to come for therapy, he said that his mother insisted that
   he come for help. He has been living with her. He also said that he has
   been arguing with everyone else in his family. He denies feeling anxious
   or depressed but does say that his sleep is not restful. You notice that his
   eyes are bloodshot and that he keeps jiggling his leg during the session.
   His affect and eye contact are normal. What else would you want to ask
   Rodrigo? What diagnoses would you consider for Rodrigo?

Chapter Ten

Professional Phone Contacts and the Initial Phone Call

As a beginning therapist, you will probably be assigned clients by a supervisor at your training site. Once the client is assigned, you will need to contact the client to set up an appointment time. This chapter will take you step-by-step through contacting the client by phone.

PROFESSIONAL PHONE GREETINGS

Before calling the client, be sure that your voice mail is set up at your training site. That way, if you need to leave a message for the client, she will get your personal voice mail when she calls back. A short professional message is best. State your full name and your position. If you are not in the office every day, include any relevant information about when you will return calls. Ask your supervisor whether to include information about emergency contacts. Avoid any overly personal or religious remarks:

> Wrong: "Hi! This is Amber. Leave a message. God Bless!"
> Right: "Hello, this is Amber Scott, psychology practicum student. I am in the office on Mondays and Wednesdays and will return your call next time I am in. If you need help before that, please call [alternate phone number at training site]. [Optional sentence: If you are having an emergency, please call 911 or go to your nearest emergency room.] Please leave me a message after the beep."

When answering the phone, again, professionalism is paramount.

> Wrong: "Hello?"
> Wrong: "Hi, this is Amber."

Wrong: "Yes?"
Right: "Hello, this is Amber Scott."
Right: "This is Amber Scott, psychology practicum student."
Right: "Hello, this is Amber Scott [or Dr. Scott if you have a doctoral degree]."

MAKING THE INITIAL CALL

If several phone numbers are available for the client, choose the one that seems the most private to call first, generally the cell phone number. You may wish to avoid leaving a message until you have tried to contact the client directly at all the numbers that you have. If the client is not available at any of them, choose the number that seems the most private and leave a message.

Sometimes you can be fairly sure that no one else has access to the voice mail that the client has given you. In these cases, the phone number the client has given you goes directly into voice mail or onto an answering machine. The client states that it is his phone number and does not name anyone else, for example, "Hi, this is Stephen. I can't come to the phone right now, so please leave a message," or, "Hello, this is Stephen Desai with ABC Manufacturing. I'm sorry I can't come to the phone right now, but please leave a message." In these cases, I would leave a brief message:

> "Hello, this is [your name]. I'm returning your call from [name of facility]. You can reach me at [phone number]. If you don't reach me directly, please leave me some times and numbers when I can reach you. I look forward to your call. Good-bye."

Issues of confidentiality are very important when making these initial contacts. Rarely will you know whether anyone else who might answer the phone knows whether the client is seeking therapy. If it is unclear whether the voice mail is just for the client or whether other might be able to pick up the messages, you might want to wait and try again later. If after trying two or three times you haven't reached the client directly, you might leave a brief and uninformative message:

> "Hi, this is [your name] returning a call from [client name]. He can reach me at [phone number]. Thank you."

IF SOMEONE ELSE PICKS UP AT WORK
AND CLIENT IS NOT AVAILABLE

When you call, always ask to speak to the client by name: "Could I speak to Stephen [or Stephen Desai if clearly a work number], please?" Because of confidentiality concerns, if you reach someone else, you must be as uninformative as possible. If you are calling a work number, it is usually okay to leave a very nondescript message:

Receptionist: "Hello, this is ABC Manufacturing, Nicole speaking."
Therapist: "Hi Nicole, could I speak to Stephen Desai please?"
R: "I'm sorry, he's in a meeting right now. Could I leave him a message?"
T: "Yes. Could you ask him to call [therapist name] at [phone number]?"
R: "Okay. Can I tell him what this is regarding?"
T: "I'm not sure. I'm just returning his call."
R: "Okay."
T: "Thanks for your help. Good-bye."
R: "Good-bye."

The client likely receives all kinds of phone messages at work, so yours won't stand out from the others. Avoid leaving any job names or titles (e.g., doctor).

IF SOMEONE ELSE PICKS UP AT HOME AND CLIENT IS NOT AVAILABLE

If you are calling a home number and someone else picks up, don't be hesitant. Speak briskly in a professional tone, and try to keep the initiative on your side in the conversation:

Relative: "Hello."
Therapist: "Hi, can I speak to Stephen?"
R: "He's not here right now."
T [speaking quickly so relative doesn't have a chance to ask questions]: "Can you tell me when he might be back?"
R: "He'll probably be home at about 3 P.M."
T: "Thanks, I'll call back then." [Then therapist hangs up, and doesn't wait for relative to ask questions.]

On occasion, the relative may succeed in asking some questions. Here are some possible questions and suggested responses:

Relative: "What is this call regarding?"
Therapist: "I don't know, I'm just returning his call. Thanks so much for your help! Good-bye!" [Then the therapist hangs up the phone, whether or not the relative has responded.]
Relative: "Would you like to leave a message?"
Therapist: "No thanks, I'll call back later when he is at home. Thanks so much for your help! Good-bye!" [Then the therapist hangs up the phone, whether or not the relative has responded.]

Relative: "How do you know Stephen?"

Therapist: "I don't know him, I'm just returning his call. Thanks so much for your help! Good-bye!" [Then the therapist hangs up the phone whether or not the relative has responded.]

When you get a curious relative, roommate, or other on the line, you will have to choose whether to be polite or whether to maintain confidentiality as much as possible. The more you stay on the line, waiting for the individual to be willing to say good-bye, the more you give the individual a chance to quiz you and become more curious because you are unwilling to give any substantive answers. It is better to say good-bye pleasantly, in an unrushed tone, and then hang up—although clearly it is not optimally polite.

Sometimes, you may try a couple times and still can't reach the client. In those cases, you have little choice but to leave just your name and number as a message. Again, state that you don't know what the call is regarding and that you are just returning a call.

WHEN THE CLIENT IS AVAILABLE

When you call, know what your goals are for the conversation. Most likely, you will just want to set up a mutually convenient appointment. You might also want or need to gather a little information about the client's presenting problem. In some settings, you might also be asked to screen the client briefly to ensure that the client is appropriate for the services that the setting offers. If there are any screening issues, talk to your supervisor for advice on how to handle them.

Let's assume that you want to set up an appointment, get a little information, and also learn what the presenting problem is so that you can talk that over with your supervisor before the first session. Here is a sample transcript:

Client: "Hello."

Therapist: "Hi, could I speak to Pamela, please?"

C: "This is Pamela."

T: "Hi Pamela, this is [trainee name] calling from [mental health facility]. I was returning your call regarding setting up an appointment. Is this a good time to talk?"

C: "Sure."

T: "Great. Let's first set up a time to meet. How about 5:00 this Thursday?"

C: "I'm sorry, I can't come then."

T: "What about 3:30 on Friday?"

C: "That sounds fine."

T: "Okay, I'll mark you down for that time. Could you come in about 30 minutes early to fill out some paperwork?"

C: "Sure."

T: "Okay. I'd like to get a little information from you before we meet. What is your date of birth?"

C: "October 20, 1970."

T: "Could you tell me a little bit about why you decided to come to therapy at this time?"

C: "I'm having some problems with my girlfriend, and I've been feeling depressed about it."

T: "Sounds like it's a good idea to come for therapy then. Do you know where the clinic is?"

C: "Yes."

T: "Good. I also need to tell you that the clinic requires that you pay your fee at the time of appointment and that you will be charged your fee if you cancel an appointment with less than 24 hours' notice. Do you have any questions about that?"

C: "No."

T: "So I'll look forward to seeing you this Friday at 3:30, and you'll come in at 3:00 to do the paperwork first."

C: "Okay."

T: "See you then."

C: "Good-bye."

T: "Good-bye."

Note here that the therapist keeps the conversation short and to the point. The therapist highlights important aspects of the payment policy to minimize any possibility of misunderstandings later. The therapist is friendly but also brisk. The therapist doesn't want to get into an extensive conversation with the client over the phone because it is very difficult, even for an experienced clinician, to properly assess or treat an unknown client over the phone.

REFRAIN FROM LENGTHY PHONE CONVERSATIONS

Sometimes your prospective client will want to talk at length over the phone; this may not be easy to stop. However, be aware that having a lengthy phone conversation with a prospective client may create a doctor–patient relationship in the eyes of the law (Simon, 2004), which is something you should avoid doing before you have had a chance to assess the client in person (although it should be noted that giving the client an appointment could be seen as creating a doctor–patient relationship as well; Simon, 2004). Creating a doctor–patient relationship with someone you can't yet properly assess in person may increase your legal liability for negative events, such as suicide, that you cannot properly assess over the phone. That said, if you do sense that the client may be suicidal over the phone, insist that the client come to the clinic or go to an emergency room immediately.

Therefore, in most cases, it is best to keep the first phone contact brief. Most people understand that health care practitioners are busy people and don't have time to talk at length over the phone. As needed, use this intervention:

> "I have to apologize. I wanted to get back to you in a timely fashion, but I don't have much time right now. I can see that all these things you are telling me are very important, but I don't have enough time right now to do justice to these issues over the phone. Can I ask you to fill me in about all of this when we meet for our first session?"

Generally, the client will readily agree to wait until the session to discuss the issues.

YOUR TONE ON THE PHONE

You will want to present yourself in a balanced manner when you are on the phone with clients. You will want to be pleasant and friendly. You will want to indicate that you are interested in what your client has to say and look forward to the session. However, maintain a professional demeanor. At times you may need to be brisk and politely redirect the client to accomplish your goal for the phone contact without veering into topics that are better addressed in therapy.

IF A CLIENT'S FRIEND OR FAMILY MEMBER CALLS YOU

Sometimes clients' friends and family members are aware that the client is seeing you. The friend or family member may then call you about the client. If this individual wants information about the client, gently inform the caller that psychotherapy is confidential and that you cannot provide any information. If this individual wants to tell you about the client's behavior outside the session, inform the caller that you can listen but cannot comment and that you will need to tell the client about the call at the next session (paragraph informed by Gabbard, 2000a).

TALKING TO YOUR CLIENT ON A CELL PHONE

You may be able to retrieve messages from your clients while away from your clinical office. At times, you may find it helpful to contact your client by cell phone. Remember that if you call the client by cell phone, it is likely that the client will then have your cell phone number at her disposal. This is not optimal. If you must use your cell phone, before you call, contact the carrier to see how to block your phone number from appearing on the client's caller ID and use this code whenever calling clients.

Generally, it is much better to just wait until you are in your office or home so that you can make a confidential call. Again, if you are calling from home, consider blocking your number from caller ID. Carefully consider any other location to determine whether you can make a confidential call securely. If you just need to call the client to confirm an appointment time, it may be possible to do that in a location that is not totally confidential:

> "Hi, this is [therapist name]. I just wanted to call to confirm that our next meeting is at 2:00 P.M. on Tuesday."

Do not say the client's name or talk about the client's problems. If the client mentions another issue during the call, you should respond this way:

> "I'm sorry, I can't talk about that right now, because I'm not in a location where I can talk confidentially. But I just wanted to get back to you in a timely manner about your question about the appointment time. Can we discuss it when we meet on Tuesday?"

While Pinals and Gutheil (2001) argue that you should always inform your clients and/or other professionals when you are using a cell phone, I disagree. They rightly point out that cell phone communications are subject to interception. However, the large majority of phones used now are either cell phones or cordless phones. Incidents of interception are unlikely.

YOUR HOME AND CELL PHONE GREETINGS

A training site supervisor is reviewing vitas of mental health trainees that might be matched to the site. She is interested in interviewing one of the candidates and calls his home phone number to leave a message. The student's voice mail replies, "Hi! You've reached Dr. Nick and Dr. Sarah at THE LOONY BIN! [Giggles, laughter, and lame jokes continue about shock therapy, meds, and so on.] Leave a message for the doctors after the beep!" The supervisor does not leave a message and decides not to offer an interview.

Be sure you have an appropriate message at your home and cell phone voice mails, as your fellow professionals may call you there at times.

NEVER SHARE YOUR PERSONAL PHONE NUMBERS

I recommend that you never give out your home or cell phone number to clients. Some experienced licensed practitioners may make exceptions when they are working with a low-risk population. In addition, some private practitioners may use their cell phone as a practice phone number. As a trainee, you should not do that. Instead, there should be a professional phone number where your clients can leave messages for you. Staff there can decide whether to contact you on your personal phone.

If you feel tempted to give out a personal phone number, talk it over with a supervisor first. You should carefully consider the relevant clinical issues together.

YOUR PERSONAL PHONE AND HOME
ADDRESS SHOULD BE UNLISTED

You should call your phone company now and change your phone number to unlisted. Your address should not be in the phone book, either. You might also want to check online directories and try to remove yourself if possible. As a therapist, you are at significantly greater statistical risk of being threatened, assaulted, or even killed (Berg, Bell, & Tupin, 2000). Keeping such data private helps keep your private life safe.

Chapter Eleven

Preparing for the First Session

A first session with the client is the most important one. This session will often determine whether the client feels trusting and comfortable. Being well prepared for this session will help you make a positive, professional impression so that the client feels that he or she is getting a good quality of care.

UNDERSTAND YOUR SITE'S
INITIAL INTERVIEW REQUIREMENTS

Sites have varying requirements and formats for initial outpatient psychotherapy client interviews. Two basic models are frequently employed. First, the client has an intake interview, and at the conclusion of the interview, the client is usually assigned to another clinician. The goal of these intake interviews is to assess the client and refer to the appropriate health care practitioner or program. You might do some of these intake interviews, you might be assigned clients who have already had an intake interview, or both.

Second, a client may be assigned to you for treatment, but very little information may be available from the client's initial (probably phone) contact with the clinic, so you will need to spend the first session getting oriented to the client's problems.

You should also know what the site's procedures are for voluntary and involuntary hospitalization should the client need it.

GET ORGANIZED

Before the session begins, be sure that you are organized. If the client has not already reviewed this information in an intake interview, have the following forms available:

- The site's informed consent form. If the site does not have a form, be prepared to address this verbally using the information in appendix 2.
- The site's confidentiality form (or this may be part of the informed consent form). If the site does not have a form, be prepared to address this verbally using the information in appendix 3.
- The site's HIPAA (Health Insurance Portability and Accountability Act) form.
- The site's interview outline, if there is one, or you can use a copy of the outline in appendix 4 or devise your own using the information and screening questions in the appendices.
- Several copies of the facility's release of information form.

Other items that you may wish to have handy are the following:

- A pad of paper and several pens.
- Sticky notes in case you want to write down any information for the client.
- A copy of the recent *Diagnostic and Statistical Manual of Mental Disorders* in case the client has a diagnosis that you are less familiar with because you may not remember enough symptoms to make a definitive diagnosis otherwise.
- Brochures, business cards, or flyers for referrals that the clinic often makes; your supervisor can help you with this.

BE PREPARED TO TAKE AMPLE NOTES

During a first session, most people benefit from taking copious notes. Otherwise, you may not remember all the details of the client's symptoms and history when you write the progress note. It always helps to write down some of the client's more unique or diagnostic statements verbatim. These give anyone reading your progress note a more nuanced view of the client. Here are some examples of statements I might write down:

- "I thought that I couldn't feel any pain, so I put cigarettes out on my arm."
- "I've always been very shy; I didn't talk at all in preschool."

- "There's high pressure from my family to do well."
- "I like to be in control."
- "My life situation sucks, and I'm sick of it."

REVIEW AVAILABLE INFORMATION ABOUT THE CLIENT

Before the session begins, you will want to take a few moments to review what you know already about the client. Review any progress notes and other documentation that already exists. You may wish to think about what you learned from any phone contact you had with the client. Think about what else you would like to learn about the client. It might be helpful to write down these thoughts to ensure that you ask about them in the intake session.

CLIENT MANAGEMENT

Some clients are very talkative and want to tell you many details about their life stories. If you see that you are likely to run out of time and the client is very talkative, think about whether it would be better to refocus or to just let the client talk and get more specific information next time. If the client is unstable or for any other reason it is essential to get the information today, you can refocus the client: "What you've just told me is very helpful in understanding your situation. Could we spend a little time focusing on some other information that I need to get from you today?" After this point, use close-ended questions as much as possible. If you need to ask an open-ended question as a follow-up, try something like this: "Could you tell me briefly what types of sleep problems you've been having?"

Certain clients are too severely mentally ill to be able to fully participate in the first session. For various reasons, they are unable to provide full historical, social, and diagnostic information in a timely manner. In these cases, try a couple of times to refocus the client, but if this is not possible, refocus yourself. Don't expect that you can get all the information you'd like to today. If the client was brought in by a friend or family member, perhaps that person can provide some useful information. Make a careful note in the chart of the symptoms that you observe and why the client is unable to participate fully. The client can be further assessed later when able to communicate more clearly. In some cases, a client may be manic, agitated, depressed, or psychotic but still be able to be coherent and participate meaningfully in an initial session. These clients may be able to be treated effectively on an outpatient basis.

Agitation in the client is important to note and is diagnostically relevant. However, agitated people are difficult to talk to. Go ahead and ask client to slow down when talking to you: "I'm sorry, but you're going so fast that I'm having difficulty following you, and you've said a lot of important things that I'd like to know more about. Can I ask you to slow down?" Redirect the client to the previous topic if it is not finished. Consider asking the client to take a few deep breaths together with you. See if the client can say why he or she feels agitated. If the client is unable to calm down and refocus, it is likely that hospitalization may be needed.

Assessing manic clients is difficult as well. The clients have pressure of speech and can talk at length about subjects that are utterly unrelated to the tasks of the first session. They are often so excited about what they are talking about or, alternatively, so irritable that it is difficult to interrupt them. Try to refocus the client a couple of times as you would with the agitated client. If this is not effective, make a note of all the manic symptoms you observe and focus on determining whether the client needs to be hospitalized (probably so if the client is that manic). Just note in the chart something like this: "Further historical information could not be gathered today since client was too tangential and displayed pressure of speech, talking about unrelated topics in response to my questions."

In cases of severe major depression, some clients will be too depressed to be able to participate fully in the first session. If this is the case, it is likely that hospitalization will be needed. Get as much information about symptoms as you can and note the depressive symptoms that you observe. Again, perhaps an accompanying friend or family member could be a source of information.

Sometimes a client will have prominent psychotic symptoms. Perhaps the client is preoccupied by delusional material and is unable to refocus on other topics. Perhaps the client is so cognitively disorganized that he is unable to answer questions in a coherent fashion; his responses may be nonsensical or tangential. Or the client could be distracted by auditory or visual hallucinations; in this case, you might observe the client looking around the room.

In all these cases, it is likely that the client will need hospitalization if he is so mentally ill that he cannot communicate effectively. You will just need to document enough information about the severity of symptoms to clarify why admission is needed. Do not feel that you need to gather all the social history and so on for a client who is too mentally ill to communicate effectively. This will be a waste of time and will contribute to the client's distress if she is unable to communicate well at present. This information can be gathered later when the client is more able to participate effectively.

TIME MANAGEMENT

Managing time during an initial interview can be challenging even for the experienced psychotherapist. Start out the interview with open-ended questions that will help build rapport and allow the client to tell you important material in her own words, which will help you know where to go next. Later, transition to more close-ended questions to help you get more information in a limited time period. Keep in mind that the four most important goals for seeing a new client are the following:

- Establish rapport
- Obtain informed consent including providing information on confidentiality (depending on the population and the specific client, this can be done in writing prior to the session, with an opportunity for questions within the session)
- Determine the presenting problem
- Evaluate the client for suicidality and other crises

Even if you run over with time, you must accomplish these four goals in each initial session. Usually the first three goals do not take much time. However, evaluating for crisis risk can take a long time, perhaps the entire session, if the client's symptomatology and history are complex.

These goals should also be accomplished in most initial sessions:

- Diagnose any mental illnesses (if the client has suicide or violence risk, you will need to do this anyway as part of the risk assessment—for more information, see chapters 19 and 20).
- Give feedback to the client about diagnoses and treatment.
- Make referrals (chapters 15–17). In order to make an appropriate referral, you will need to understand the severity of the client's symptoms and his level of distress.

Finally, if you have enough time, it is helpful to gather this information:

- Get an overview of current life problems the client may be having (if the client has suicide or violence risk, you may have had to gather this information already as part of the risk assessment—for more information, see chapters 19 and 20)
- Obtain social, medical, and mental health histories, including getting relevant information about psychological symptoms over time and past involvement in mental health care (outline in appendix 4)

With experience, you will be surprised about how much important information you can get in an hour. Consider how much time you have left for the interview as you complete each goal. When you see that you have only 5 to 10 minutes left in the session, start to wind it up—conclude your discussion, make referrals, and schedule the next session.

EXERCISES AND DISCUSSION QUESTIONS

1. What policies and procedures does your training site have regarding intake sessions?
2. Does the site prefer that you continue the intake session as long as needed to gather all information or gather the most important information within a 45- to 50-minute intake session? What is the most important information?

Chapter Twelve

The First Session: Tasks and Structure

Two situations can arise during the first session. First, you may see an intake client whom you will evaluate and then refer to other treatment. This type of first session is generally also your last with the client. Alternatively, you will have a first session with an ongoing psychotherapy client, then schedule regular psychotherapy appointments to continue to see the client. I address both of these scenarios in this chapter.

TASKS OF THE FIRST SESSION

Often, as clinicians, we are asked to see an intake client in about a 45-minute session. We are then expected to be able to make a diagnosis and send the client to whatever treatment is appropriate for his problems. Sometimes this is a realistic goal, sometimes it isn't. Some of your psychotherapy clients will have very complex psychiatric histories and social histories, and you will need two to three sessions to get all the information you need. Sometimes you have a limited time to see an intake client for just one session and refer to other treatments. In all these cases, it is important to prioritize carefully during the session.

Here is an outline of all the tasks you would ideally want to accomplish in the first session:

- Start the session.
- Obtain informed consent, including providing information about confidentiality and HIPAA (Health Insurance Portability and Accountability Act).
- Obtain this verbally if it hasn't already been obtained in written form and provide an opportunity for questions (chapter 7).

- Establish rapport.
- Determine the presenting problem.
- Get an overview of current life problems the client may be having.
- Diagnose any mental illnesses (chapter 9).
- Evaluate the client for suicidality and other crises (chapter 19).
- Obtain social, medical, and mental health histories, including getting relevant information about psychological symptoms over time and past involvement in mental health care. (Because of time constraints, you will often address these historical issues in subsequent sessions; see outline in appendix 4.)
- Give feedback to the client about diagnoses and treatment.
- Make referrals (chapters 15–17).
- End the session.

In many cases, you will not gather all this information in the first session. Remember that the four most important aspects of seeing a new client are the following:

- Establish rapport
- Informed consent, confidentiality, and HIPAA
- Presenting problem
- Evaluating the client for suicidality and other crises

Since you have undoubtedly learned about rapport-building skills in other course work, I do not address basic rapport-building skills in this chapter. Instead, only specific rapport-building issues that are pertinent to the initial session are discussed: client ambivalence, fears, and expectations. Addressing all the details of doing an accurate and complete initial interview is far beyond the scope of this book, as entire books have been written on this subject alone (see Craig 2005; Morrison, 1995).

START THE SESSION

Salma El Sayad is a mental health trainee working at a college counseling center. She goes to the waiting room to meet her new client, Tara Morris. She sees just one client in the waiting room and approaches her. "Hello, are you Tara?" Tara nods yes. Salma says, "I'm Salma El Sayad, it's good to meet you. Let's go to my office." Salma guides Tara through the hallways to her office. They make small talk about the women's basketball team, which has been very successful this year, in the hallway. When they reach her office, Salma gestures to indicate which seat Tara should take. "If you wouldn't mind sitting here." Salma then orients Tara to the tasks of the first session. "Today, I would like to focus on getting an overview of what is going on with you. So, I will be asking you some questions about how things have been for you lately and any symptoms you might be experiencing. This will be helpful so that we can plan what treatment will be most effective for you. How does that sound?" Tara indicates her agreement.

Joel Mitchell is a mental health trainee working at a community mental health center. He is doing intakes today with walk-in clients. When he finishes each intake interview, the client will be assigned to another clinician for ongoing treatment. The receptionist informs him that a new client, Sharon Yang, has walked in. He checks the electronic medical record, but Sharon is new to the clinic, and there is no old chart to review before seeing her. He goes to the waiting room, which has a dozen clients in it. He says, "Ms. Yang?" Sharon gets up and comes toward him. He reaches out to shake her hand. "Hi, I'm Joel Mitchell, I'll be meeting with you today. Could you follow me to my office?" Sharon indicates her agreement and follows him. Joel indicates which chair is hers and then tells her, "Today, I'd like to talk to you and try to understand what is going on with you so that I can refer you the treatment that is right for you. When we are done today, I will be referring you to another therapist or treatment program where you can get help on an ongoing basis. I'll be taking some notes as we go along so that I don't lose track of anything important."

At the time of the session, go to get your client from the waiting room. Depending on the setting, you might prefer to ask for the client by first name (e.g., college counseling center) or by title and last name (e.g., older populations). Do whatever other clinicians in your setting do in this regard.

Keep in mind that the client, if anything, is more anxious than you are. You might want to begin with just a minute or two of chitchat to make both of you more comfortable. If you talk with the client in the waiting room or the hall, it should be superficial, such as, "Did you have any difficulty getting here?" or, "How was traffic getting here?" Brief remarks about general impersonal topics, such as the weather, parking, or traffic encountered today, can break the ice. You might also riff off of something about the appearance or possessions of the client. For example, it might be morning—you are drinking coffee, and the client has brought coffee—so you might commiserate about needing it in the morning. Or if the client is wearing a sports logo, you could share some brief remarks about sports. Others prefer to avoid any chitchat and move directly to the interview (Morrison, 1995); both approaches are appropriate. Be sure not to chat too long, as this deemphasizes the professional nature of the relationship.

You can then segue into starting the session. Many clients know little about the therapeutic process or how psychotherapy sessions typically proceed. So it can help to spend the next few minutes of the session orienting the client to the session's tasks, as Joel and Salma do in the previous vignettes. Note that Joel carefully informed the client from the start that he would not be the on-going therapist. Most clients do not mind if you take notes as long as you can maintain good eye contact at appropriate times.

INFORMED CONSENT, CONFIDENTIALITY AND HIPAA, AND CLIENT QUESTIONS

Salma asks Tara if she brought in her intake forms. Tara printed them out off of the counseling center's website and has them. Salma asks for a moment, then looks over them briefly. She sees that Tara's signature indicates that she understands the confidentiality, informed consent, and HIPAA forms but still asks, "Do you have any questions about therapy?" Tara asks, "What type of treatment do you recommend for depression?" Salma suspects that Tara is asking about herself. She does not know enough about Tara yet to know whether she does actually does have depression, how severe it is, or what type of treatment might be appropriate. So she says, "It depends on the particular individual and how serious the depression is. How about if I try to understand what is going on with you, and then at the end, I can give you my input about what treatment I would recommend for any depression you might be experiencing?" Tara indicates her agreement. Salma then tells Tara, "I also want you to know that, since I am a student, I need to discuss all my work with a more experienced therapist. I will need to audiotape our sessions after today. My supervisor will sometimes listen to those tapes. Do you have any questions about that?" Salma then answers a couple questions about the role of the supervisor in Tara's psychotherapy.

Joel asks, "Do you have any questions?" Sharon indicates that she doesn't have any questions yet. Joel then uses the outlines in appendices 2 and 3 to verbally review informed consent and confidentiality. He gives her a HIPAA form to sign. Joel tells Sharon, "After we talk, I will be discussing your situation with a more experienced therapist. Do you have any questions?" Sharon does not have any questions about that.

Salma's client has already reviewed information about informed consent and confidentiality in written form. After orienting the client to the tasks of the session, she gives the client an opportunity to ask questions about informed consent, confidentiality, or any other therapy topics she is curious about. Joel's client, on the other hand, has not been given any written materials, so he reviews informed consent, confidentiality, and HIPAA at the beginning of the session.

Some clients will have many questions, but many will have few or none. Do the best you can to answer whatever questions arise. If you don't know the answer, it's okay to say so. Be sure you address informed consent and confidentiality at the beginning of the session since it is difficult to return to it later. In addition, this prevents a very difficult situation: the client informs you of abuse that needs to be reported *before* you have educated the client about limits to confidentiality. Further information about informed consent, confidentiality, and HIPAA was presented in chapter 7.

ESTABLISHING RAPPORT—ADDRESSING AMBIVALENCE, FEARS, AND EXPECTATIONS

Tara indicates that she is uncertain whether it was right to come to therapy. Salma tells her, "It was very wise of you to come to therapy right now. I can see that this breakup is really getting you down, and you have been having a lot of trouble coping lately. I'm very hopeful that together we can figure out how to help you feel better." Tara says that she has been trying not to let her friends know how bad she feels. Salma says, "You've been very brave to talk about this; I can see that it must be difficult for you."

Joel asks Sharon whether she has had any mental health treatment before. She indicates that she has seen five or six different therapists, "but none of them did me any good." He asks her how long she attended treatment and finds that she went for no more than a few sessions. She also says that she has been given medication before but that "I didn't need it." Joel says, "I see that you've tried therapy a number of times, but you feel that it has not worked for you. But I think that I'm noticing a problem. I don't think that you've been giving it enough time. You've been coping with your problems for a long time, and none of them are going away overnight. So I have to tell you that you will have to make a commitment to come for many sessions in order for your therapist to get to know you so you can feel better. This may take a lot of time and commitment on your part. You will probably need to go very regularly for a month or two before you start to see any improvement. Be sure to keep that in mind, okay?" Sharon indicates her understanding. Joel also suggests that she talk to her therapist if she is thinking of stopping therapy again instead of not showing up anymore.

During the initial session, the client is likely to be quite anxious and might also be somewhat ambivalent about therapy. The client might be fearful to talk about things that she has kept secret for a long time. She may not have told even her closest friends or family how upset she has been. You can help the client engage in the therapeutic process by being alert to these concerns and addressing them as they come up. Your client might indicate that she has not been telling anyone how bad she feels. Clients who are secretive about their difficulties often feel ashamed. You can imagine how difficult it would be for a client who has been secretive to talk about her problems. It takes desperation but also courage to do so. Emphasize the positive with her. Complement her on the courage that she has displayed in talking about these very personal and painful difficulties, as Salma does in the previous vignette.

Sometimes you get a client who has been in and out of therapy. This type of client may begin therapy hopefully but may expect too much too soon and, as a result, will drop out of therapy. In these cases, it can be helpful to identify the pattern and educate the client about treatment as Joel has done in the previous vignette.

PRESENTING PROBLEM

Salma asks, "What has made you decide to come to therapy at this time?" Tara says that she has recently been "dumped" by her girlfriend and that she has been crying for hours every day. She goes on to describe sleep disturbance, overeating, and social isolation. She also says that she hasn't been doing well in school this year (she is a freshman) and that even before the breakup she was having problems concentrating and getting all her schoolwork done.

Joel says, "Please tell me what problems made you decide to come for treatment." Sharon says that she has been arguing with her elderly parents and that she doesn't like living with them anymore. Joel asks how this living arrangement came to be. Sharon says that she is on disability and has a low income. Joel asks her if she could tell him why she gets disability, but she is unable to tell him. She does tell him that it was difficult for her to get to the clinic because all the people on the bus were criticizing her on the way there.

Often the presenting problem can include clues as to the life problems and symptoms that the client is having, so it is wise to further explore whatever symptoms are suggested by the presenting problem first. Your questions about the presenting problem should be open ended (like Salma's or Joel's in the previous vignettes) and allow the client to talk for several minutes. Encourage the client to keep talking with open-ended questions as needed and use your active listening skills to get whatever information you feel is relevant.

OVERVIEW OF CURRENT LIFE PROBLEMS

Salma asks Tara, "Has anything else been stressing you out lately?" Tara talks about her grandmother, who she is very close to. Her grandmother has terminal lung cancer. Tara says she has been wondering whether she has at-

tention deficit disorder because of her school problems and is worrying that she will never finish college.

Joel asks Sharon, "Have any other things been bothering you lately?" Sharon says that she had been going to a community support program but that it was closed because of a lack of funds. She has a boyfriend whom she met there, but her parents do not approve since he has a history of cocaine use and psychiatric hospitalizations.

Asking about current life problems can help you further assess the client's level of distress. This is helpful to put the client's symptoms in context; in addition, it is helpful to have this information when evaluating crisis risk.

DIAGNOSE ANY MENTAL ILLNESSES AND EVALUATE CRISIS RISK

Salma observes Tara as they talk. She sees that Tara has poor eye contact and that her eyes are red from crying. Her speech is slow, and she looks sad. These symptoms are clearly suggestive of depression. At this point, Salma continues the interview by systematically asking Tara about depressive symptoms. She screens Tara for a history of manic episodes to rule out bipolar disorder and asks her about any history of depressive seasonality because it is November. Salma notices that she just has 15 to 20 minutes left in the therapy session. She says, "I need to take a few minutes to ask you some standard questions. It is okay if we do that now?" Tara indicates her agreement. Then Salma screens Tara for suicidality, homicidality, substance abuse, psychotic symptoms, and post-traumatic stress disorder (PTSD). She knows that she has not asked about every possible disorder, but she has followed up on the presenting problem and her observations, she has asked about crises, and she has screened for diagnoses that are often comorbid with depression. Tara denies all these symptoms but has been having some passive suicidal ideation lately. Tara denies any suicidal intent or history of suicidal behavior.

Joel observes Sharon as they talk. He sees that she sometimes looks around the room distractedly. Her affect is flat despite the fact that she clearly verbalizes that she is upset about her living situation with her parents. These symptoms are suggestive of psychosis. At this point, Joel systematically asks Sharon about psychotic symptoms as well as depressive and manic symptoms. He asks about the duration of all these symptoms so that he can make a differential diagnosis between schizophrenia, schizoaffective disorder (depressed or bipolar types), and other disorders with psychotic features. Joel needs to finish the intake interview. He tells Sharon, "Now, I need to ask you some standard questions. Can we do that now?" Sharon agrees. Sharon denies past or current suicidal or homicidal ideation. Joel had already asked her about psychotic and mood symptoms, but he screens her for trauma history and PTSD since he knows that psychotic symptoms have a high comorbidity with PTSD. Sharon indicates that she experienced date rape from a boyfriend in high school and was also raped by an acquaintance 20 years after that. He assesses PTSD symptoms and determines that she has mild symptoms of PTSD, sufficient for a diagnosis.

The process of making a diagnosis was reviewed in chapter 9. The above vignettes are provided to assist you in following these cases throughout the first interview. Asking about certain symptoms—such as psychosis or suicidal and homicidal ideation—can be problematic. Some clients can have these symptoms while appearing speaking and behaving appropriately, so the clinician should routinely ask screening questions. However, certain clients can get upset if they draw the mistaken conclusion that they have said something that has led you to think that they are have serious difficulties of this sort. Prefacing your questions with a statement that they are "standard questions" as Salma and Joel do can be helpful (Moline, Williams, & Austin, 1998).

GIVING FEEDBACK ABOUT DIAGNOSES AND TREATMENT

Salma says, "I'm going to try to summarize some of the things that you've told me. It sounds as though you are having some significant problems with depression. You told me about sleep problems, eating problems, crying, and feeling down; these are all symptoms of depression. Depression is very treatable, so I am hopeful that you will be feeling better soon. Right now, the best thing for you would be to resume your usual activities, even if you don't feel like it. Staying alone in bed and crying is just making your depression worse. Try to get out with your friends over the next week and go to class, okay?" Tara agrees to try. Salma says, "I'm not sure why you've been having these problems with school. It may be related to your depression, or it may be a separate problem. For now, I'd like you to fill out this questionnaire and bring it back to me next week. I'll ask you some more about how school has been going then." Tara agrees to fill out the questionnaire on attention-deficit/hyperactivity disorder for next week.

Joel says, "Sharon, it seems as though you have been hearing voices for some time. You also talked about your difficulties with feeling that the neighbors are spying on you. It sounds like you and your parents have been arguing about whether to confront the neighbors about this." Sharon nods. Joel continues, "I think that you have a mental illness called schizophrenia. Have you ever heard of that?" Sharon indicates that she knows she has been given that diagnosis before. She asks, "I'm not crazy, am I?" Joel replies, "I don't really like the word 'crazy,' but if you're asking whether you've lost touch with reality, I'd definitely say you have, at times. Schizophrenia is actually a very common problem; about one out of every hundred people has it. Chances are excellent that you can feel much better if you are able to stick with treatment and work closely with your therapist and your doctor."

Giving a diagnosis validates to the client that there is a problem that deserves to be addressed. It allows you to provide information about specific treatments that are helpful. You appear competent and knowledgeable, which is reassuring to the client. As the clinician, if you know the diagnosis, you can access a large body of professional literature that will help you treat the client effectively.

Many clients, because of their social isolation, have developed the idea that their problems and symptoms are "crazy" and totally unique and cannot be treated. They have tried to cope alone, but this has been ineffective. These clients may make remarks such as, "I'm not crazy, am I, Doc?" or "Have you ever seen anybody like me before?" Often, they fear that you will not know what their problem is or how to help them. They may fear that their problem is so unique that you have never seen it before. They may have developed a belief that their problem cannot be treated because they have not been able to make progress with it alone.

A client with these worries generally does have a diagnosable mental illness. As Joel does in the previous vignette, tell her about her diagnosis, let her know that her difficulties are definitely not unique, and give her hope that there is an effective treatment for her. This is an opportunity to educate the client about her illness so that she can cope more effectively in the future. Depending on the client's comprehension and functioning level, it can also be helpful to talk to the client about her feelings about being stigmatized and to discuss cultural biases against persons with mental illness as treatment progresses.

Allay your clients' fears through assurances such as the simple ones in the previous vignettes. Talk in a calm and matter-of-fact voice. This gives an implicit message that you don't think that their problems are shameful. Reassure them that their difficulties can improve and that they can be treated. If their problems are more common than they think, let them know. Give them a chance to ask you questions about your feedback to them.

MAINTAINING RAPPORT AND GIVING
FEEDBACK WITH SUBSTANCE-ABUSING CLIENTS

Giving feedback about substance use is complex. Early in therapy, it is best to avoid putting any labels on the client's substance use (W. R. Miller & Rollnick,

2002). Instead, identify the client's concerns, reflect them back, and ask the client to elaborate on what the client has already said.

At the end of the session, you might say to the client,

> "You mentioned that you are concerned about your alcohol use. You said that you recently got a DUI and that you are embarrassed to admit that you are still driving under the influence. I am very concerned for you as well. I'm glad that you brought this issue up, and we can definitely discuss it further when we meet next. For now, what are your plans for dealing with this issue?"

At this point, because the client has already expressed his concern about the issue, he will often volunteer a plan for avoiding driving drunk. Here you can use a motivational interviewing approach (W. R. Miller & Rollnick, 2002) with the client and use the client's own statements to nudge him to be safer between now and the next session. In this type of situation, carefully document that he has agreed to take action to avoid driving drunk in the future and what that agreed-on action is (e.g., take cabs when going out with friends to bars).

ENDING THE SESSION WITH
ONGOING PSYCHOTHERAPY CLIENTS

Salma asks, "How has it been to come in and talk about these things today?" Tara says, "I feel relieved. It wasn't as hard to talk about everything as I thought it would be." Salma indicates that she is glad to hear that. She says, "I see that it is about time to wind up today. Let's talk about schedules. I'd like you to come in twice a week until you are feeling better. What times will work for you?" They agree on a time. Salma says, "Okay, I will save 4 P.M. on Tuesdays and 1 P.M. on Thursdays for you. Those will be your scheduled times every week. When you are feeling better, we will go down to once a week. If you have to cancel, please let me know as soon as possible. Please try to give me at least 24 hours' notice. Can you do that?" Tara indicates that she understands. Salma says, "Thank you so much for coming. I enjoyed meeting you, and I'll see you next week, okay?" She leads Tara to the door, opens the door, and says good-bye.

If the client is starting individual psychotherapy, you will want to accomplish several important goals at the end of the session. Ensure that you have gathered the most important information. Then allow about 10 minutes to finish the session. During this process, make referrals for any adjunctive treatments that you would recommend (chapters 15–17), check in with the client about his perceptions of the session, and schedule your next appointment. Be sure that the agreed-on appointment is convenient for both of you. Never schedule an ongoing psychotherapy client at a time that is inconvenient for you. If the client proposes a time that is inconvenient, just state, "I'm sorry, I'm not available then." Reiterate the clinic's cancellation policy as needed. If the clinic does not have an explicit cancellation policy, feel free to clarify your expectations about cancellation to the client. Even if the clients at your site tend to be lower functioning, some will still be able to comply with a request to call to cancel. As the client leaves, shake hands if you like or if the client extends a hand. Provide directions out of the building if you think it would be helpful.

ENDING THE SESSION WITH INTAKE CLIENTS

Joel says to Sharon, "I think it is about time to end our session. I'd like you to go back to the waiting room and wait to see the psychiatrist who is on call before you leave today. I suspect that he would like to give you some medication that will help you with the voices. Are you willing to do that?" Sharon agrees. Joel says, "Please wait in the waiting room until Dr. Moore comes to get you, okay? Also, I am giving you an appointment with Ms. Cho for next Monday at 2 P.M. Can I count on you to come in then?" Sharon says that she will be there. Joel continues, "I'm glad you came in today. I'm really hoping that Ms. Cho will be able to help you with your problems. Good luck with everything." Joel leads Sharon to the door, opens the door, shakes hands, and says good-bye. He then walks over to the psychiatrist's office to brief him on his interview with Sharon.

If the client is an intake client who you are referring for individual psychotherapy, you should allow about 5 to 10 minutes to finish the session. You might not want to ask for feedback about how the intake session went since you will not be working with the client on an ongoing basis, or you might ask for more general feedback: "How are you feeling about coming in for treatment now?" Set a follow-up appointment for the client or tell her how that will be done.

In some settings, part of your job as an intake worker is to decide which treatment is most appropriate for the client. Making the appropriate referrals from the intake interview is called *making a disposition*. Before seeing any intake clients in this type of setting, you and your supervisor will want to have a detailed discussion about the various treatments and who is appropriate for each one. Sometimes you will know what the most appropriate referral is, and sometimes you will want to include input from the client and/or your supervisor in making the disposition. You will want to allow plenty of time to discuss the options. A client who needs a treatment that she might not have been expecting or a more intensive treatment, such as inpatient or intensive outpatient, will need more time to ask questions and decide what to do.

The first few times you make a disposition, you may need to excuse yourself from the room and discuss the case with a supervisor. The supervisor will help you decide on the appropriate referrals. You can then go in and discuss these recommendations with the client. Be open to the client's input and willing to make some adjustments as needed.

Sometimes a client will request a treatment that you feel is inadequate to meet his needs. You should state this explicitly. Reference the client's past: "I see that you have been in individual therapy for a year, but you are still very depressed. I would like to see you get better as soon as possible. I am not sure whether individual therapy is enough for you right now since it hasn't been helping enough so far. I would like you to consider a partial hospitalization program instead. We have a good one affiliated with our clinic. How about if I set up an appointment for you to meet some of the staff there so that you can learn more about it and make a more informed decision?" Few clients will refuse a request stated in this way. You are just encouraging them to gather more information so that they can make a better decision; you are not demanding that they make any particular choice. Once they learn more, it is likely that they will accept the recommended treatment.

THE THERAPIST'S REACTION TO THE FIRST SESSION

First sessions with a client are often the most difficult and draining, even for experienced clinicians. Of course, they are far more stressful for a beginning therapist. Often, it is difficult for beginning clinicians to realize that they have been helpful. Let me assure you that you have, indeed, been helpful. Just talking about problems to someone who cares is a very healing and validating experience. Think about how much better you feel after talking to your friends about your problems. With training, you will grow in your ability to heal the emotional pain of others. With experience, you will gain faith and trust in the therapeutic process. With time, you will become confident that psychotherapy really can help.

RECOMMENDED READING

Morrison, J. (1995). *The first interview: Revised for DSM-IV.* New York: Guilford Press. *This should be the next book you read about interviewing. Morrison provides an excellent introduction to making diagnoses according to the* Diagnostic and Statistical Manual of Mental Disorders *(4th ed., text revision) during the first session, which is a very challenging task for beginning therapists. He adeptly addresses many of the clinical challenges that can arise during a diagnostic interview.*

EXERCISES AND DISCUSSION QUESTIONS

1. What do you anticipate (or what have you found) to be the most challenging aspects of meeting a client for the first time?

Chapter Thirteen

Progress Notes and the Chart

Writing a good progress note is an essential professional skill. If you ever are accused of malpractice or need to make a deposition or your notes are subpoenaed for any reason, good progress notes will save you from professional embarrassment and worse.

PROGRESS NOTES AND THE STANDARD OF CARE

Julie Chen is a mental health trainee who is working for a group practice that treats high-functioning clients. She sees a marital case that ends in divorce. After the case is closed, the husband leaves her a number of threatening messages demanding that she return the fees he has paid the practice. In consultation with her supervisor and the practice's lawyer who specializes in mental health issues, she does not return the calls or the fees. The husband files suit against the group practice for malpractice, and the case goes to trial. It turns out that Julie has not maintained any progress notes after the initial session, nor did she document the threatening phone calls. She is not certain of the dates of the sessions, either, as the practice collected some payments in cash and the records are muddled. Julie's supervisor did not review Julie's (lack of) written documentation for the case contemporaneously. In court, Julie's verbal report of her treatment of the couple is found to be up to professional standards, but her supervisor and the practice are found negligent because of Julie's lack of appropriate professional record keeping, and the husband was given a substantial monetary award.

Zachary James is a mental health trainee working in a pain clinic. He runs many treatment groups together with his supervisor and does evaluations of

153

pain patients. He is very busy and procrastinates writing the progress notes that his supervisor has assigned to him. An internal review of documentation found that Zachary was behind on group therapy notes by 6 weeks. Both Zachary and his supervisor were written up by the review committee for providing an inadequate standard of care. When his supervisor insists that he complete the documentation, Zachary is able to deduce what psychoeducational information he presented from his files but is embarrassed to admit that he no longer remembers any personal issues that the group members brought up in the sessions 3 to 6 weeks ago.

Progress notes should always be written on the day of interaction or the following day. Your memory will fade if you postpone the note more than 1 day after the session. Even better, organize your schedule to write your progress notes immediately after each session so that you don't forget important details (Cameron & turtle-song, 2002). Remember, from a legal perspective, "if it isn't written, it didn't happen" (Gutheil, 1980).

Follow the record-keeping standards and guidelines advocated by your professional association. As indicated in the previous vignettes, no matter what you did in the session, if you don't chart the session, you are providing an inadequate standard of care.

THE USES OF PROGRESS NOTES

Keep in mind that there are many potential audiences for the progress notes you write: (a) you, who may need to look back on what you've done; (b) other members of the treatment team; (c) emergency coverage clinicians; (d) reviewers, such as insurers and utilization and quality assurance reviewers; (e) the legal system; and (f) the client (Gutheil & Hilliard, 2001). If the care of your client is ever transferred to another clinician, the notes will be an invaluable source of information about the client's progress.

ELECTRONIC CHARTS

In many facilities, there is now an electronic medical record (EMR) available. If your site uses an EMR, your supervisor can educate you in how to use the EMR software and to sign the note electronically. An EMR allows for improved documentation since notes are always legible. However, with an EMR system in a medical center, psychotherapy notes may become part of the general medical record, so you should determine whether other clinicians throughout the facility will have ready access to them.

With an EMR, you can contribute to improved continuity of care. It is wise to skim all the recent progress notes, including your own, before seeing the client. If there are any emergent psychological issues, even if brought up by a different clinician, the EMR can inform you and you can address them as needed with the client. With an EMR, be aware that other clinicians will be reading your notes and be especially mindful of the level of detail. Since other clinicians can easily see your notes in your setting, you might add more detail that could be helpful to them:

Instead of this: "Ms. R stated that she was having problems with her medication; I suggested that she call her psychiatrist."

You might write this: "Ms. R stated that she was having dizziness, nausea, and headaches. She believes that this is due to her medication. I suggested that she call her psychiatrist."

The second note would be much more helpful to your psychiatrist colleague.

Occasionally, everyone will make errors when charting. If you have an EMR at your facility, it is unlikely that you will be able to change notes after they are signed. If you mistakenly put a note in the wrong chart, talk to the computer experts to see if the note can somehow be made unreadable. If you have made an error in a note, you can probably put an addendum onto your previous note with the new date and the corrected information.

PAPER CHARTS

Make an effort to write legibly in a paper chart. On each new blank page, write or stamp the client's full name, date of birth, and any numerical identifier. When you are signing a paper note, sign with your first initial or first name, your last name, and your degrees (if any). Add your title underneath your name. If your signature is not legible, I recommend that you print your name underneath the signature. As a trainee, your supervisor should be reviewing and cosigning all your notes, so leave space for the supervisor's signature below yours. Do not include any blank lines inside the body of the note or between the end of the note and your signature.

Write with black pen only in a paper chart. Black pen makes better photocopies than other colors. Do not use felt pen, as it can smear if something is spilled on the chart, or pencil, which is legally problematic because of its ease of erasure (Cameron & turtle-song, 2002).

If you make an error in a paper chart, ensure that your corrections are not done in a way that would arouse suspicion of inappropriate alteration of the chart should the chart ever be reviewed in a court of law. Cameron and turtle-song (2002) suggest the following: "Never erase, obliterate, use correction fluid or in any way attempt to obscure the mistake. Instead, the error should be noted by enclosing it in brackets, drawing a single line through the incorrect word(s), and writing the word 'error' above or to the side of the mistake. The counselor should follow this correction with his or her initials, the full date, and time of the correction. The mistake should still be readable, indicating the counselor is only attempting to clarify the mistake not cover it up" (p. 291).

CONTENTS OF THE CHART

There is no definitive list of information that should be included in a client's chart (Moline, Williams, & Austin, 1998). However, here is a helpful list of chart items compiled from various sources (Moline et al., 1998; Rivas-Vazquez, Blais, Rey, & Rivas-Vasquez, 2001). This first list is comprised of documents that the psychotherapist would generate or gather from the client:

- Intake forms filled out by client (if required)
- Informed consent form, including legal limits to confidentiality (if there is no written form, the first progress note should document discussion of these issues)
- HIPAA (Health Insurance Portability and Accountability Act) form
- Mental health insurance company, policy number, and phone number
- Initial note that includes the following:
  - Referral source and reason for referral
  - Identifying data, including name, phone number (work and home), date of birth and age, gender, ethnicity, physical description, marital status, occupation, school or education, children living with client (ages and names), and other persons living with client (ages, relationship to client, and names)
  - Background/historical data
  - Functioning level, adequacy of coping, social support, and strengths
  - Diagnosis and prognosis
- Release of information forms that you and the client generate (make a copy to send out and keep the original in the chart)
- Treatment plans
- Progress notes, cosigned by a supervisor if you are being supervised
- Termination summary

If these items come to you from the client or other sources, they should also be included in the chart:

- Release of information forms sent from other health care professionals
- Any legal documents pertaining to the client, such as subpoenas
- Any correspondence, writings, or drawings given or sent to you by the client
- Printouts or electronic copies of any e-mails sent between you and the client containing any clinically pertinent information
- Communications sent to you by other professionals regarding the client
- Chart information that other sites sent you in response to a release of information
- Any questionnaires administered to the client
- Any other documents pertaining to the client

A separate chart should be opened for each client being treated, even if they are being treated jointly in marital or family therapy. This preserves the confidentiality of each family member. Many clinicians use abbreviations in the chart, and many common mental health abbreviations are listed in appendix 17. However, note that some experts recommend that no abbreviations be used because of the possibility of confusion or misinterpretation (Simon, 2004).

FORMAT

Arun Singh is a mental health trainee practicing at an outpatient clinic. He treated a client, Kenneth Lewis, for 2 years for adjustment disorder and relationship problems. About a year after therapy is terminated, Kenneth is arrested for murdering his girlfriend, which he had done during the period of treatment with Arun. Arun's progress notes are subpoenaed, and he is required to testify at the murder trial. The defense is claiming that Kenneth is not guilty by reason of insanity. Arun was not aware of the murder at the time. He is anxious about testifying but knows that he had thoroughly documented the client's stability at each session. The fact that Kenneth was emotionally stable throughout the treatment turns out to be a crucial piece of evidence.

This vignette illustrates the importance of documenting an assessment of the client at every psychotherapy session. For that reason, I always write progress notes in the SOAP (Cameron & turtle-song, 2002) or DAP format. The sections for this type of note are as follows:

- S/O is an abbreviation for "subjective and objective," which are generally combined into one section, or you can use D for "data" instead:
  - Subjective is what the client says.
  - Objective is what you observe about the client; include any significant behavior.

- ○ This section should include any interventions that you have made and how the client responded.
- ○ You should also include any advice that you gave to the client and the client's response. ("I advised the client not to drive after he had consumed more than two drinks, and the client stated that he understood the risks and agreed that he would call a cab on those occasions.")
- ○ These two are generally combined into one section by most clinicians but can be written separately.
- A is an abbreviation for "assessment," which includes the following:
  - ○ Whether the client is stable today
  - ○ If the client has been struggling with emotional stability, a statement about whether the client is worse or better than the previous session
  - ○ Any important emotional tone to the session
  - ○ Any risk management evaluations you had to make in this session
- P is an abbreviation for "plan," which includes the following:
  - ○ Any homework you have given the client (e.g., "Mr. F agreed to keep a sleep diary over the next week.")
  - ○ Any important steps the client states he or she will accomplish by next week (e.g., "Ms. G agreed to go to an Alcoholics Anonymous meeting tomorrow.")
  - ○ Any referrals that you have made and how they will be accomplished (e.g., "Mr. R agrees to contact his internist to be evaluated for his chronic headaches.")
  - ○ Anything you will be doing to manage the case between now and then (e.g., "I will fax release of information to Dr. Q.")
  - ○ Issues or interventions to consider for the next session (e.g., "Ms. K brought up her frustration with her best friend at the end of the session. We agreed to discuss this next week.")
  - ○ When the client will next be seen.

This progress note format forces the clinician to remember to include the assessment and the plan after each session. These crucial bits of information are often forgotten by clinicians who do not use this format. As you can see from the vignette, this information can be crucial if the notes are ever involved in litigation or in any internal review.

Progress notes should be well organized and easy for other clinicians to skim. Put different topics (e.g., depressive symptoms, anxiety symptoms, and family history) in separate paragraphs. Use simple, clear topic sentences, even if it seems a bit repetitive: "Ms. K. displayed numerous symptoms of depression."

TONE

Progress notes should be neutral and professional in tone. Avoid any implied criticism of the client or of any other clinician. It is most respectful to refer to adult clients in the notes by their title and last name, such as "Ms. Rodriguez," or you can abbreviate this as "Ms. R."

Never make negative comments about the client or observations about the client in the chart that could be seen as value laden or overly opinionated (Cameron & turtle-song, 2002; Gutheil, 1980). Here is an example:

Wrong: "Ms. S. was very manipulative again today. She was making her typical suicide threats in order to get more attention from the staff on the inpatient unit."

Right: "Ms. S. made suicidal statements on the unit today. However, on questioning, she denied any active suicidal intent. We discussed how she might verbalize her requests for help in a more prosocial manner."

I appreciate Gutheil's (1980) suggestion that, while writing progress notes, you always imagine that there is a hostile lawyer looking over your right shoulder and imagine how the lawyer might belittle you in court. I would add to this advice that you should also imagine that the client is looking over your left shoulder, ready to take offense at any tactless or careless remark you make in the chart that would lead to therapeutic disruption.

CONTENT

Chaniya Wilson is a psychotherapy trainee working in an outpatient clinic. The clinic is part of a large academic medical center that requires all clinicians to post progress notes in the EMR (electronic medical record). She is seeing a client, Teresa Baker, who has borderline personality traits. One week, Teresa comes into the office in a rage, brandishing a printout of her progress notes. She has marked what she deems to be inaccuracies in red ink throughout the notes.

Progress notes document whether the psychotherapy is appropriate and effective, and they are a tool to help keep psychotherapy on track. Document the client's emotional status and symptoms. Document the issues that were addressed. Use the progress notes to remind yourself of the homework assigned to the client the past week. If you make treatment recommendations, note whether the client agreed to comply. Note any plans that you have for the next session. It is wise to establish the habit of reviewing the recent chart notes before each session, as this will help you keep track of your client's progress, any homework you gave, and the goals for the client's treatment.

Progress notes should include an appropriate amount of detail. Major topics that were discussed during the session should be noted, but the details of the discussion are generally unnecessary, unless there is a crisis. Keep in mind that malpractice attorneys say, "If it isn't written, it didn't happen" (Gutheil, 1980), so anything of clinical importance must be documented. Here are some examples:

> Too much detail: "Ms. B came in upset and said that she had another fight with her brother. He said something that she thought was insulting, then she yelled at him, then they had a shoving match again, and he called her a 'bitch on wheels.' She said that she hates him. After some discussion, she calmed down and was able to hear some input about how to talk to her brother more effectively."

> Right level of detail: "Ms. B discussed interpersonal conflict with brother. We worked on effective communication skills."

Many psychotherapists have extensive training in how to interpret the meanings of the interactions between the therapist and the client. We call this "process." The actual topics discussed are referred to as "content." Progress notes should stick to documenting content and behavior and should avoid process (Gutheil, 1980). Do not document hypotheses, dynamic issues, suppositions, or interpretations. The vignette at the beginning of this section indicates one of the benefits of keeping your notes focused on content. Another example might clarify:

> Instead of writing: "Ms. N took her shoes off and put her feet up on the couch during the session. This unusual behavior symbolizes a crucial attachment change regarding her relationship with the therapist."

> You might write this: "Ms. N took her shoes off and put her feet up on the couch during the session. She had not engaged in this behavior during a session before."

As is implied by this example, it can be helpful to note any unusual behavior in the chart, even if its meaning is not totally clear. However, even if you think you know the meaning of the behavior, the meaning is usually not appropriate to write in the chart. Again, don't include speculations, psychodynamics, or clinical insights in the progress notes.

SAMPLE PROGRESS NOTE FOR INTAKE SESSION

7-5-20xx
90801

S/O. Ms. Ava Reid is a 26-year-old single White female who works as a waitress at Diner Z and attends community college classes. She lives by herself in an apartment; she has no children. She is tall and thin with straight medium brown hair and has a ring through her right eyebrow.

Ms. R reports a history of chronic depression with poor self-esteem, feelings of guilt, and chronic sadness. She reported that this has worsened within the past month. Now she has difficulty falling asleep because she is ruminating about a failed relationship. She feels tired "all of the time" and has had little appetite. She has lost about 10 pounds without trying and is now markedly thin.

Although she states that she "can't take it anymore," Ms. R has been continuing to go to work and class and has apparently been coping adequately with these responsibilities. She denied any suicidal ideation and also denied ever being suicidal in the past or ever engaging in any suicidal behavior. She denied feelings of hopelessness and has no relatives who committed suicide.

Ms. R has a history of childhood sexual abuse by an older cousin and has had nightmares off and on over the years but in the past year has had only about one per month. She reported that she rarely thinks about the traumatic incidents and has discussed them in therapy before as needed.

Ms. R denies any symptoms of psychosis or mania now or in the past. She denies significant symptoms of anxiety. She denies any past or present violent ideation or behavior.

Ms. R said that she attends Unitarian church on a weekly basis. She has a number of friends from her church group as well as two good friends whom she has relied on for support since she was in high school. She stated that in the past week, she has been talking about her difficulties with her friends and that this has been very helpful to her.

Ms. R stated that she drinks about two times per week when with friends. She consumes between one and three drinks each time.

Ms. R comes from an intact family. Her parents live in a nearby suburb, and she has one younger brother. She characterizes her family relationships as supportive but distant.

Ms. R has been in treatment once in the past and stopped after about 6 months. She stated that she had addressed her history of childhood sexual abuse in those sessions and had stopped because she had been feeling much better.

A. Ms. R is suffering from symptoms of increased depression. She is not at risk for suicidal behavior, as she has no suicidal ideation or intent. She has social supports that she is using well, she states that her involvement with her friends and her church sustains her, and she has no previous history of suicidal behavior or ideation.

P. I talked with Ms. R about the importance of ongoing treatment for chronic depression. She stated that she understood. She accepted appointments next week with a psychiatrist for medication evaluation and a social worker for supportive counseling. Staff will further assess PTSD symptoms as tolerated.

| /signed/ | Fatimah Abdul, B.S.W. |
| /cosigned/ | Nathaniel Wood, L.C.S.W. |

In the heading, the progress note is dated and given a CPT code of 90801, indicative of an initial mental health evaluation session. CPT stands for "current procedural terminology" and indicates what type of health care appointment the client had.

In the first paragraph of the S/O section, the clinician gives basic information about the client's demographics, appearance, and life situation so that future readers of the progress note are oriented to Ms. R. The clinician uses indentations for each paragraph and uses topic sentences that introduce the reader to the content that will be detailed in each paragraph. You can see that the clinician screened for PTSD, depression, mania, substance abuse, and psychosis. The client may need further evaluation to determine whether PTSD is also a current diagnosis since sometimes it is difficult to determine whether a client has sufficient PTSD symptoms for a diagnosis during an intake session. The clinician also briefly described the client's functioning level, which is adequate despite the severity of her depression, and assessed the client's social supports. She briefly described the client's family of origin and will probably need to gather more data on that later.

In the A section, the clinician makes whatever conclusions she can about the client's diagnosis. She clearly documents that the client is not at risk for suicidal behavior at this time.

In the P section, the clinician documents the follow-up plan of ongoing psychotherapy and medication management and the client's agreement with that plan. The clinician clarifies that staff will need to further assess PTSD symptoms in the future as tolerated by the client. As this is an electronic progress note, it is signed electronically.

SAMPLE PROGRESS NOTE FOR PSYCHOTHERAPY

7-1-20xx
90806
S/O. Ms. Njembe came in today feeling very upset. A close friend was concerned that he might have cancer.

Discussion of this issue led to the conclusion that Ms. Njembe can be more concerned about others and not have concern about her own health problems, which include poorly controlled asthma and arthritis pain. She stated that she avoids talking about her problems with others, thinking that they cannot tolerate them and will think negatively of her.

A. Stable but somewhat tearful today. Indicating that she often feels very depressed and anxious under stress, tends to ignore these feelings otherwise.

P. Return for appointment as scheduled next week. Will continue to address self-esteem and mood issues. Ms. Njembe agreed to homework of talking to a different friend about some of her concerns. She agreed to contact the physician referrals I gave her.

| /signed/ | Fatimah Abdul, B.S.W. |
| /cosigned/ | Nathaniel Wood, L.C.S.W. |

This note is similarly formatted to the intake note, although the CPT code of 90806 is for a 45- to 50-minute individual psychotherapy session. Note that the session summary includes significant topics discussed but is brief. The A section consists of an assessment of current emotional functioning today. The P section documents all plans agreed to in the session. Note that the clinician did not include the names of either of Ms. Njembe's friends in the progress note.

WHAT TO DOCUMENT: FULL STORY
OF ATTENDANCE AND TREATMENT

Ahmad Hakim is a mental health trainee. He is managing a very suicidal client, Rachel Nghiem. Lately, Rachel has been missing her sessions. Ahmad diligently calls her after each missed appointment and leaves her a message indicating his concern and when she could come in next. Rachel's attendance continues to be irregular. Then, after two missed sessions, Rachel commits suicide. The institution that Ahmad works for has a formal review of the case. Ahmad had thoroughly documented his outreach efforts with Rachel before her death. Here are the notes that Ahmad wrote:

8-5-20xx
90806

S/O. Ms. N talked at length about her troubled relationship with her son. She stated that her antidepressant medications appeared to be helping her this time. She said that she had no suicidal thoughts over the past week.

A. Less depressed. Her suicidal thoughts have always been passive, and today Ms. N reports that she hasn't had any in the past week.

P. Attend scheduled session next week.

/signed/	Ahmad Hakim, M.S.
	Psychology Practicum Student
/cosigned/	Lydia Strong, Ph.D.
	Licensed Clinical Psychologist

8-12-20xx
No-show
  Ms. N did not show up for her scheduled appointment. I called her home number and left a message asking her to call me. I reminded her to come in for her next session scheduled for 8-19-xx at 2:00 P.M.

/signed/	Ahmad Hakim, M.S.
	Psychology Practicum Student
/cosigned/	Lydia Strong, Ph.D.
	Licensed Clinical Psychologist

8-19-20xx
No-show
  Ms N. again did not attend her scheduled appointment. I called her home number and her cell phone number and left messages expressing my concern and asking her to call me as soon as possible. I reminded her to attend her next session scheduled for 8-25-xx at 2:00 P.M.

/signed/	Ahmad Hakim, M.S.
	Psychology Practicum Student
/cosigned/	Lydia Strong, Ph.D.
	Licensed Clinical Psychologist

The management of the case was found to be appropriate by Ahmad's supervisors and peer reviewers. Later, this documentation in the chart deterred Rachel's relatives from filing a lawsuit for wrongful death against the institution.

Your notes should tell the full story of the client's treatment and attendance, as Ahmad's did in the previous examples (Cameron & turtle-song, 2002). You can see from the notes that Ahmad was aware of Rachel's difficulties with suicidal thoughts and had been monitoring them regularly. He appropriately documented his outreach efforts to this client, whom he knew had some suicide risk.

Beginning therapists are often uncertain what interactions and clinical activities should be documented with progress notes. I have provided a partial list here:

- Psychotherapy sessions
- Cancellations by client (briefly note why, if known)
- Cancellations by therapist
- No-shows
- Outreach phone calls following missed sessions
- Any phone call with significant clinical content
- Some treatment team meetings
- Some consultations between professionals
- Any clinically significant e-mails from the client (print out the e-mail and put it in a paper chart or copy and paste it into an electronic chart)

An example of a phone call or e-mail that need not be documented would be a client asking a routine question such as the time of the next appointment. An example of a phone call or e-mail that *should* be documented is a contact from a client who missed two sessions, states that she has been depressed, and agrees to come in later in the week. Check with your supervisor if you are unsure. It is possible that your supervisor will want you to document every e-mail, whatever the content.

Clinically relevant phone calls are difficult to remember to document since only a tiny percentage of them turn out to have any important clinical signif-icance in the long run. However, we cannot predict in advance which phone call might be the one that it is crucial to document.

Occasionally, there may be other interactions of significance that should be documented that I have not included here. For example, under certain cir-cumstances, a therapist at a Veterans Affairs medical center might attend a benefits hearing for one of her clients. The therapist would then document that this meeting had been attended and why.

WHAT TO DOCUMENT: CLINICAL MANAGEMENT OF TREATMENT-INTERFERING BEHAVIORS

4-23-20xx
90806

S/O. Mr. U attended his appointment for the first time in a month. We re-viewed our initial goals for him to attend weekly psychotherapy sessions. Mr. U. stated that he was having financial and child care problems that were interfering with his ability to attend. We brainstormed about getting some help from his mother. After some discussion, he agreed to ask his mother to babysit every week during his scheduled appointment time. He also said that he knew she would contribute to his transportation costs if he asked her to do so. He verbal-ized his intent to attend on a weekly basis from now on.

A. Mr. U was open to discussing his attendance problems. Stable.

P. Attend scheduled appointment next week. Mr. U agreed to discuss child care and transportation with his mother before then.

/signed/	Ahmad Hakim, M.S.
	Psychology Practicum Student
/cosigned/	Lydia Strong, Ph.D.
	Licensed Clinical Psychologist

6-19-20xx
90806

S/O. Ms. Q and I discussed her difficulties taking her psychotropic medications regularly. I educated her again about how regularly taking her medication will help prevent future manic and depressive episodes and will help keep her out of the hospital. We reviewed several strategies for medication adherence. After a discussion, she agreed to keep them with her toothbrush and take them every morning before she brushed her teeth.

A. Stable.

P. Ms. Q's next appointment is scheduled in 2 weeks. We agreed to check in on her progress with taking her medications regularly then.

/signed/	Arun Singh, M.A.
	Psychology Intern
/cosigned/	Lydia Strong, Ph.D.
	Licensed Clinical Psychologist

Be sure to address treatment-interfering behaviors during the psychotherapy session and in the chart. These behaviors could include lack of attendance and lack of adherence to treatment recommendations. You can't effectively treat a client who doesn't attend appointments or who doesn't take needed medications and is therefore at significant risk of rehospitalization. In these situations, it is incumbent on you to demonstrate in the progress notes that you are making an effort to address these issues so that you can provide an effective treatment. In the previous progress notes, the trainees have helped the clients with problem solving and have documented their efforts.

WHAT TO DOCUMENT: SAFETY AND RISK ISSUES

Christina Jones is a mental health trainee in a community mental health center. Her new client has intense suicidal ideation and is on many psychotropic medications. Some of the medications have a risk of overdose. The treatment team discusses the case and agrees to give medications out on a weekly basis until the client is more stable. Christina documents this discussion in a separate note in the client's chart:

6-25-20xx
Treatment Team Meeting
   Present at today's treatment team meeting were Dr. Gilford, Dr. Victor, Ms. Thomas, and myself. We discussed the client's risk of overdose as well as her need for medications. The team agreed that medications are warranted because of the likelihood that they will help her depression and reduce the risk of suicide in the long term. To reduce short-term risk, Dr. Gilford agreed to prescribe a less toxic medication whenever possible and give medications out on a weekly basis. I will reinforce the suicide prevention plan with the client again at our next meeting.

/signed/	Christina Jones, M.D.
	Psychiatry Resident
/cosigned/	Laura Gilford, M.D.
	Psychiatrist

   Most settings have ways of documenting routine treatment team meetings that mental health trainees do not need to worry about. However, if a therapist's client is exhibiting risky behavior and the team discusses the case and comes to an agreement about it, then the team's assessment and treatment plans should be documented, as in the case of Christina's client.
   Progress notes concerning a crisis situation should be written as soon as possible and definitely should be completed before the clinician leaves to go home for the day. Stay late if you have to. See chapters 18 to 21 for further information on documenting crises.

WHAT TO DOCUMENT: CLIENT'S HOSTILE OR THREATENING BEHAVIOR

Fatimah Abdul, a mental health trainee, is treating a client who has schizophrenia. The client expresses anger and violent ideation toward Muslims. Fatimah is Muslim herself and wears a head scarf. While the client never makes any negative comments about her and is always pleasant toward her personally, she feels threatened by his remarks. She wisely discusses her concerns with her supervisor. After this consultation, she carefully documents all the inappropriate comments that the client made in the last session. She also goes back and makes an addendum to several previous notes on occasions where she remembers his angry remarks but had not documented them. Fatimah and her supervisor do a careful risk assessment of the client. After determining that he has no known history of violent behavior and consulting with the psychiatrist about adjusting his medication to reduce paranoid ideation (which had been increasing in other settings as well), Fatimah decided to continue to see the client for now. However, she and her supervisor decide that, when he is more stable, they are determined to give the client feedback about his inappropriate remarks.

Fatimah is interviewing a different client in the emergency room. The client stands up and begins to yell at her. Fatimah gently asks the client to calm down and asks him to lie back down on the gurney. The client complies with these requests. She carefully documents the behavior in his chart.

If you feel threatened by a client or if the client's behavior or statements are hostile, you should document carefully and thoroughly, as Fatimah has done. This behavior is highly clinically relevant and may be crucial information in evaluating risk factors and stability of the client in the future.

WHAT TO DOCUMENT: CLIENT'S SEXUAL STATEMENTS OR BEHAVIOR

Jared Russell is a mental health trainee treating a female client with borderline personality disorder. At one point in a session, the client stands up and asks, "Should I take off my blouse?" Of course, Jared tells her not to do so. At the end of the session, he carefully documents in her chart exactly what she had said and his response to her. He discusses this issue very carefully with a supervisor and documents the discussion in the chart. During the next session, he carefully explores the client's inappropriate behavior from last time. He emphasizes to her the professional nature and professional boundaries of their relationship. Again, he carefully documents this discussion in the chart.

There is one important exception to the rule to avoid documenting process: document any statements or behavior that suggests that the client has sexual feelings toward you. On rare occasions, clients may make blatant or subtle inappropriate sexual remarks toward you. This behavior should always be documented as well as what you say in response to the client. This documentation must be contemporaneous in case there is ever any question about whether your response was appropriate in the future. Jared also documents the steps he takes to address the client's behavior in supervision and in the next session.

WHAT TO DOCUMENT: YOUR INTERVENTIONS AND RECOMMENDATIONS

1-6-20xx
90806

S/O. Ms. G. admitted to cutting herself with a razor, leaving superficial scratches on her arm, when she was home alone with her 2-month-old baby. I asked her to show me the scratches, which were indeed superficial. She was able to identify a feeling of loneliness and emptiness that triggered the behavior. I suggested that we review some alternative behaviors. However, she refused, stating that this has worked well for her for years and that she had no intentions of changing. After some discussion, she was willing to acknowledge that this behavior could be scary to her baby when the baby was older.

A. There is no evidence that the baby is in any danger; in fact, she verbalizes her desire to take good care of the baby frequently. Ms. G denied any suicidal intent during today's session. She continues to appear depressed, however.

P. We agreed to further discuss the issue next week. Will discuss the issue with the treatment team.

	/signed/	Christina Jones, M.D.
		Psychiatry Resident
	/cosigned/	Laura Gilford, M.D.
		Psychiatrist

1-13-20xx
90806

S/O. I asked Ms. G about cutting again. She admitted to cutting herself with a razor and again showed me superficial scratches on her arm. She was able to identify that feelings of loneliness and emptiness triggered the behavior. She verbalized her desire to stop engaging in cutting, stating, "It's such a bad influence on my daughter." We discussed some alternative behaviors that she could engage in when feeling lonely and empty. These included calling a friend, praying, writing in her journal, and refocusing her attention on her baby. She agreed to attempt these changes and follow up on her progress next week.

A. While Ms. G's cutting is of concern, at this point, the scratches she has made on her arm are superficial, and she denies making any other scratches in other areas of her body. She verbalizes her intent to address the behavior.

P. Attend scheduled appointment next week. Ms. G agreed to try some alternative behaviors and discuss how that went. She agreed that if she does cut, she

will pay attention to her thoughts and feelings at that time so that we can discuss
them further.

/signed/	Christina Jones, M.D.
	Psychiatry Resident
/cosigned/	Laura Gilford, M.D.
	Psychiatrist

While writing a progress note, many therapists do not document any of the
remarks or suggestions that they have made to the client during the session.
This is a mistake. You will often make important interventions and therapeutic recommendations, and these should be documented. In the two previous
notes, Christina documented the attempts that she made to help the client substitute more effective coping strategies for cutting. As Christina does, document when the client agrees with your recommendations and when the client
doesn't. If the client refuses, document how you plan to deal with the refusal
(e.g., in the first session, Christina gets the client to agree to discuss the issue
again next week). Note that Christina also carefully assessed the safety of Ms.
G and her baby as needed.

WHAT *NOT* TO DOCUMENT

Some things should not be documented in the chart. You should avoid including the names of the client's friends or significant others in the chart. If a
client is criticizing another clinician at the facility where you work, this information should not be included in the chart (Cameron & turtle-song, 2002).
Here is an example:

> Wrong: "Mr. R. talked about how he feels that his psychiatrist is 'a mean bitch
> who's out to get me.'"
> Right: "Mr. R. and I discussed how he can communicate more effectively with
> his psychiatrist."

If the client uses curse words, it is unprofessional to use them in the chart.
If you feel it would be illustrative to quote a phrase of the client's when she
uses a curse word, "bleep" it out:

> Right: When I asked Ms K. whether she had taken the medication prescribed by
> her psychiatrist, she stated, "F— — that s— —!"

Finally, do not include information that could be seen as slander toward others in the chart; this could expose you to legal liability (Simon, 2004):

Wrong: "Mr. J. talked about how he suspects that his coworker Joe S. is the one stealing from the till at work. He thinks it may be blamed on him instead."
Right: "Mr. J. talked about his worries regarding allegations that someone had been stealing on the job."

WHEN THERE IS PRIOR MENTAL
HEALTH DOCUMENTATION

A client who is new to you may not be new to your training site. My recommendation is that you review the entire chart of the client at your current facility before seeing the client for the first time. If there is significant information in the chart, you will want to indicate in a progress note that you are aware of this. For example, a new client might have a history of inpatient hospitalization following a suicide attempt at the facility. You will want to indicate your own awareness of this important historical information in your first note. For example, "The client indicated that he had been previously hospitalized at this facility for acute depression. His report of this incident was consistent with the chart documentation."

Alternatively, this client may be new to both you and the site but may have a prior mental health history at other facilities or with other practitioners. In these circumstances, it is incumbent on you to be aware of the content of the previous mental health treatment notes. Get a release from the client during the first session and send a copy of this release to the previous practitioner or facility. Document in the chart that you sent the release. Ignorance of their content is no excuse if you are sued for risk issues (Baerger, 2001).

Unfortunately, some facilities are negligent about responding to requests for information. Give the facility 2 to 3 weeks to respond. Then if you haven't gotten anything, document that in the chart, send another copy of the release, and document that you have done so. Again, if you don't get anything, document that the facility has not responded. Talk to your supervisor and possibly also the site's legal counsel for further advice at this point.

WHEN YOUR CLIENT WANTS
TO READ THE PROGRESS NOTES

Your client may want to read the progress notes you have been writing. Generally, state law and professional association guidelines indicate that the client has a right to read the progress notes (Moline et al., 1998), so agree to let the client read the notes. Before you show the notes to the client, it would be wise to explore in therapy why the client wants to look at the notes. Then suggest that the client read the notes *during* the next scheduled session. Indicate that you recommend this so that you are immediately available to answer any questions as they come up.

Often, clients have unrealistic expectations about their progress notes. After agreeing to let the client look at the notes and providing a structure to do so, this is a good time to explore what the client's worries, ideas, and fantasies are regarding the content of the progress notes. The client may expect that you have written sparkling and brilliant insights. However, if you limit yourself to content rather than process, this will not be the case. Most clients will actually find the progress notes quite boring. Consider warning them ahead of time, "I'm happy to show you the notes, but I have to tell you it will probably be a bunch of facts that you already know." Document that the client has reviewed the notes in the chart, along with any significant statements or affect.

Sometimes the client requests changes in the chart after reading it. You must gently refuse to make changes to the chart (Gutheil & Hilliard, 2001). The chart is a contemporaneous record of what happened in therapy. However, if you think that the client has a valid point about inaccuracies in the chart, you may agree to make an addendum, dated today, to a previous note.

HOW TO DOCUMENT: SENSITIVE ISSUES

Jared Russell, a mental health trainee, is meeting with a long-term client who has PTSD. The client has not been talking to anyone on the treatment team about his traumatic experiences. During this session, the client tells Jared about being sexually abused by his uncle. Then the client asks Jared not to document anything that he has just said in the chart. Jared explains to the client that other clinicians need to know that the client has a history of trauma because they will want to provide a treatment that meets the client's needs. Jared also explains that it is unnecessary to include all the details. He tells the client what he is likely to write: "Mr. R reported that his uncle would fondle him on occasions when his parents were not at home. He cannot remember the frequency of these abusive episodes but stated that they were too frequent to count between the ages of 6 and 10." The client says that this is okay.

Christina Jones, a mental health trainee, is meeting with a new client. The client reveals that her husband drinks to excess and hits her when he is very drunk. She also stated that she is afraid that the husband might some day hit her children, although she states that he hasn't yet. The client then asks Christina not to document any of this information in the chart. Christina says, "I know that you are bringing this up because you are concerned about it. I am concerned as well. Since this issue concerns safety, I am ethically bound to document it. The other people who are working with you need to know about this so that they can help you, too. However, I will be happy to make it clear in the note that I know you are bringing it up because you are concerned about the issue and you are seeking help to work on it. How does that sound?"

Sometimes clients will ask that you not document certain things they tell you in their charts. In some situations, the client may be aware that there is just one chart at the facility that is shared by all the health care practitioners.

Before responding, think about the client's situation carefully. Ask yourself these questions: Is this information a critical piece of historical information that other clinicians should know? Is this information related to suicidality or other potentially risky situations? Is there any other strong reason for this information to be documented? In the first vignette, Jared feels that the information must be documented, but he is sensitive to the client's concerns and reassures the client that his note will be brief. In the other vignette, the client told Christina information that is related to important risk and safety issues. Do not skip charting a safety issue, even if the client requests that you do so.

Often clients will tell us about upsetting experiences from the past, such as childhood abuse, rape, other traumas, or atrocities committed in the military. When they are ready to address these difficult issues, they may tell us considerable detail about the episodes of trauma. Unless there is a pressing reason to do so, it is wise not to include details. Nonetheless, it is often clinically relevant to document that the client did experience this particular trauma. In addition, certain aspects of the trauma might be of clinical relevance, such as the age at which it occurred, how long, and so on. An example might clarify this:

Instead of writing: "Mr. O stated that when the Vietnamese women did not cry enough while being raped, [additional explicit details about Vietnam wartime atrocities]."
You might write: "Mr. O talked about his experiences seeing Vietnam War atrocities."

At other times, the issue at hand is embarrassing to the client but has no major bearing on any risk issues or other aspects of the treatment. In those cases, it is fine to either record the issue in vague generalizations (Gutheil & Hilliard, 2001) or, if it is more embarrassing than clinically relevant, to even skip documenting the issue.

HOW TO RELEASE RECORDS

In most circumstances, you must have a valid signed release of information to release chart materials. Then check with your supervisor before you release any records. Do not release more than is asked for. If you have some concerns about how the release of these records might impact the client, discuss this with the client before records are released. The client has the right to revoke the release at any time.

In general, you should not release information that you have obtained from other facilities or practitioners; they should be contacted directly for their chart material on the client. In certain instances, you can refuse to provide records if you consider this detrimental to the client (Moline et al., 1998); however, if you have followed the guidelines for writing progress notes provided in this chapter, you are unlikely to be faced with this possibility.

On rare occasions, information can be released without a written release from the client. These situations were discussed in the "Confidentiality" section of chapter 7.

ENSURE SECURITY OF CLIENT INFORMATION

DoD [Department of Defense] Personnel Info Part of VA [Veterans Affairs] Data Theft. As the investigation into the stolen Department of Veterans Affairs (VA) data continues, the full extent and ramification of the theft has grown. It was learned last month that, aside from the information of approximately 26 million veterans contained on the laptop and external hard drive stolen from a VA employee's home, the personal information of 2.2 million military personnel was included, as well. And, while law enforcement agencies have stated that the theft was a simple burglary and that the computer equipment was likely erased and resold before its contents were ever made public, government overseers say that such a theft could easily happen again. (Spotswood, 2006)

The security of client information must be guarded at all times. Do not take written or electronic records home. They must remain on-site at all times. The true incident in the previous quote regarding VA and DoD records illustrates why. You cannot vouch for the security of records off-site.

ENSURE APPROPRIATE DISPOSAL
OF CLIENT INFORMATION

Hundreds of Patient Records Found in Pharmacy Dumpster. Drugstores are not supposed to put your personal health information into open dumpsters. But 13 Investigates [Indianapolis television station WTHR] has shown it happening at pharmacy after pharmacy as drug stores all across Indianapolis failed our recent test. Store workers admit if even one patient record gets into the trash, that's one too many. But what we discovered in just one trash bag this week surprised even us. It didn't contain just one patient record—it had 732 of them. That's right—732 patient records on labels, receipts, prescriptions, order forms and pill bottles, all in one garbage bag behind one pharmacy. (Segall, 2006)

Occasionally, we have client information that needs to be disposed of. Here are some examples:

• Fax cover sheet with name of patient, accompanying release, or other document
• Extra copies of chart notes (perhaps printed out from electronic chart to fax in response to a release of information)
• Written phone message to call client
• Brief jotted notes as a reminder of what to document, which are now unnecessary since you completed the progress note

This information must be shredded. Do not ever throw it in a trash bin unshredded. You might put the privacy and safety of your clients at risk. The investigation into pharmacy privacy that was cited previously began when the station found out that thieves had masqueraded as pharmacy employees to get an elderly woman's Oxycontin (Tucker, 2006). The thieves had found her prescription information in the pharmacy trash bin.

HIPAA AND PROGRESS NOTES

Throughout this chapter, I have been discussing how mental heath charting is traditionally done. However, there is another option described by the HIPAA Privacy Rule. It is possible to keep very sketchy notes in the clinical record and also keep more extensive progress notes (called "psychotherapy notes" by HIPAA) that contain more detailed and personal information in a separate location.

The HIPAA Privacy Rule allows these "psychotherapy notes" to have special privacy protections when they are kept separate from the rest of the clinical record. "Psychotherapy notes" are defined as follows: "notes recorded (in any medium) by a health-care practitioner, who is a mental health professional documenting or analyzing the contents of conversation during a private counseling session or a group, joint, or family counseling session and that are separated from the rest of the individual's medical record." Psychotherapy notes exclude "medication prescription and monitoring, counseling sessions start and stop times, the modalities and frequencies of treatment furnished, results of clinical tests and any summary of the following items: diagnosis, functional status, the treatment plan, symptoms, prognosis and progress to date," so this would be the information that would be in the general medical record (American Psychological Association Practice Organization, 2007, p. 8).

As Brendel and Bryan (2004) indicate, what HIPAA refers to as "psychotherapy notes" are essentially what most therapists would call "process notes." As I'm sure you've noticed, I have been advising you throughout this chapter not to document process issues in the chart anyway. When you reread the progress note before a session, the content will remind you of the process issues sufficiently so that you do not need process notes. I recommend that you try to do without them, unless your supervisor wants you to keep process notes as a teaching tool.

Apparently, the main point of this aspect of the HIPAA Privacy Rule was to bar insurance companies from having access to process notes on clients *if* we keep them separate from the rest of the chart. Ask your supervisor whether these kinds of notes are kept separate from the rest of the clinical record at your facility.

There are many valid clinical reasons why you would *not* want to separate your progress notes into these two categories (as allowed by HIPAA) and instead keep just content notes in the one and only clinical record, as I have advised in this chapter. First, the "psychotherapy notes" or process notes can be subpoenaed (Brendel & Bryan, 2004), and most clinicians would not like to have their notes on the therapeutic process scrutinized in court; if these notes do not exist, they cannot be subpoenaed. Given the collaborative nature of much mental health treatment, it is often clinically useful to have important psychotherapy information available to other mental health practitioners at the same facility; critical information could be lost by keeping separate process notes. In addition, the facility may have an EMR system that does not allow two separate sets of notes. As trainees come and go and certain clients come and go as well, it can be helpful for later treatment practitioners to have a more complete record of the client's past psychotherapy. Finally, important issues such as risk management must be thoroughly documented in the clinical record anyway.

TREATMENT PLANS

Mental health professionals in medical centers and clinics and those working with certain managed care organizations are required to produce written treatment plans. Interestingly, physicians in other health specialty areas rarely have to produce any treatment plans (V. Nee, personal communication, February 23, 2007).

The format of treatment plans varies according to requirements of the site and the managed care organization (Zuckerman, 2003). However, in general, treatment plans typically include the following:

- *Diagnostic and Statistical Manual of Mental Disorders* diagnosis, usually all five axes

- Behavioral description of symptoms and/or behaviors that are targets of treatment
- "Objectives," meaning shorter-term goals, again as behaviorally described as possible
- "Goals," meaning longer-term goals
- Target dates or number of sessions for accomplishment of objectives and goals
- Interventions and treatments that will be employed
- Who is responsible for implementing each intervention/treatment
- Referrals made and adjunctive treatments employed

Your supervisor can show you some examples of treatment plans made according to the format and requirements of your site.

RECOMMENDED READING

Cameron, S., & turtle-song, i. (2002). Learning to write case notes using the SOAP format. *Journal of Counseling and Development, 80*, 286–292.
A short and helpful article about how to write appropriate progress notes.
Gutheil, T. G. (1980). Paranoia and progress notes: A guide to forensically informed psychiatric record-keeping. *Hospital and Community Psychiatry, 31*, 479–482.
Despite its age, this classic article provides timeless, wise, and succinct advice about writing progress notes.
Moline, M. E., Williams, G. T., & Austin, K. M. (1998). *Documenting psychotherapy: Essentials for mental health practitioners.* Thousand Oaks, CA: Sage.
The authors provide a thorough discussion of documentation issues, including why good documentation is essential, what belongs in a clinical record, documenting crises, and other topics.

EXERCISES AND DISCUSSION QUESTIONS

1. Your client reveals that she has been taking money and drugs for sex, then asks you not to document this in her chart. Would you document it? Why or why not? What would you tell the client?
2. Your client states about his wife, "I could just kill her sometimes, I'm so angry." The client then asks you not to document this in the chart: "My psychiatrist will think I'm crazy if you write that in there." Your client has denied any history of violent behavior, and you think he wasn't literally that angry—he was just being dramatic. Would you document it? Why or why not? What would you tell the client?
3. Write progress notes for the clients in the two vignettes in chapter 12.

Chapter Fourteen

Starting Psychotherapy

Depending on the complexity of the client, you may need one session, two sessions, or even parts of the third session to fully evaluate the social history and symptoms and to make referrals that are needed. In this chapter, I am referring to the sessions that follow your evaluation in which psychotherapy really starts taking place. Instead of teaching you to *do* psychotherapy, which encompasses many hundreds of books, my goal is to help you think about how to *prioritize and structure* the early psychotherapy sessions. At the end of this chapter is a list of helpful books to further your journey on the path of learning about doing psychotherapy.

HIERARCHY OF PSYCHOTHERAPY ISSUES

Beginning psychotherapists often work in settings, such as community mental health, where the clients are very complex. The sheer number of problems and diagnoses for just one client can be overwhelming. In this section, I provide a hierarchy of psychotherapy issues to help you determine where to start treatment with these very complex clients. Start at the top of the hierarchy and work your way down. In general, you should not address lower-ranked issues until the higher-ranked issues are resolved or have already been addressed sufficiently earlier in the session. I have modified and added to Linehan's (1993) treatment hierarchy to address the needs of a general client population (which is also informed by Courtois, 1997). Italicized sections are addressed in this chapter:

1. Address immediate threats
   - Immediate threats of bodily harm to self or others, such as active suicidality, homicidality, and physical abuse of significant others (chapters 18–21)

2. Ensure regular attendance (chapter 3) and attend to the *therapeutic al-liance*
3. Start therapy
   * *Set goals for therapy*
   * *Psychoeducation* about diagnosis and course of treatment
4. Stabilize and reduce distress: make referrals for needed adjunctive treatments and address behaviors with high risk of negative consequences
   * Referrals for psychotropic medication and other treatments (chapters 15 and 17)
   * Referrals to stabilize client's situation, such as health-related referrals (chapter 16), housing, income, legal, treatment for family members, and so on
   * Treat and/or refer for substance abuse or dependence (chapter 17)
   * Reduce self-harm and suicidal gestures (chapter 19)
   * *Reduce high-risk dysfunctional behavior*
5. *Increase behavioral skills*, such as the following:
   * *Behavioral interventions: improve sleep and relaxation training*
   * *Normalize activity level and socialization*
   * *Encourage client-initiated activities, such as self-help, exercise, or meditation*
6. Psychotherapy focused on other present-day difficulties
7. Psychotherapy focused on past issues as needed

Like any hierarchy, this will not work for every client in every situation. At times, items lower on the hierarchy will need to be addressed first or simultaneously. However, this should give you a rough idea of how to prioritize treatment topics when many complex issues are present.

FOSTER THE THERAPEUTIC ALLIANCE

The therapeutic alliance refers to the bond and the quality of the relationship between the therapist and client, which includes agreement on the goals and tasks of therapy (Crits-Cristoph, Gibbons, & Hearon, 2006). Multiple studies have confirmed that better therapeutic alliances lead to more improvement in therapy (Crits-Cristoph et al., 2006). How does one foster a good therapeutic alliance? Clearly, the active listening skills you have learned in other course work are essential. Personal characteristics such as warmth and genuineness clearly contribute to the therapeutic alliance (Bachelor, 1995). But for now, the scientific literature does not have definitive further answers to this question. However, some experts provide us with useful advice in this matter.

Sue and Zane (1987) talk about *giving*, using interventions early in therapy that help the client achieve significant gains. All clients benefit from your efforts to stabilize them and alleviate distress early in therapy. This will build your credibility as a therapist, demonstrate your concern and attention to the client's distress, and help foster the therapeutic alliance.

J. S. Beck (2005) talks about the importance of a therapeutic attitude of hopefulness: "Patients generally respond positively when their therapist maintains a consistently upbeat attitude about the probability that therapy will help" (p. 66). However, she points out that this must be done in the context of a relationship in which the client feels understood so that the client does not feel that you are being unrealistic. Often, you can integrate your psychoeducation of the client (see later section in this chapter) with verbalizing your expectation that the client has an excellent chance of recovery.

It is okay and, in fact, quite therapeutic to be soothing to your client (Gabbard & Westen, 2003). Being soothing can simply mean that you are accepting of the client. You can soothe by maintaining a calm attitude in the face of the client's emotional storms. You can also be soothing by your attitude, interventions, and problem solving that show that the client's distress can be alleviated. Psychodynamic theory suggests that the client will start to internalize some of your reactions toward him or her (e.g., being accepting of self) in substitution for those the client already has (e.g., being hypercritical of self).

WHEN YOU NEED TO SET THE
AGENDA FOR PSYCHOTHERAPY

Amelia Peterson is a 35-year-old woman in individual therapy. Amelia has a history of multiple suicide attempts and chronic suicidal thoughts. Her diagnoses are borderline personality disorder, panic disorder, recurrent major depression, and post-traumatic stress disorder (PTSD). Currently, Amelia is living with a new boyfriend who is verbally abusive. When the boyfriend is abusive, Amelia's suicidal thoughts return, and she scratches herself with a razor blade. Amelia's therapist has left the agency, and she is assigned to a new psychotherapy trainee, Daniel Cox. Daniel has reviewed the chart carefully, and he is aware of her risk factors. During the first session, Daniel assesses Amelia's current level of symptoms. Amelia has not been actively suicidal for about 6 months, but she has passive suicidal ideation on at least a weekly basis. She usually scratches herself at least twice a month. Her depressive and panic symptoms are not well controlled by her medications, so Daniel consults with the psychiatrist, Dr. Torres, between sessions. At the beginning of the second session, after asking Amelia how she has been doing,

Daniel states, "Amelia, I'm very concerned about how you have been doing, and I'd like us to do everything we can to help you feel better. I'm especially concerned about your suicidal thoughts since I can't help you with your other issues if you're not alive. Can we start our therapy by focusing on these thoughts? I want to know when you are most likely to be thinking suicidal thoughts, what feelings you are having then, and so on."

There are specific situations when you must set the agenda for the psychotherapy session and other situations in which it is best for the client to do so. If you have a client who is unstable, low functioning, and/or high risk, these are situations in which you must set the therapy agenda. When there are immediate threats, such as active suicidality, intent to hurt others, or child abuse, you are ethically and legally required to take action to prevent harm to the client and others. In these cases, you must take charge. You need to be sure that psychotherapy is started and maintained appropriately, and you need to take the lead in stabilizing the client and referring to appropriate adjunctive treatments.

Ensure at the beginning of the session that you have checked in with the client to see how he or she is doing this week. If there is a crisis, this may need to be addressed first.

SET GOALS FOR THERAPY

Client: "My daughter is driving me crazy. She's only 3 years old, but the tantrums she has in stores are humiliating. When she behaves that way, I feel that I'm the worst mother in the world, and I think about suicide all over again."

Therapist: "I can see that your daughter's tantrums are very upsetting to you. You're also concerned about her, and you know that, for her own good, her behavior needs to improve. It sounds like you haven't been able to figure out how to get her to stop. I'd be happy to help you with that. This is a very solvable problem, and I believe that we can figure out to improve her behavior if we work together on it. So one of our goals is to improve your daughter's behavior and get her to stop having tantrums."

Client: "Yes, absolutely."

Therapist: "Lots of parents have this problem, and it is wise of you to seek help before she gets any older. I think we also need to explore why you are so negative about yourself, calling yourself 'a bad mother,' even though here you are asking for help with this problem, which is doing exactly what you need to do about it."

Client: "Yes, I'm very hard on myself. I've always said that I'm my own worst critic."

Therapist: "We also need to work on your suicidal thoughts. You know, I'm wondering whether, in this situation, these thoughts may mean that you feel out of control and helpless in the situation. Is that right?"

Client: "Yes, I have no idea what to do, and I think I'm never going to get it right. It's an awful feeling."

Therapist: "So I'm thinking that maybe if we can help you figure out some things you can do to calm down when you are distressed, it might help you feel more in control and less suicidal."

A patient who says her goal is a satisfying romantic relationship leading to marriage has every right to seek that in life. However, the therapist can't realistically promise that she will find a suitable partner and end up happily married following therapy. The therapist can, however, offer the possibility of exploring the patient's conflicts about intimacy, her inhibitions about giving herself fully to another person, and any problematic relational styles that might interfere with her romantic pursuit. (Gabbard, 2000a, p. 82)

When therapy starts, you will want to help the client translate the presenting problem(s) into goals for therapy. Questions such as these can help focus the client (J. S. Beck, 1995, pp. 31–32):

"Can you tell me specifically what problems you've been having?"
"What would you like to accomplish in therapy?"
"How would you like your life to be different?"

The client provides information on what her problems are, you use your knowledge and expertise at treating these problems, and together you and the client can arrive at a formulation of the treatment goals. In the previous vignette, the therapist uses the client's statement about her daughter to help formulate three goals of treatment: eliminate her daughter's tantrums, address negative self-talk, and improve client's coping with emotional distress. As Gabbard (2000a) indicates in the previous quote, your conceptualization of the goals for therapy may differ somewhat from the client's life goals that bring her to therapy.

PSYCHOEDUCATION

Client: "All my family says I'm crazy, and sometimes I feel like I am, too. I can't concentrate and I can't hold a job."

Therapist: [after thoroughly evaluating client] "I can see that you have been suffering from a combination of depression and attention deficit disorder and that this has had quite a negative impact on your life."

Client: "Is there anything that can be done for me?"

Therapist: "Absolutely! Both of these conditions can be treated, and if you stick with treatment, I don't see any reason why you can't be feeling significantly better soon. Let me fill you in some more about how we usually help people with these kinds of problems."

Many clients do not have a framework for conceptualizing their difficulties, although they are aware that there is a problem. As you talk to the client, you will gain an understanding of the client's difficulties, and if the client has a mental illness, you will be able to identify it. Surprisingly, even clients who been in treatment for years may be unable to identify what their mental illness is and how it is effectively treated.

Effective psychoeducation will inform the client (a) about what diagnoses the client has and why you think the client has that diagnosis, (b) different treatment options that can be effective, and (c) your recommendations for treatment—taking into account the client's feedback about options. After effective psychoeducation, the client will usually feel understood, reassured, and more hopeful about the future.

Often clients with *serious mental illness* (often defined as schizophrenia, bipolar disorder, and schizoaffective disorder although sometimes more broadly) have a limited understanding of their situation. However, research has shown that when clients with serious mental illness have insight, they can work collaboratively with their caregivers and have a better treatment outcome (Rusch & Corrigan, 2002). Assess the client's level of insight by asking some simple questions, such as "What is your diagnosis? What have doctors said is your diagnosis when you were in the hospital? Do you know what that means? Tell me what you know about it. Do you believe that the voices are real? Do you think that people are really out to get you?" These types of responses are common:

Client 1: "They say that I have schizophrenia, but I have only one personality." (In this case, you would want to explain what schizophrenia really is and get the client to articulate whether he has the symptoms.)

Client 2: "They say I'm manic depressive, but I feel fine without my medications, and I don't think I need them. I've gone for months, and I've been fine." (In this case, you would want to explain that most people with bipolar disorder have only one or two mood episodes per year and feel just like everyone else most of the time.)

As you can see from these examples, clients can have a very poor understanding of their mental illnesses. Psychoeducation can go a long way in improving treatment adherence, symptomatology, emotional functioning, and outcome (Lukens & McFarlane, 2004).

REDUCE HIGH-RISK DYSFUNCTIONAL BEHAVIOR

Clients may be engaging in a multitude of high-risk behaviors that threaten to interfere with emotional and physical health. These include the following (modified from Linehan, 1993):

- High-risk or unprotected sexual behavior
- Excessive spending
- Gambling
- Poor financial management (such as unpaid bills, poor budgeting, or not following through to get disability checks)
- Criminal behavior (such as shoplifting or embezzling)
- Staying with abusive partner
- Dysfunctional employment-related behavior (such as quitting suddenly, getting fired, or not looking for a job when unemployed)
- Dysfunctional school-related behavior (such as not going to class or not studying)
- Poor management of physical illness (such as not taking medications, avoiding seeing doctors, or refusing to treat physical illness)
- Housing-related problems (such as inappropriate or unstable living environments or dysfunctional or abusive roommates)
- Inadequate concern for personal safety (such as going to crack houses or walking in dark alleys at night)

Psychotherapy about other life problems is often futile in the presence of these destabilizing behaviors. The client will not be able to achieve emotional stability with these chaotic, dysfunctional problems. Help the client problem-solve and refer the client to appropriate community resources to address these problems. A motivational interviewing approach can be helpful in assisting the client to gain motivation for change (W. R. Miller & Rollnick, 2002).

INCREASE BEHAVIORAL SKILLS

Therapist: "It sounds as if you have been drinking a lot of coffee throughout the day and that your sleep has not been restful. I would suggest that you try not to drink any caffeinated beverages after 12:00 noon. Also, I'd suggest

that you try to keep the amount of coffee to no more than two cups in the
morning. Would you be open to making that change? Let me know next week
how your sleep is between now and then."

Increasing behavioral skills entails working collaboratively with the client.
The client will indicate what symptoms are of concern, and you will provide
guidance to him about how to effectively address these symptoms. Then the
two of you will work out an individualized behavioral plan. The previous vignette illustrates a simple behavioral intervention to help a client's sleep
when the client has been drinking coffee in the late afternoon; the half-life of
caffeine is about 6 hours for a healthy adult (Statland & Demas, 1980) but can
be much greater, depending on the health status and age of the individual.
Since it is such a common issue, guidance on improving clients' sleep hygiene has been supplied for you in appendix 18.

Relaxation training is another effective behavioral intervention that can be
learned relatively quickly by the clinician (see Bernstein, Borkovec, & Hazlett-
Stevens, 2000). Relaxation training can help reduce chronic pain and anxiety
(Symreng & Fishman, 2004) and anger (Deffenbacher, Oetting, & DiGiuseppe,
2002).

NORMALIZE ACTIVITY LEVEL AND SOCIALIZATION

Scott Mladnik is a psychotherapy trainee at a large mental health clinic. A new
client, Antoine Bryant, calls in a crisis, and Scott tells Antoine to come in later
that day. Antoine has been depressed for 2 weeks and has been lying in bed all
day ruminating about his problems. He has been calling in sick and telling
everyone that he threw out his back. He hasn't been returning anyone's calls. Fi-
nally, he realized that something was wrong and called for help. Scott assesses
Antoine for a history of manic symptoms as part of his routine assessment and
finds that Antoine had a manic episode earlier this year. He has never been di-
agnosed with bipolar disorder before. Antoine is referred for medications imme-
diately. Scott educates Antoine about bipolar disorder and recovery from de-
pression. He urges him to go back to work and to call his family members and
friends, who have been leaving him frantic messages. Antoine does these things,
even though they are very difficult. Two weeks later, Antoine is much better. His
medications are helping, he is back at work, and he has told everyone what hap-
pened. He is surprised at how supportive everyone has been. Therapy then fo-
cuses on understanding bipolar disorder and accepting the diagnosis.

When people are feeling depressed, they tend to behave as Antoine does in the
previous vignette. They withdraw from their family and friends. They don't

tell anyone about what they are going through. They avoid their coworkers and may even be missing work. They stop going to their religious group, their book group, their bowling league, or any other group function. Often they think that they are not feeling up to engaging in these activities. Or they may be thinking that they need to rest and that resting will help them feel better and be able to cope eventually. *This is not true.* In actuality, continued social isolation and withdrawal increases the risk of long-term social and vocational disability (Kawachi & Berkman, 2001). In addition, the client is avoiding the very things that will improve mood: the support of friends and family, enjoying the company of others, spiritual sustenance, feeling productive, being distracted from her problems for a while, and maybe even having a little fun.

Behavioral activation "emphasizes structured attempts at engendering increases in overt behaviors that are likely to bring the patient into contact with reinforcing environmental contingencies and produce corresponding improvements in thoughts, mood, and overall quality of life" (Hopko, Lejuez, Ruggiero, & Eifert, 2003, p. 700). In other words, one early goal of therapy, especially with depressed clients, can be to help the client normalize social and vocational functioning as well as personal activities as soon as possible. The focus is to help the client accomplish behavioral goals *even when feeling depressed.* This normalization will lead to feeling better emotionally, thinking more positive thoughts and fewer negative thoughts, and having an improved quality of life. This type of treatment has been found to be as effective for treatment of depression as cognitive-behavioral therapy in a meta-analysis (Cuijpers, van Straten, & Warmerdam, 2007).

Help the client brainstorm about how to cope with returning to work (e.g., how to leave early if necessary or whether it would be helpful for you to supply a letter for the Human Resources Department if any accommodations are needed). Help the client brainstorm about some goals for the next week that improve socialization and support (Client: "Okay, this week, I'll call my best friend in Arizona and tell her how I've been feeling, and I'll go over to my sister's house and visit with her and my niece, then Saturday I'll go to the synagogue with Mom"). Help the client brainstorm about adding some enjoyable activities into her schedule (Client: "This week, I will spend half an hour doing watercolors, even if I don't feel very inspired, and I'll make an appointment for a massage").

After the client does these things, ask how it went. Sometimes clients will complain that they didn't feel any better afterward. Then your next question should be, "Did you feel any better *while* you were [doing the activity]?" Generally the client will say yes, providing you an opportunity to point out that it is helpful to have had that time when she did feel better because if she hadn't engaged in the activity, she probably wouldn't have felt very good during that time period. Knowing what helps the client feel better provides an opportunity to change her schedule and activities to feel better more often, which will eventually help overall mood and functioning.

A rapid return to previous level of activities is likely to be most effective with clients such as Antoine, who very recently had a high-functioning level. Clients who are low functioning will need to work on these issues steadily over time.

ENCOURAGE APPROPRIATE CLIENT-INITIATED ACTIVITIES

With your input or on their own, clients often like to take the initiative to start activities that contribute positively to their mental health. Research suggests that these activities can be particularly helpful: self-help groups and books, exercise, and meditation.

Extending your client's psychoeducation and treatment through books and film can be helpful for certain clients. See Norcross (2006) for helpful lists of the following: top-rated self-help books, top-rated self-help autobiographies, and top-rated self-help films.

Your client may be interested in attending self-help groups. There are traditional substance-related self-help groups, such as Al-Anon and Alcoholics Anonymous (and others like these, such as Cocaine Anonymous and Narcotics Anonymous). Other self-help groups for various other personal problems exist as well. As a whole, research has found self-help groups to be an effective adjunct to individual therapy (Norcross, 2006). However, carefully ask your client about any self-help groups attended because, on rare occasions, some of them can be counterproductive to treatment (e.g., a group for "survivors of Satanic abuse" or an online group where individuals write at length about how much they appreciate cutting themselves).

Exercise has been shown to have antidepressant effects (DiLorenzo et al., 1999; Fox, 1999) and may be helpful with anxiety disorders as well (Fox, 1999; Lancer, Motta, & Lancer, 2007). Exercise may help increase the client's resilience to stress (Salmon, 2003). Exercise may be particularly beneficial for clients with symptoms of fatigue or low energy (Puetz, O'Connor, & Dishman, 2006). Generally, cardiovascular exercise has been studied in this research. However, the possible benefits of yoga have been studied as well; yoga involves both exercise and mindfulness components. Despite methodological inadequacies, a number of studies suggested that yoga could be helpful with anxiety disorders, especially obsessive-compulsive disorder (Kirkwood, Rampes, Tuffrey, Richardson, & Pilkington, 2005). A trauma expert also suggests yoga for alleviating anxiety in PTSD clients (van der Kolk, 2002).

Research to date suggests that regular meditation can have emotional, physical, and cognitive benefits, similar to but somewhat different from those from relaxation training (Davidson et al., 2003; Jain et al., 2007; Ramel, Goldin, Carmona, & McQuaid, 2004). Depressed or anxious clients who ruminate may be especially good candidates for trying meditation (Jain et al., 2007; Ramel et al., 2004). If you meditate regularly or you have in the past, you may be able to teach it to your client. If you do not meditate yourself, do not attempt to teach it; instead, refer the client to community resources.

Some "alternative" treatments are ineffective at best and harmful to the client at worst. A licensed mental health practitioner should not provide or recommend these treatments. If needed, you may want to educate the client about their lack of empirical support. See appendix 19 for a partial listing of "treatments" to avoid. In addition, the licensed practitioner should be aware of the scientific reasons that certain "alternative" practices may seem to work but remain unproven (see Beyerstein, 1997, which is readily available online).

LETTING THE CLIENT SET THE
AGENDA FOR PSYCHOTHERAPY

In their work with stable and high-functioning clients, many therapists prefer to let the client set the agenda for the psychotherapy session. When the client sets the agenda, he or she will generally choose an issue that that is particularly salient that week, giving you an opportunity to explore continuing themes—such as anxiety, anger, or self-esteem—in light of that issue.

Some therapists start each session with whatever question or comment feels right at the time; others use a standard opening line. Here are some opening lines (*Independent Practitioner*, 2007, p. 22, and various personal communications):

"What brings you here today?"
"What seems important today?"
"Let's talk about what's on your mind."
"So, how are things going?"
"Well, where do we pick it up?"
"What problems can I help you solve today?"

At times, you and the client may have closed the prior session by noting that you had more to discuss regarding a topic, or you might have realized that there was a related topic that you didn't have time for. In those cases, I might open with something like this:

"So, last time you said that you were bothered by how you were getting along with your coworkers, but we didn't have time to discuss that. I'm wondering if you'd like to discuss that or something else today?"

EDUCATE YOURSELF ABOUT PSYCHOTHERAPY

Many beginning therapists, paradoxically, have been thoroughly educated yet feel unready to start seeing clients in psychotherapy. You have learned a lot in graduate school. Yet for true psychotherapeutic competence, even more knowledge and reading is essential above and beyond what is provided in school. What you have learned so far has provided you with the tools you need to understand and put into context what you learn from now on.

Often, beginning therapists complain that they know a lot about theory but have no idea how to apply it. Books are often the best resources at this stage, as they often start at a more basic level than journal articles and can provide a comprehensive treatment description. The list of recommended readings at the end of this chapter provides you several suggestions of very readable books to get you started. Integrative approaches are becoming more important. Because of that, I have recommended books that illustrate a variety of approaches. These readings will help provide you with the cognitive framework that you need to be an effective psychotherapist.

EDUCATE YOURSELF ON THE MOST
RECENT UPDATES AND SPECIAL ISSUES

Stephanie Long is a mental health student who has a new client with chronic migraine headaches and major depression. The client states that he would rather not take medications for the headaches since he already has a multitude of complex medical issues and a complicated dosing schedule. Stephanie tells the client that she will research the issue. Looking through journal articles, with the assistance of PsychInfo and Google Scholar, she finds that thermal biofeedback has some supporting evidence for treating migraines. She networks with colleagues and finds a health psychologist at a local medical center who is trained in administering thermal biofeedback. Next time she sees the client, she refers him to the health psychologist for adjunctive treatment. They continue to discuss the client's major depression as well as the emotional issues that sometimes trigger his migraine headaches.

While books are essential for learning about basics of psychotherapy practice, journal articles can be helpful for learning about the most recent updates and research as well as specialized topics, such as the one researched by Stephanie in the previous vignette. Of course, the professional literature is vast, so some suggestions about how to find information may be helpful. A combination of Google Scholar and PsychInfo often yields good search results. Many of the articles can be easily obtained online through your university. Note that this search strategy will probably overrepresent cognitive-behavioral and pharmacological interventions, as these have had the greatest amount of scientific research. If you want to review how another theoretical orientation approaches the disorder, it often works to search using the name of the orientation (e.g., *psychodynamic*) with the disorder (e.g., *panic disorder*) or to look for a book on the topic instead. To be able to put what you learn from the research literature in an appropriate context, it is helpful to be knowledgeable about the empirically supported treatments debate (for an introduction, see the American Psychological Association Presidential Task Force on Evidence-Based Practice, 2006).

RECOMMENDED READING

Kawachi, I., & Berkman, L. F. (2001). Social ties and mental health. *Journal of Urban Health: Bulletin of the New York Academy of Medicine, 78,* 458–467.
  This article provides a helpful overview of the relationship between socialization and mental health.
Lukens, E. P., & McFarlane, W. R. (2004). Psychoeducation as evidence-based practice: Considerations for practice, research, and policy. *Brief Treatment and Crisis Intervention, 4,* 205–225.
  This article provides a useful review of the evidence for psychoeducation as an effective treatment modality.
Norcross, J. C. (2006). Integrating self-help into psychotherapy: 16 practice suggestions. *Professional Psychology: Research and Practice, 37,* 683–693.
  Norcross provides a helpful review of how mental health professionals and clients can use various modalities of self-help (books, films, groups, and the Internet) to further treatment.

HELPFUL BOOKS ABOUT DOING PSYCHOTHERAPY

Beck, J. S. (1995). *Cognitive therapy: Basics and beyond.* New York: Guilford Press.
  This book provides a helpful description of the therapeutic process in cognitive therapy.
Beck, J. S. (2005). *Cognitive therapy for challenging problems: What to do when the basics don't work.* New York: Guilford Press.
  Judith Beck extends the reach of cognitive therapy in this helpful volume.
Epstein, M. (1998). *Going to pieces without falling apart: A Buddhist perspective on wholeness.* New York: Broadway Books.
  Eastern philosophy has made a powerful impact on the practice and theory of mental health in the past two decades. This very readable volume introduces important concepts.

Gabbard, G. O. (2004). *Long-term psychodynamic psychotherapy: A basic text.* Arlington, VA: American Psychiatric Publishing.

This book is written specifically for the beginning psychotherapist. Important modern principles of psychodynamic psychotherapy are outlined remarkably clearly in this text, along with ample references to research literature. Highly recommended.

McWilliams, N. (2004). *Psychoanalytic psychotherapy: A practitioner's guide.* New York: Guilford Press.

Dr. McWilliams writes about complex psychotherapeutic issues in highly accessible prose. Her advice is highly practical and down-to-earth.

Miller, W. R., & Rollnick, S. (2002). *Motivational interviewing: Preparing people for change* (2nd ed.). New York: Guilford Press.

If you read one thing about working with substance-abusing clients, read this book. This book provides helpful guidance in establishing rapport and an effective treatment alliance with this difficult population, and the lessons are applicable to any client with ambivalence about change.

WEB RESOURCES

http://scholar.google.com

As of this writing, this is a beta version of Google Scholar. It picks up different things than other professional literature search engines, so is a valuable adjunct.

http://www.nami.org

This website for the National Alliance on Mental Illness provides reliable information on mental illness.

http://www.ncptsd.org

This is the website for the National Center for PTSD, part of Veterans Affairs. This excellent website provides useful information about PTSD for both clients and clinicians.

http://www.nimh.nih.gov

This website for the National Institute of Mental Health (part of the U.S. government) provides reliable information on a multitude of mental illnesses.

http://mentalhelp.net/selfhelp

This website provides client referrals to all sorts of self-help groups by type of problem.

EXERCISES AND DISCUSSION QUESTIONS

1. What interventions might you use for each of the high-risk dysfunctional behaviors listed in this chapter? If you don't know what interventions to use, how would you find out?
2. Think about the types of problems that clients at your training site often have. Make a list of psychoeducational materials (websites, books, and brochures—many can be found online) that would be particularly helpful with your client population.

Section III

REFERRALS

Chapter Fifteen

Psychotropic Medication Referrals and Adherence

This one chapter is insufficient to describe all the psychotropic medications available today and their uses, side effects, and so on. Instead, I will focus on how psychotropics can help the symptoms of your clients and when a referral for psychotropics should be made. Web resources are listed at the end of this chapter to help you learn more about classes of psychotropics and individual medications.

As of this writing, psychotropic medications can be prescribed by psychiatrists, other physicians, and master's level nurses. Psychiatrists have intensive advanced training in prescribing psychotropic medication for clients with mental illness. However, primary care physicians also often prescribe psychotropics as well. There is also a movement to allow psychologists with advanced training to prescribe psychotropic medications, which is controversial even within clinical psychology itself (Robiner et al., 2002), although it is supported by the American Psychological Association. However, generally, psychiatrists will be prescribing medication for your clients, so for simplicity's sake, I refer in this chapter to practitioners prescribing the clients' medications as "psychiatrists."

MYTHS ABOUT PSYCHOTROPICS

Outlined next are some myths that persist about psychotropic medications.

Myth: Psychotropic medications are supposed to be sedating.

Fact: This is simply not true. Decades ago, when there were few medications available, some of the medications that were used were quite sedating. However, modern medications are developed with the goal of preserving or increasing alertness. A few medications are sedating, and these are generally prescribed at bedtime, so the sedative effect will assist with sleep and will mostly wear off by the next morning. In addition, the sedating effect of many medications can often wear off as the client takes the medication for a longer time period.

Myth: Using psychotropic medications is wrong, cruel, or ineffective. (There is even a whole religion—Scientology—that insists that all mental health treatment is just plain wrong. Yet, peculiarly, they proffer pop-psych-type offerings on their website.)

Fact: I can assure you that knowledgeable professionals, who know about the scientific literature on psychotropic medication, are in full agreement that they can be therapeutic and should be used as needed. One of your jobs as a mental health professional is to understand the potential benefits of psychotropic medications and use this knowledge to determine when it is appropriate to initiate a referral for a medication evaluation.

Myth: Schizophrenia is best treated without psychotropic medications.

Fact: This is totally inconsistent with the psychological and psychiatric research literature. Even with psychotropic medication, only a minority of clients with schizophrenia have attained a full recovery of social and vocational functioning (Robinson, Woerner, Delman, & Kane, 2005). That said, after some years, a few individuals do seem to recover from schizophrenia (Robinson, Werner, McMeniman, Mendelowitz, & Bilder, 2004). In addition, there is some preliminary evidence that selected clients who have had one episode of psychosis can be kept fairly stable over the short term by prescribing antipsychotic medication only when *prodromal* symptoms occur (suggesting a looming psychotic relapse); however, much more study is needed (Robinson et al., 2005).

Myth: Antipsychotic medications cause people to look and behave in an odd manner.

Fact: This is misinformation, coupled with outdated information. Decades ago, thorazine was the only medication that was available to treat schizophrenia. Thorazine had severe and distressing side effects, including muscle stiffness—which gave people a strange gait, sometimes called "the thorazine shuffle"—and a high level of sedation. I don't know anyone who still prescribes thorazine. Currently available antipsychotics are superior, with fewer and less severe side effects. Since there are many antipsychotics to choose from, if the client has a negative reaction to one, the client can be easily switched to another. Most of clients' odd behavior (e.g., flat affect and eccentricity) is due to the underlying mental illness. In actuality, most people who take antipsychotic medication look relatively normal on casual observation; they blend into a crowd, and you would never notice them.

Myth: A client says, "If I really need my medication, I'll be able to tell right away after I stop taking it."

Fact: This is wrong in two ways. First, the client's mental illness may not recur immediately after medication discontinuation, but continued medication is essential to prevent relapse and rehospitalization. This is the case for bipolar disorder and also for some clients with schizophrenia and other psychotic disorders. Bipolar clients are notorious for stopping their medications; however, they may not understand that the main purpose of ongoing medications is to *prevent recurrence* of infrequent but acute mood episodes. Second, the client who suddenly discontinues medication may have negative reactions that could have been avoided had the client collaborated with the psychiatrist. For example, antidepressants should never be stopped suddenly, as this can lead to *discontinuation reactions*, such as dizziness, insomnia, impaired concentration, irritability, and suicidal thoughts or behavior (Otis & King, 2006). Instead, they should be tapered under the supervision of a physician or master's-level nurse. In addition, some antianxiety medications will lead to withdrawal symptoms if discontinued suddenly, and—if the client is taking a larger dose—sudden discontinuation might even be lethal (M. Mills, personal communication, January 29, 2008).

CONTROVERSIES ABOUT PSYCHOTROPICS

There are a number of current controversies about psychotropic medications that you should be aware of. There is concern that psychotropics are overprescribed for children (Bonati & Clavenna, 2005) and for the elderly (Mort & Aparasu, 2002). Many professionals are concerned about the influence of prescription drug companies over physicians who practice in the current health care climate (Coyle, 2002). And there continues to be some concern about the effectiveness of antidepressants compared to placebos (Kirsch, Moor, Scoboria, & Nicholls, 2002).

CAUTIONARY ISSUES ABOUT PSYCHOTROPICS

Primary care physicians are often urged to treat mental illness with medications. However, research has shown that physicians who do not specialize in psychiatry vary considerably in their ability to effectively prescribe psychotropics, with many of them prescribing at too low a dose to be effective (Donoghue & Hylan, 2001). In addition, primary care physicians often do not schedule needed follow-up appointments or ensure that the client has refills (E. H. B. Lin et al., 2000).

Women who are pregnant, who want to become pregnant, or who are breast-feeding should be sure to share that information with their health care practitioner any time they are going to take medication. Sometimes medications are unsafe for the fetus, or the safety of the medication has not been sufficiently assessed.

Like any type of medication, psychotropics can have side effects and, in certain rare circumstances, can be dangerous. Some psychotropic medications can be fatal if the client ingests the entire bottle during a suicide attempt. Other medications carry a small risk of potentially dangerous complications and must be monitored carefully.

SIDE EFFECTS

You will usually meet more often with the client than the psychiatrist does. The client may not distinguish, as we do, between the specialties of various treating clinicians. The client may tell you about the side effects of medications even if you don't prescribe them. You may wish to have a reference work on hand so that you can look up common side effects (see suggestions at the end of this chapter). The best response to complaints about side effects is to urge the client to discuss the concerns with the psychiatrist. This is especially important if the client finds the side effects to be intolerable; urge the client to call the psychiatrist on the phone immediately to address the issue. Otherwise, the client is at risk of stopping the medication. If needed, assure the client that no one wants him or her to be uncomfortable with the medication and that the psychiatrist will want to know about these problems.

Selective serotonin reuptake inhibitor (SSRI) antidepressants, such as Prozac and Zoloft, are well known for their high rate of sexual side effects. You might want to screen your clients who are taking SSRIs for sexual problems. Urge clients to discuss any sexual side effects with the psychiatrist. Consult with the psychiatrist, as there may be ways to ameliorate the side effects while maintaining the gains from the medication.

If you are working with clients who take antipsychotics, discuss side-effect issues with the psychiatrist so that you understand some of the specific issues with that population. Here are some of the additional things you will want to learn about antipsychotics: neuroleptic malignant syndrome, tardive dyskinesia, akathesia, and how weight gain from certain antipsychotics can lead to type II diabetes.

MENTAL ILLNESS AND BIOLOGY

Many different methodologies have been used to study the biological basis of mental illness over the years. Many earlier studies focused on heritability and analyzed data from studies with twins and first-degree relatives. In recent decades, with scientific advances, researchers have looked for genetic abnormalities that might predispose one to mental illness and have looked inside the workings of the brain with functional magnetic resonance imaging (fMRI), photon emission tomography (PET) scans and so on.

We commonly think of psychotherapy as helping the client cope with the environmental and developmental factors that contributed to the client's mental illness, while we think of medications as affecting the biological basis of the mental illness. However, biological changes—due to psychotropic medication—can change thinking and self-image, and psychotherapy can measurably change the functioning of the brain (Gabbard, 2000b). Clearly, our traditional Western ideas of the mind–body dichotomy are insufficient to understand the complexities of mental illness.

As far as I know, research has shown that every mental illness that has been sufficiently studied so far has some evidence of biological and genetic basis. In addition, as far as I know, research has shown that every mental illness is more likely to occur with certain life situations and stressors. As a general rule, the more heritable or genetically influenced a disorder is, the more necessary psychotropic medication is to treat it (for more information about heritability of mental illnesses, see chapter 9). For example, bipolar disorder and schizophrenia cannot be treated effectively without medications, while depression and anxiety disorders often can. In conclusion, "environmental and developmental factors must interact with genes to produce psychiatric illness" (Gabbard, 2000b, p. 117).

COMORBID SUBSTANCE ABUSE

People who abuse substances are more likely to have rehospitalizations if they have bipolar disorder (Keck et al., 1998) or schizophrenia (G. E. Hunt, Bergen, & Bashir, 2002). Thus, recognizing and treating the substance abuse is an important step in stabilizing the client and preventing rehospitalization.

General cautions for medicating the mentally ill substance-abusing client include these: The substance-abusing client is unlikely to take medications regularly. Using illegal drugs can reduce the effectiveness of psychotropic medications. Finally, dangerous drug interactions between the illegal drugs and the psychotropic medications could occur.

Antianxiety medications (benzodiazepines like Valium and Xanax) can be quite addictive and should be used with great care if substance abuse is present. In those cases, ensure that you have a release of information and talk to the psychiatrist *before* the client gets a psychiatric evaluation. Nonetheless, appropriately treating anxiety can help the individual who is motivated to do so stop self-medicating through substance abuse. Most other psychotropics don't have much potential for abuse, but ask a psychiatrist if you are unsure.

WHEN PSYCHOTHERAPY IS NECESSARY

Psychotherapy is often a necessary part of treatment, especially when the client has the following:

* Chronic interpersonal problems
* High level of emotional distress
* Deficits in ability to cope
* Maladaptive coping strategies
* Risk of violence or suicide
* Feelings of stigmatization by a diagnosis of chronic mental illness and thus being at risk of stopping psychotropic medications

Many people think of disorders such as schizophrenia or bipolar disorder as primarily biological and thus do not provide psychotherapy for those clients. However, on the contrary, psychotherapy is essential for these clients to achieve the highest possible level of functioning and to reduce the overall cost of their mental health care (Gabbard, Lazar, Hornberger, & Speigel, 1997).

WHEN TO REFER A PSYCHOTHERAPY
CLIENT FOR MEDICATION

Whether or not you prescribe psychotropic medications, you will often be the first clinician the client sees. Thus, you will have the responsibility of determining whether a referral for psychotropic medications is needed. You need to understand when medications are optional and when they are necessary for effective treatment of your clients. As competent, effective, and ethical clinicians, it is our responsibility to ensure that our clients improve as quickly and as completely as possible. Therefore, treatment may need to include medications as well as psychotherapy. Here are some guidelines for making this decision.

Carefully consider the severity of the symptoms, determine how much the symptoms are affecting functioning, and then make a mutual decision about medications with the client. Discuss the pros and cons with the client, including when the issue should be revisited.

For many depressed and anxious clients, psychotherapy alone is sufficient treatment. If a client has some depressive symptoms but the diagnosis is adjustment disorder, psychotropics would probably be unnecessary. In cases when the client is distressed by depressive symptoms but functioning is adequate, psychotherapy can be effective alone, but progress can be quicker with the addition of medications. For occasional panic attacks or mild obsessive-compulsive disorder (OCD), you can discuss the pros and cons of medication, psychotherapy, and combination treatment with the client and make a decision together, depending on the client's preferences.

A medication evaluation is recommended if the client has any of the following:

- High level of subjective distress
- Sleep disruption from depression, anxiety, or posttraumatic stress disorder leading to exhaustion
- Poor concentration or motivation leading to deteriorating performance at work or school
- Strained interpersonal relationships because of distress and symptomatology
- Disabling panic attacks or severe OCD
- Impaired ability to fulfill obligations with work, schoolwork, or relationships

Antidepressants can help disturbed sleep in depression (Saletu-Zyhlarz, Anderer, Arnold, & Saletu, 2003) and PTSD (Maher, Rego, & Asnis, 2006). Other mental illnesses, such as attention deficit/hyperactivity disorder, eating disorders, and others, can be helped to some extent with medications. Discuss these issues with your supervisor and with a psychiatrist.

WHEN MEDICATIONS ARE NECESSARY

If your client has ever had an episode of hypomania, mania, or a mixed-mood episode, the client should be referred to a psychiatrist. Continued maintenance on mood-stabilizing medications (and possibly other medications, depending on the symptomatology) is essential in preventing future mood episodes and increasing the probability of functional recovery (Keck et al., 1998).

If your client is having psychotic symptoms, medications are also essential to return to a healthy state as quickly as possible. Continued medication is essential for individuals with schizophrenia and schizoaffective disorder.

The distressing and disabling symptoms for these disorders cannot be controlled by psychotherapy alone. Medications are generally considered necessary for severe major depression, especially if the client has psychotic features. *In conclusion, any client with current or past mania, hypomania, or psychotic symptoms must be referred for an evaluation for psychotropic medication.* Clients with severe anxiety and depressive disorders are likely to require psychotropic medications as well.

WORKING WITH PSYCHIATRISTS

If you don't prescribe medication, you will need to develop good working relationships with mental health practitioners who do. If you and the psychiatrist work in the same clinic or facility, you can discuss the client's treatment freely. If you don't, you will need to get a release of information from the client to talk to the psychiatrist to coordinate care. Once you make the referral for psychotropic medications, get a release signed and fax it over to the psychiatrist along with a request to call you at the psychiatrist's earliest convenience.

You may wish to contact the psychiatrist prior to the first session with the client to provide your impressions. If there are significant risk issues or complex diagnostic issues, a call is especially warranted. Then contact the psychiatrist after the first appointment with the client to compare impressions and coordinate care. Ideally, the psychiatrist will be open to your input and will be responsive to the client during and between sessions.

In some settings, you will be expected to present oral information to the psychiatrist you are working with. Be brief and to the point. Describe the client succinctly and list all the diagnoses. Instead of suggesting any medications or types of medications, highlight any symptoms that you are concerned about.

Wrong: "Elle lives with her two daughters and their kids. Would you believe it— there's 10 people living in a three-bedroom house? Anyway, she's feeling pretty depressed lately and kind of anxious too. I think that some Valium might do her a world of good. She doesn't know how she can continue to support all these people on her income from being a bus driver."

Right: "Elle is a 64-year-old White female bus driver with recurrent major depression and panic disorder. Her depression and panic attacks are negatively impacting on her work functioning. In addition, her sleep is very poor with frequent awakenings."

The information about Elle's stressors and social situation is important, but it is more pertinent to your work as the psychotherapist than it is to the psychiatrist's choice of psychotropic medications.

ASSESSING MEDICATION ADHERENCE

Taking medications as prescribed is sometimes called *adherence* and sometimes called *compliance*; I use these terms interchangeably. Cramer and Rosenheck (1998) found that, on average, patients with physical disorders took 76% of their prescribed medications, while patients taking antidepressants took only 65%, and patients taking antipsychotics took only 58%. Bipolar clients' adherence rates can be as low as 35% (Osterberg & Blaschke, 2005). Thus, medication nonadherence is an even more serious problem with mental illnesses than physical illnesses.

Given these findings, *we must assume that a large proportion of our clients are not taking their medications as prescribed.* Some of them will not be taking their medications at all, whereas others are taking their medications sporadically or just missing occasional doses. Thus, all clients taking psychotropic medications should be screened repeatedly and regularly for medication compliance. One method to determine whether the client is taking medications is to simply ask. Avoid questions such as this: "Are you taking all your medication?" This question will probably elicit a reassurance from the client that all the medications are being taken rather than elicit the client's difficulties with adherence. Instead, try these questions:

"How are things going with your medication?"
"What kinds of difficulties are you having with your medication?"
"Are you having any problems with taking your medication?"
"How often are you forgetting your medication?"

Assure the client that occasional forgetting is common and that your goal is simply to help problem-solve. Osterberg and Blaschke (2005) describe some other ways to determine medication adherence.

If you can find out when the client has refilled the medication (perhaps if you are working in a health maintenance organization or a Veterans Affairs facility), this information can provide a rough measure of compliance. For certain medications, a blood test is routinely done to see whether the blood level of the medication is at the therapeutic dose; a trained physician can often determine whether the client has been adherent from that information.

IMPROVING MEDICATION ADHERENCE

Claire Carter is a mental health trainee working with Sheena Moore, a client with bipolar disorder. When asked, Sheena admits to not taking her medication regularly. She has good understanding of why she needs to take it and is willing to do so. After some discussion, Sheena agrees to put a note next to her tooth-brush reminding her to take her medication before she brushes her teeth in the morning and evening. She agrees to keep a small pill bottle with some spare pills in her purse in case she forgets to take her medication and then remembers later when she is out of the house or in case she stays over at her mother's house.

In the literature, no single intervention for improving medication compliance has been found to be superior (Peterson, Takiya, & Finley, 2003). Thus, I recommend that you try to gain an understanding of what unique factors are contributing to this client's nonadherence (for a helpful list of factors contributing to nonadherence, see Osterberg & Blaschke, 2005). Then take a personalized approach to the client's medication adherence difficulties and tailor the intervention appropriately.

Sometimes there are barriers to treatment (Osterberg & Blaschke, 2005). The client may have difficulty paying for the medications. Or the client may have impediments to attending appointments. Try to problem-solve with the client and help the client tap into personal and community resources to address these barriers.

Many clients may have impaired concentration, attention, and memory because of their mental illnesses. This can result in difficulties with reading comprehension or poor receptive listening skills. These cognitive difficulties may mean that the client did not understand fully why the medication is important and why it needs to be taken on an ongoing basis. You can contribute to adherence by patiently explaining these issues to the client as slowly and as often as needed.

On the other hand, the cognitive difficulties or just plain disorganization may be contributing to forgetfulness about taking the medication. In this case, you might try interventions that aim to improve adherence to the dosing schedule (Osterberg & Blaschke, 2005). You might urge the client to put the medication into a pillbox with separate compartments for days of the week (or times of the day if there is a more complex dosing schedule or multiple medications at different times). These are readily available in any drugstore. If the client uses a pillbox, it is obvious which medications were missed, and it gives you an opportunity to problem-solve around those incidents:

"You always miss when you go over to your sister's house for the day? How about putting a few pills in a small container in your purse so that you'll have them when you realize that you missed your medications? Would you mind asking your sister to help you remember your medicine on those days?"

Suggest that the client keep a few pills of each medication in a purse, backpack, or briefcase that he or she carries around throughout the day in case the client later remembers a missed dose.

Another intervention for the forgetful client is to use cues to improve adherence (Osterberg & Blaschke, 2005). You could urge the client to identify an activity performed every day at the time that the medication needs to be taken ("I brush my teeth every morning," "I turn off the television every night before I go to bed," or "I have lunch") and have the client leave a little note by the toothbrush (or television or dining room table) to take the medication *before* brushing teeth (or turning off the television or having lunch) because if the client takes medications afterward, he or she may still forget. Emphasize the importance of medication becoming a routine, like the toothbrushing (or whatever) is.

In certain cases, these interventions with the forgetful client are ineffective in improving adherence despite your and the client's best efforts. In these cases, you might want to involve any family members living with the client to assist with the medication. If the client is taking certain antipsychotic medications, it could be administered in a shot rather than pills, thus ensuring adherence (Osterberg & Blaschke, 2005).

Psychiatrists will sometimes prescribe a medication (or two or more medications) on a complex dosing schedule. Complicated medication dosing schedules (e.g., three or more times per day) are inherently difficult to remember, and many clients will miss doses (Cramer & Rosenheck, 1998). Try to work with the client to improve adherence, but you can also consult with the psychiatrist. Perhaps a different medication or dosing schedule can be tried. Be aware that clients will sometimes set difficult dosing schedules for themselves unnecessarily: "I'm trying to take my blood pressure medication in the middle of the morning because I'm afraid that it won't mix with my Prozac." Assure the client that, as long as the psychiatrist knows about both medications, it is okay to take them together.

INSIGHT AND ADHERENCE

Bethany Gonzalez is a mental health trainee working with Luiz Ortiz, a 50-year-old client with schizophrenia. She is trying to educate him about his mental illness and asks him if he thinks he has schizophrenia. He says, "Well, my doctor says I have schizophrenia, but I don't think so." Bethany says, "It sounds like people are telling you that you have schizophrenia, but you are uncertain and need to decide for yourself. I have a list of symptoms here, so how about if we go through them and see if you have any? Maybe it will help us sort this out." She pulls out the Diagnostic and Statistical Manual of Mental Disorders, *reads through each symptom, and describes it in layman's terms. Then they discuss whether Luis has the symptom. They determine that he has hallucinations and delusions. Bethany says, "So those are the symptoms that made your doctors think that you have schizophrenia. What are your thoughts about that?" Now that Luis understands what schizophrenia is, he agrees that he probably does have it.*

Clients can have poor insight into the fact that they have a mental illness. This contributes to poor medication adherence. A gentle, nonconfrontational inquiring approach, such as Bethany's in the previous vignette, can be effective in fostering greater agreement between the client and the therapist. Further insight and adherence to recommended treatments can also be fostered by using motivational interviewing techniques (Rusch & Corrigan, 2002).

Insight may also be lacking when the client finds that she is asymptomatic when she stops her medication. In certain cases, this is relatively okay (e.g., depression or panic disorder) and the client just needs to be monitored carefully. In other cases (e.g., schizophrenia, schizoaffective disorder, or bipolar disorder), many clients can be asymptomatic for some time periods, but the symptoms will almost certainly recur, probably leading to hospitalization and/or great emotional distress. Taking the medications during even asymptomatic periods greatly increases emotional and functional stability in the long run. This issue is especially pertinent to bipolar clients, who may have one or fewer mood episodes per year (on average, if unmedicated, four mood episodes would occur in 10 years, according to the American Psychiatric Association, 2000) and can have limited insight into the need for consistent medication even when they are asymptomatic. Provide additional education about the course of the illness to the client, including that there may be periods of being asymptomatic, even if the underlying illness is still present. Discuss the importance of regular medication for keeping the client out of the hospital and as functional as possible over the long run.

STIGMA AND ADHERENCE

Blake Richardson is a mental health trainee working at a Veterans Affairs medical center. Blake is working with an Iraq War veteran, Todd Kelly, who has PTSD from combat. Todd says, "I don't want to take my medication be-

cause I think I should be able to snap out of it." Blake responds, "I wish you could snap out of PTSD too, but I haven't ever met anyone who was able to do that. You didn't ask for the trauma to happen to you, but it did, and I think that it's having a powerful effect on how you're feeling. Is that right?" Todd agrees. Blake continues, "I think that there's a good chance that you won't need the medicine at some time in the future, but for right now, you're not feeling very well, you're having nightmares every night, and I think the medicine will help you feel better. I think that if you feel better, you will be more able to get along with your wife and hold down your job. You can also get more rest so that you can think clearly and not feel so tired all the time. If you make progress in therapy, there's a good chance that later on the medicine won't be needed. What do you think about that?"

Sheena Moore comes in to see her student therapist, Claire Carter, the week after they talked about taking her medication regularly. Sheena says, "Every time I take my lithium, I realize that I'm manic-depressive, and I get upset about that." She and Claire talk at length about her feelings about bipolar disorder. Claire says, "It seems that you are discriminating against yourself for having bipolar disorder, but you can't help having it, and you didn't ask for it."

Sometimes the client has strong feelings about taking medication, and these feelings should be explored in therapy. Spend as much time as you need to thoroughly explore and examine the client's feelings and thoughts. Once you have done that, further psychoeducation about the biological basis of mental illness disorder can help the client reframe the issue. Note that Claire, in the previous vignette, has reframed Sheena's negative feelings about taking her medication as internalizing a societal discrimination and stigma against those who have chronic mental illness. Further discussion of this issue can continue at whatever depth is appropriate for the particular client.

ETHNICITY AND ADHERENCE

Research into psychotropic medication adherence has found lower adherence rates among Latinos and African Americans than among Whites (Diaz, Woods, & Rosenheck, 2005). Reasons for this difference have not become clear from the research to date.

Cultural mistrust could be contributing to nonadherence among African American clients. African American clients who are high in cultural mistrust have been found to have more negative attitudes about mental health, to terminate psychotherapy prematurely (especially if with a White counselor), and to disclose less with White counselors than African American ones (Whaley, 2001).

Why mistrust of the health care establishment exists is clear, when we explore this from a historical perspective. In 1972, a story broke about 399 African American men with long-standing histories of syphilis. These men had been studied for decades to understand the natural progression of the disease (Centers for Disease Control and Prevention, 2007). The men were misled about the study and never given an opportunity for appropriate informed consent. The men suffered for decades with progressing syphilis that was never treated, even though the disease could have been cured. This highly unethical and horrific experiment caused a major scandal. Even in recent years, I have had African American clients refer to the Tuskegee study when talking about their reluctance to take psychotropic medications.

Be attuned to any statements that may suggest concerns or mistrust on the part of your client. Ask questions to elicit further information about the concerns and validate your client's feelings. Be open to discussing these issues and avoid defensiveness. Provide more information as needed; also consider directing the client to reputable websites for further information.

RECOMMENDED READING

Gabbard, G. O. (2000). A neurobiologically informed perspective on psychotherapy. *British Journal of Psychiatry, 177*, 117–122.
Gabbard presents a clear and sophisticated discussion of the current knowledge on the interaction between biology and psychology.
Osterberg, L., & Blaschke, T. (2005). Adherence to medication. *New England Journal of Medicine, 353*, 487–497.
Osterberg and Blaschke provide a thorough discussion of the issue of adherence problems regarding medication for various groups of health care patients.
Otis, H. G., & King, J. H. (2006). Unanticipated psychotropic medication reactions. *Journal of Mental Health Counseling, 28*, 218–240.
Otis and King provide a thorough discussion of the psychotherapist's role in collaborating with the psychiatrist and client when psychotropic medications are involved. Emotional and physiological reactions are discussed.

RECOMMENDED WEBSITES

http://www.fda.gov/cder/drug/DrugSafety/DrugIndex.htm
This Web page is from the U.S. Food and Drug Administration website and provides consumer information sheets for many commonly prescribed medications.
http://www.epocrates.com
This website offers free information on drug dosage and side effects. In addition, if you have a Palm or Windows Mobile personal digital assistant (PDA), you can

download a program that will keep updated medication information on your PDA every time you sync it.

http://www.nami.org/Template.cfm?Section=Policymakers_Toolkit&Template=/ContentManagement/HTMLDisplay.cfm&ContentID=18971
This is a page on the website of the National Alliance for the Mentally Ill that has a handy list of commonly prescribed psychotropic medications by trade and generic names. To find it easily, conduct a Web search for "NAMI psychotropic medications."

RECOMMENDED VIDEO

Zwerin, C. (Director). (1988). *Straight no chaser* [Motion picture]. (Available from Warner Home Video)
If you are interested in observing someone who is probably taking thorazine, you might want to watch this documentary about Thelonious Monk. As you may know, he was a brilliant jazz piano player and composer who also happened to be mentally ill. From written accounts (e.g., De Wilde, 1996), it is not clear whether he had schizophrenia or schizoaffective disorder. Nonetheless, it is documented that when he was functional, his wife helped him remember to take his thorazine. He was famous for "dancing" during breaks in the music when he was not playing. In actuality, he may have had severe akathesia—a common side effect of thorazine (much less common with newer antipsychotics) that causes a person to feel an irresistible impulse to move around—moving the legs in particular. Additionally, he was known for his stiff-fingered piano-playing technique, which he may have developed because of muscle stiffness from his medication.

EXERCISES AND DISCUSSION QUESTIONS

1. Have you ever had difficulty taking a medication regularly or completing a prescription? (Be honest! Just about everyone has.) What factors do you think contributed to this? Are there other reasons why people might not take their medications besides the ones discussed in this chapter?

Chapter Sixteen

Health-Related Referrals

Since you will often be the first health care professional whom the client has seen in a while, perhaps years, it is important that you see the client holistically. You will need to recognize when to make a referral to other health care professionals, and you will need to be able to explain to clients why getting additional treatment is important.

Untreated medical issues add to the client's pain and suffering, which has a negative impact on emotional health. Untreated sleep disorders or insomnia will cause poor concentration, poor memory, and exhaustion. Unrecognized cognitive problems will impede the client's recovery. Of course, you can't be an expert in all these areas of practice. However, if you think any of these referrals is warranted, talk to your supervisor to see what resources are available in your area and how to make a referral.

MEDICAL REFERRALS

Travis Sanders is 57-year-old man who presents with depression. His energy level has been very poor for months. He is coming at the insistence of his wife. He has gained about 10 pounds in the past 2 months and is wearing a turtleneck, although it is 77 degrees outside. He indicates that he has been feeling depressed and irritable for several months and doesn't know why. He reports that he has never been depressed before. The therapist asks him when he last saw a physician. He said that he hasn't seen a doctor in over 10 years. The therapist recommends a complete physical exam. The physician finds that Travis is suffering from hypothyroidism and puts him on oral hormones, which improve his mood and returns him to his prior level of functioning.

Be alert to whether your client has been in appropriate and regular contact with a physician. In the case of Travis in the previous vignette, a medical exam was definitely needed and resolved the problem. A client can present for a mental health issue but may have unidentified medical issues contributing to and/or causing the mental health symptoms. There might also be unidentified medical issues that should be treated even if they do not impact mental health per se. Be alert to any behaviors that may be indicative of medical problems. These can include the following:

* Unsteady or halting gait
* Tremor
* Swelling of the extremities
* Shortness of breath
* Chronic cough, wheezing, or any difficulty breathing
* Skin abnormalities
* Clothing that is inappropriate to the climate (Morrison, 1997)

When you notice anything that would be suggestive of a physical symptom of a physical disorder, ask your client about it: "I've noticed that you have a small hand tremor. Have you discussed this with your physician? Do you know what is causing this?" Your client is used to being asked about such things by health care practitioners and is unlikely to take offense. If the client cannot identify a known medical problem that causes the symptom, inform the client that it is essential to obtain an evaluation from a physician to pinpoint the reason for the symptom.

Any unexplained symptom reported by the client should be fully evaluated by medical staff. This would include but not be limited to the following:

* Nausea and vomiting
* Pain
* Weakness
* Fatigue or lethargy
* Feeling too hot or too cold
* Feeling too thirsty
* Vision problems
* Rashes (Morrison, 1997)

Individuals with eating disorders also need to be evaluated by a physician for potential medical complications. There are a multitude of medical issues that your client might mention to you, and it is impossible to list all the possible symptoms. But again, ask your client whether the symptom has been reported to a physician and, if not, recommend an appointment in a timely manner. Do not hesitate to send the client to the emergency room if you feel it might be needed (e.g., uncontrolled gasping, shortness of breath, or chest pain); it is better to err on the side of caution than to allow a client to put off evaluating an urgent problem too long.

CHRONIC PAIN

Melanie Diaz is a mental health trainee who is doing a practicum in a medical center outpatient therapy clinic. She has been doing intake interviews. Today Melanie is interviewing Jorge Rodriguez; her diagnostic impression is generalized anxiety disorder. She asks him whether he has any medical problems; he states that he does not. She asks him whether he has had any pain recently. He states that he often has headaches. Melanie determines that he has severe tension-type headaches almost every day. Jorge states that over-the-counter pain medications have not helped him. She refers him to a health psychologist on staff who will evaluate him for biofeedback treatment.

As in the previous vignette, many clients deny any medical problems but then will say that they have pain if asked directly. People may deny any medical problems yet have chronic headaches, chronic back pain, arthritis, or other pain issues. You may ask a client to rate the severity of the pain on a scale from 0 (no pain) to 10 (the most severe pain they have ever had). Keep in mind that one client's rating of 10 may differ from another's. For example, a young man with a history of few medical issues may have a relatively low 10, having experienced very little severe pain in his life, while an older woman who has given birth to three children and has chronic pain will have experienced more severe pain and will have a higher 10. You might also want to ask the client how bothersome the pain has been. If it appears that pain has been contributing to your client's distress or interfering with daily functioning, you should address the issue.

Although many definitions of chronic pain exist, researchers do agree that chronic pain is "one of the most disabling and costly afflictions in North America, Europe, and Australia" (Harstall & Ospina, 2003, p. 1). A review of multinational studies of chronic pain found a mean weighted prevalence of chronic pain, using a standardized definition, to be about 12% of the population (Harstall & Ospina, 2003). Chronic headaches and chronic back pain are common pain conditions in the United States. Since pain conditions are so frequent and because pain has a profound impact on emotional and adaptive functioning, pain should be briefly assessed in all initial psychotherapy sessions.

The current prevailing model of pain is the biopsychosocial model. This model hypothesizes that pain is multiply determined by biological, psychological, and social factors. Pain can exist with no known physical cause. The biopsychosocial model recognizes the reality of this pain and does not just assume that it is "all in the patient's head." Often it is helpful to educate your client about this model and offer assurances that you understand that the pain is real and distressing even if the doctors cannot find a physical cause.

Recent research findings have indicated that short-term chronic pain can cause the nerve pathways to be altered so that long-term chronic pain becomes more and more likely (Woolf & Salter, 2000). In other words, the client may be completely healed but still have chronic pain due to maladaptive modifications of the nervous system. This pain is very real and is caused by the nervous system becoming hyperalert to pain signals.

Treatment of pain can be simple or complex. In the simplest situations, the patient's primary care physician can help the patient manage the pain through use of medications. This, together with psychotherapy encompassing stress management and relaxation training, may be sufficient to alleviate the pain significantly. A health psychologist, as outlined in the next section, can help you with more complex or treatment-resistant cases.

Chronic headaches that interfere with functioning should always be evaluated and treated. There are several types of headaches that respond to different types of treatment. A full discussion of this issue is beyond the scope of this book. For further information, see the resources listed at the end of this chapter. However, migraines are headaches that have a distinct pattern of symptoms: pain around the eyes, sensitivity to light, and more. When they are distressing and/or impair functioning, refer the client to a physician because there are many helpful medications that can prevent migraines from occurring and/or that can treat them quickly when they occur (Schoenen, 2001).

HEALTH PSYCHOLOGY

Tyler Butler is a mental health trainee evaluating Nancy Miller. Nancy is very concerned about her history of smoking because her mother has just died from emphysema. Nancy has tried to quit many times and has not succeeded. Tyler refers her to the health psychologist on staff who evaluates her and treats her in conjunction with a physician. A combination of medications, group therapy, and individual behavioral therapy finally help Nancy quit smoking.

Health psychologists are licensed psychologists who have extensive additional training in the psychological management of health issues. A qualified health psychologist has received specialized pre- and postdoctoral training. Health psychologists often work in large academic medical centers and provide "psychological therapies to enhance health behaviors, manage symptoms and sequelae of disease, treat psychological symptoms and disorders, prolong survival in the face of a life-threatening illness, and improve quality of life" (Compas, Haaga, Keefe, Leitenberg, & Williams, 1998, p. 89). Compas et al. (1998) divide the field of health psychology into four broad intervention groups: (a) decreasing health risk behaviors, such as alcohol use and smoking, along with increasing health promoting behavior, such as exercise and a healthy diet; (b) managing specific symptoms, such as chronic pain and insomnia; (c) interventions that facilitate effective coping with chronic or life-threatening conditions, including cancer, HIV, diabetes, asthma, arthritis, and so on; and (d) addressing health-related psychological conditions, such as eating disorders and body dysmorphic disorder. Health psychologists employ a wide variety of psychological treatment techniques, including stress management training, psychoeducation, cognitive-behavioral therapy, biofeedback, hypnosis, and other specialized treatments. Health psychologists also provide psychological insight and expertise on multidisciplinary medical treatment teams.

Refer your client to a health psychologist when you identify that the client has one of the previously mentioned health-related problems and that this problem is having a negative impact on adaptive coping and/or emotional functioning. The health psychologist can treat the client concurrently with the client's psychotherapy with you and will focus specifically on the health-related issue. Have the client sign a release so that you and the health psychologist can consult and coordinate care.

Referral to a health psychologist should be considered for severe pain and/or any pain that interferes with functioning. A health psychologist has the expertise to help the client with specialized techniques, such as cognitive therapy of pain (Tan & Leucht, 1997), hypnosis (Tan & Leucht, 1997), biofeedback (Symreng & Fishman, 2004), and other techniques. Health psychologists are often found in multidisciplinary pain clinics, which are usually based at major medical centers. At that clinic, interventions at all levels of the biopsychosocial model will be employed by a multidisciplinary team working collaboratively to get the best results in pain control and functional improvement.

One modality that some health psychologists use is biofeedback, which is the practice of giving the client auditory and/or visual feedback about a physiological process in order for the client to learn how to consciously make physiological changes. The biological feedback can be blood pressure, heart rate, the electrical conductivity of the skin, muscle tension, and others. Biofeedback is used for tension headaches, stress management, and other conditions where achievement of relaxation improves the client's pain or functioning. Biofeedback is well validated, but other methods of relaxation training may be as effective for many clients (L. Miller, 1994).

INSOMNIA

Amit Patel is a graduate student in biology. He has come to the clinic because he has insomnia and acute anxiety. He tends to ruminate at night before sleeping, and then he naps during the day. His sleep schedule is not fixed, and he is exhausted all the time. After working with a therapist, he has learned the importance of maintaining a regular sleep schedule, and his sleep has improved.

Chronic insomnia occurs in about 10% of the adult population (Roth & Roehrs, 2003). It is generally a symptom of a medical or emotional disorder; many clients with depression and anxiety have problems with insomnia. They tend to ruminate when getting into bed at night, which keeps them alert and awake. They may have poor sleep habits (such as sleeping with the television on or taking long naps during the daytime). They may awaken at night and have difficulty getting back to sleep.

Insomnia can often be treated through simple sleep hygiene and stimulus control instructions by the psychotherapist (see appendix 18 for a basic instruction sheet on treating insomnia) with the addition of relaxation training as necessary. The client may also be helped by discussing the issues he or she is ruminating about and by learning techniques to reduce rumination.

If these interventions have not been effective in improving the client's sleep, consider these options. If you wonder whether the client has a sleep disorder, refer for evaluation by a physician who is a diplomate in sleep medicine. Alternatively, you could consider a referral for medication to help with sleep or a referral to a health psychologist.

SLEEP DISORDERS

Jennifer Wright, a psychiatry resident, has been treating Linda Kress in individual psychotherapy for 4 months. Initially Linda's sleep had been very disrupted by depressive symptoms, and she had difficulty getting to sleep because she was ruminating about her problems. She was sleeping only about 6 hours a night when she began therapy. After 4 months, Linda had significantly reduced depression. In addition, Linda was going to sleep promptly and getting about 7 to 8 hours of sleep every night. However, she still stated that her sleep was poor. Jennifer asked whether Linda felt rested in the morning. She stated that she did not, and in fact she never does. She also volunteered that her husband complains that she tosses and turns all night and that she kicks him when she sleeps. Jennifer referred Linda for a sleep evaluation, which confirmed that she has periodic limb movement disorder, a common sleep disorder.

Mike Murphy talked to his therapist, John Henderson, about having difficulty with concentration and distractibility. While this was consistent with his history of depression, John also noted that Mike looked sleepy during the session, which was in the late afternoon. When asked, Mike indicated that he was sleepy much of the time and took frequent naps. John also noted that Mike was a middle-aged male who was somewhat obese and had a thick neck. John asked if Mike's wife complained about his snoring, which, in fact, she did. John sent Mike for a sleep evaluation, which confirmed that he has sleep apnea.

Sleep disorders are much more prevalent than most people imagine. Two common sleep disorders are sleep apnea (occurring in up to 5% of the population of Western countries: Young, Peppard, & Gottlieb, 2002) and periodic limb movement disorder (about 4% prevalence in Europe: Ohayon & Roth, 2002). Both of these sleep disorders are underdiagnosed and undertreated in the general population (Ohayon & Roth, 2002; Young et al., 2002). Both groups of clients often report daytime sleepiness and lack of restful sleep.

In *sleep apnea*, the airway is periodically blocked during sleep, which keeps rousing the client (who may or may not be aware of this), so the client never gets enough deep sleep. Sleep apnea clients will usually say that their bed partners have complained about their loud snoring. They may know that they snort or gasp during sleep. Sometimes they know that they stop breathing during sleep (Maislin et al., 1995), or they may not be aware of their sleep breathing problems. Sleep apnea is commonly treated through the use of a *CPAP* (continuous positive air pressure) device. The device increases the air pressure through the nose to prevent the breathing interruptions that characterize sleep apnea.

In *periodic limb movement disorder* (PLMD), individuals move frequently during sleep; the cause for PLMD is unknown but is suspected to be neurological in origin. Bed partners complain about clients tossing and turning all night or kicking when asleep. Clients may note that their bedcovers are a mess in the morning. PLMD is treated with medications. These medications might include antiseizure medications and dopamine agonists. It is often but not always associated with restless legs syndrome. Both PLMD and restless legs syndrome can be exacerbated by certain antidepressant medications, such as selective serotonin reuptake inhibitors.

Other sleep disorders include narcolepsy (falling asleep unpredictably during normal daytime activities), bruxism (grinding teeth while asleep), REM behavior disorder (leading to sleepwalking or talking in one's sleep or other seemingly alert behavior, possibly violent if acting out distressing dreams, while asleep), and sleep-related eating disorder (the individual gets out of bed and eats, then goes back to sleep, later having a poor memory of the incident) (MedlinePlus, 2007; National Sleep Foundation, 2007).

If you have any suspicion of a sleep disorder, ask the client to talk the issue over with a primary care physician or make a referral to a sleep clinic yourself (ask your supervisor which is most appropriate). Sleep clinics can be freestanding or associated with a major medical center. At the sleep clinic, the client will be given paper-and-pencil screening instruments. The client will probably be interviewed by a physician who specializes in sleep medicine and then will have a sleep study that entails an overnight stay in a sleep lab while being monitored for symptoms of sleep disorders.

NEUROPSYCHOLOGICAL TESTING AND NEUROLOGY REFERRALS

Joe Preap, a clinical psychology graduate student, is treating Dorothy Peters for chronic depression. Joe notes that Dorothy never seems to complete her homework assignments. When asked, she rarely even remembers what they were. Joe also knows that Dorothy lives with a friend, is not working, and has no source of income. He is puzzled because she seems to have so little motivation. The more Joe gets to know her, the more she does not seem like a typical client with depression. Joe discusses the case with his supervisor, Dr. Gomez, who reminds him of Dorothy's history of a car accident. Dorothy had told Joe that she did not remember the actual accident itself. She regained consciousness when she was in a hospital. It was likely that she had hit her head against the windshield. Dr. Gomez told Joe that Dorothy's lack of motivation was characteristic of clients with brain damage from a closed head injury. They referred Dorothy to a neuropsychologist and a neurologist for further evaluation.

Brain injuries can be underdiagnosed and undertreated. Many people have little understanding of how a brain injury can profoundly affect the behavior, emotions, personality, and functioning of an individual. As can be seen in the previous vignette, symptoms of brain injury can be subtle and difficult to diagnose, sometimes looking like depressive symptoms. Often the client and the client's family may have no idea that the brain injury is still having a profound impact on functioning.

Strangely, a brain injury in which the skull is not penetrated can sometimes cause quite severe impairment. This type of brain injury is called a *closed head injury* since the skull is not breached. During the injury, the brain rams against the skull, then it may bounce back and ram against the skull on the other side. This can result in profound but diffuse deficits. Brain injuries in which the skull is breached usually result in a different, more focal pattern of cognitive deficits that vary depending on the location of the injury.

Symptoms of brain damage or other neurological disorders can initially be mistaken for symptoms of common emotional problems. If your client has a history of being knocked on the head or any significant injury to the head, consult a knowledgeable physician, nurse, or psychologist about the possible contribution of brain damage to the client's difficulties. Be aware that evaluating brain injury is especially pertinent in the treatment of many veterans of the wars in Iraq and Afghanistan (Warden, 2006).

The client may also have an undiagnosed neurological disorder that is not caused by brain damage. Some symptoms that would warrant an evaluation by a primary care physician or neurologist would be weakness, tingling, numbing, trouble walking, tremor, involuntary movements, dizziness, and blurred or double vision (Morrison, 2007).

REMEMBER THE MIND–BODY CONNECTION

Many medical problems, such as irritable bowel, migraine headaches, asthma, and others, are worse when the client is under stress because of the mind–body connection. Therefore, psychotherapy that alleviates distress may also alleviate the severity of many medical conditions. Given these considerations, concurrent treatment of mental illnesses and medical issues is highly recommended.

Pain and mental disorders influence each other. For example, pain appears to increase the likelihood of depression, anxiety, and stress; in addition, depression, anxiety, and stress appear to increase the likelihood of pain (for a more complete explanation of the relationship, see Keefe, Dunsmore, & Burnett, 1992; Symreng & Fishman, 2004; Worz, 2003). Thus, psychotherapy addressing the client's emotional problems should help your client cope with the pain and perhaps even decrease the pain's intensity. Conversely, if you help your client get appropriate medical treatment for the pain, the client's emotional problems have a greater chance of improving.

RECOMMENDED READING

Symreng, I., & Fishman, S. M. (2004). Anxiety and pain. *Pain: Clinical Updates, 12*, 1–6.
   This article delineates the most recent understanding of the relationship between anxiety and pain. See the first website listed next to find it online.

Turk, D. C., & Burwinkle, T. M. (2005). Clinical outcomes, cost effectiveness, and the role of psychology in treatments for chronic pain sufferers. *Professional Psychology: Research and Practice, 36,* 602–610.
The authors provide a discussion of the effectiveness of various state-of-the art treatments for chronic pain, providing a helpful overview of pain treatments for the beginning psychotherapist.

WEB RESOURCES

http://www.iasp-pain.org
This website of the International Association for the Study of Pain hosts a series of helpful articles under the title "Pain: Clinical Updates."
http://health.nih.gov
This website provides helpful information for the medical patient on a wide variety of medical diseases. It can be helpful for you as well if you have a client with a medical problem that you are unfamiliar with.
http://www.merck.com/pubs/mmanual
This is the website for the Merck Manual of Diagnosis and Therapy. *Although it is a bit technical for nonmedical practitioners, it can still be very informative about many medical conditions.*

Chapter Seventeen

Mental Health Referrals

Clients will sometimes need more intensive mental health treatment than you can provide in weekly individual psychotherapy. In these cases, you need to understand the range of treatment options available and make an appropriate referral given the client's level of distress and level of risk to self and others.

INPATIENT PSYCHIATRIC HOSPITALIZATION

Sean Foster, a mental health trainee, is working in an outpatient mental health clinic. He is running a support group for clients with chronic schizophrenia. One of the clients, Miguel Flores, looks more depressed than usual. Sean asks him how he is doing. Miguel states that he is thinking of hurting himself. Sean asks him if he has a way to do that. Miguel states that he has a gun at home. Sean knows that Miguel is an Iraq War veteran and knows how to use a weapon. Sean escorts Miguel to the psychiatrist's office. Together, the psychiatrist and Sean further evaluate Miguel and decide that he should be hospitalized. Sean escorts Miguel to the emergency room while the psychiatrist fills out the necessary paperwork for admission.

Any client who is a danger to himself or others should be referred to an inpatient psychiatric unit. Specifically, this includes a client who is having suicidal thoughts and cannot assure the clinician that he or she will refrain from acting on them. Finally, clients who have symptoms that are so severe that they are unable to care for themselves should be hospitalized. This final group would include acute psychosis and acute mania. In some instances, highly agitated clients or clients with extreme psychomotor slowing will also be admitted because of an inability to care for themselves.

If you believe that your client needs hospitalization, you should immediately get the advice of a supervisor. Agencies and medical centers have differing policies on coping with psychiatric emergencies. Most often, clients who need hospitalization will agree and cooperate. However, sometimes a client needs hospitalization but refuses. In those instances, you must be familiar with state law regarding involuntary hospitalization, and you must be aware of the procedures for involuntary hospitalization at your facility.

PARTIAL HOSPITALIZATION

Rebecca Bennett is a female grocery clerk who comes to the clinic feeling acutely anxious and depressed. Both her mother and her grandmother, who were her primary sources of emotional support, have died within the past 3 months. Rebecca is not suicidal, but she has had difficulty coping. She has been crying and spending every day in bed. The intake worker suggests that Rebecca attend the partial hospitalization program.

A partial hospitalization program is a program that provides intensive mental health treatment for most of the days of the week while allowing the client to stay at home at night rather than in the hospital. When clients are having an acute exacerbation of mental illness and emotional distress but the client is not a risk to self or others, partial hospitalization is an appropriate referral. Outcomes for these clients were no different from inpatient treatment and satisfaction is higher (Horvitz-Lennon, Normand, Gaccione, & Frank, 2001).

OUTPATIENT COMMITMENT AND INVOLUNTARY MEDICATIONS

In some states, clients can be committed by the court to attend outpatient treatment and take medications even if they do not want to (Hiday, 2003). Typically, these are clients who have a history of chronic mental illness and/or dangerousness; they are frequent users of intensive services, with a history of subsequent noncompliance with follow-up care. Talk to your supervisor to see what the state laws regarding outpatient commitment are in the state where you are practicing.

ELECTROCONVULSIVE THERAPY AND EMERGING MEDICAL TREATMENTS

Lakisha Washington, a mental health trainee, has been working with Erin Fitzgerald for about 6 months. Erin is married and has three young children in the home. She is married to her high school sweetheart, who is a dentist. The plan was for Erin's husband to earn the family income while she cared for the children. However, Erin has been too mentally ill with schizoaffective disorder in the past year to care for the children effectively. Erin has chronic suicidal ideation and sometimes scares the children by talking about her wish to be dead. Erin's psychiatrist, Dr. Pryor, has tried many different medications over the past 9 months and meets with Erin frequently to monitor her response. Lakisha meets with Erin and her husband frequently as well to monitor the suicidal ideation and do psychotherapy. Dr. Pryor and Lakisha have had to hospitalize Erin four times in the past 9 months. Finally, Dr. Pryor recommends electroconvulsive therapy (ECT). Erin is fearful, as she has heard negative things about ECT. However, the family is suffering greatly and so Erin is willing to try it. Lakisha goes to visit Erin on the inpatient psychiatric unit between treatments. Erin's mood is dramatically better, and Lakisha sees her smile and joke for the first time ever. She sees her repeatedly over the next couple weeks. Later Lakisha alludes to their first conversation immediately after the ECT. Erin does not remember any of it. However, she says that her memory is getting back to normal and that she feels much better.

You might find yourself some day working with a client who is not responding to medications, as in the previous vignette. In these cases, the psychiatrist working with the client may recommend the use of ECT. ECT is considered an effective treatment for severe major depression, especially depression with psychotic features or prominent risk of suicide, but it is rarely used as a first-line treatment (Royal Australian and New Zealand College of Psychiatrists Clinical Practice Guidelines Team for Depression, 2004).

Unfortunately, most of us have been exposed to ECT through overly sensational movies. The actual process of ECT is nothing like that. If you ever have a chance to observe it, whatever your feelings or beliefs about the treatment, I encourage you to do so. The actual process of ECT is as follows:

- The client is brought into the surgical suite with the medical staff.
- The client is anesthetized and also given a short-acting medication that relaxes the muscles. A simple pumping machine is used to keep air going in and out of the lungs.
- ECT is generally administered to the right hemisphere only to induce a seizure. The client moves very little or not at all during the procedure.
- The client awakens shortly thereafter in the recovery room, remembering nothing of the procedure.

ECT must be administered repeatedly over a course of days to be effective. The client can be an inpatient or an outpatient. Be aware that considerable controversy remains about how often and how much ECT affects memory in clients over the long term (Challiner & Griffiths, 2000; Rose, Fleischmann, & Wykes, 2004).

There are other medical approaches that show promise for clients with severe, intractable depression, including vagus nerve stimulation and transcranial magnetic stimulation. The field is changing rapidly, so talk to trusted psychiatrists to get information on the latest techniques.

SUBSTANCE ABUSE PROGRAMS AND COMMUNITY RECOVERY RESOURCES

Since substance abuse is comorbid with so many mental health issues, you will make many referrals for adjunctive substance abuse treatment over your career. A large sample of British community mental health clients with mental illness found that 44% had a problem with alcohol or drugs within the past year (Weaver et al., 2003). In addition, substance use can cause unusual symptoms, such as cocaine psychosis, that mimics other mental illnesses, so substance abusers need to be evaluated with great care.

The client will first need to be motivated to seek treatment. A confrontational approach is rarely productive (Stanton, 2004). Do not tell the client that he or she is an addict or alcoholic and must seek treatment. Instead, carefully assess the client's readiness for change and tailor your intervention appropriately (Prochaska & Norcross, 2001). If the client is not yet ready, take a motivational interviewing approach (W. R. Miller & Rollnick, 2002) in which you gently assist the client in discussing concerns about the substance use.

When the client is ready for help, you will need to consider the options together. Perhaps the client is more interested in community resources such as Alcoholics Anonymous (AA). If you are unfamiliar with the principles of AA, see its website at http://www.alcoholics-anonymous.org. AA can be an effective resource for clients, and frequent attenders are more likely to abstain (Gossop et al., 2003), but your client may need additional treatment and support to meet all the mental health and addiction recovery needs.

When the substance abuse problem is more severe and there is a physical addiction, the client may need to be medically detoxed as an inpatient. Inpatient substance abuse or dual diagnosis (e.g., both substance abuse and mental illness) programs can be helpful for many clients who have more severe addictions and need help getting sober. Some clients also benefit from living in a recovery house or other residential program for weeks or months.

Your supervisor and colleagues can help you learn about the other recovery resources available in your community and how to refer to them. Clients who have both mental illness and substance abuse problems should have both of those difficulties treated concurrently and with an integrative approach (RachBeisel, Scott, & Dixon, 1999).

COMMUNITY RESOURCES

In certain cases, you may find yourself doing more case management at first than actual psychotherapy. A client's basic needs for safety, food, housing, and so on may not be met. Under those circumstances, the client will not be able to concentrate on addressing emotional problems. Your client then needs referrals to community resources. Depending on how the facility is organized, you might make the referrals, or a staff social worker might assist you with this. Ask your supervisor for an overview of some of the resources that are most helpful for the client population you are working with.

RECOMMENDED READING

Challiner, V., & Griffiths, L. (2000). Electroconvulsive therapy: A review of the literature. *Journal of Psychiatric and Mental Health Nursing, 7*, 191--198.
Challiner and Griffiths provide a remarkably evenhanded review of the literature on the efficacy of ECT and the controversies around it.

EXERCISES AND DISCUSSION QUESTIONS

1. As a health care professional, even if you are not medically trained, you will often be the point of entry into the health care system for your clients. Do you feel comfortable referring clients to other health care professionals as needed? Do you need further training? Are there any rules of thumb you can use to know when to make a referral?
2. Have you ever seen a client who might have benefited from ECT? Would you be willing to refer a client for ECT? Why or why not?
3. Does your state allow for outpatient commitment? If so, what is the procedure to do that?

Section IV

CRISIS READINESS

Chapter Eighteen

Managing Crises Step-by-Step

Luisa Garcia, a 28-year-old Latina female, is attending her regular psychotherapy session with Katherine Mahoney, a mental health trainee. Luisa tells Katherine that she has been thinking about suicide.

Robert Moore, a 25-year-old White male, comes to the intake clinic. He tells the intake worker, Shane Abel, a mental health trainee, that he needs treatment since he is thinking about killing his brother over a financial disagreement.

Ryan Fernandes, a 55-year-old East Indian male, is brought to the clinic by his elderly parents. All of them are Catholic and first-generation immigrants. The intake worker, Brandi Williams, a mental health trainee, reviews the chart and sees that Ryan has a long history of schizophrenia. His parents tell Brandi that Ryan has been pacing all night for the past several nights and that he is talking to himself.

The focus of this chapter is to assist you in conceptualizing the overall process of crisis management. These three detailed vignettes are elaborated throughout the chapter to illustrate the steps in crisis management with very different clients as well as the process of interacting effectively with the crisis client. The chapter also focuses on common issues that occur with all crisis clients, such as deciding whether to hospitalize, formulating a crisis management plan, and documenting appropriately. Specific issues that are pertinent to particular crises are discussed in subsequent chapters.

Managing crises is the most anxiety-provoking work that psychotherapists do. Here are the steps in doing so:

- Establish rapport
- Assess

- ○ The current situation
- ○ Historical and demographic risk factors
- Plan and implement
  - ○ Give and elicit feedback
  - ○ Consult supervisor
  - ○ Consider whether hospitalization is appropriate
  - ○ Make a crisis management plan and secure client's verbal agreement
  - ○ Implement plan
- Document

Throughout, you will need to figure out how to cope effectively with the crisis. You should consult with other professionals as needed throughout this entire process.

ESTABLISHING RAPPORT: COPING WITH CRISES AND THE THERAPIST'S EMOTIONS

Katherine feels very anxious about talking with Luisa about her suicidal thoughts. She has never actually assessed a real client for suicidality before, although she has done role plays in class. Katherine takes a deep breath and reminds herself that she does know how to do this. She also reminds herself that more experienced staff are available to help her at any time if she needs to ask for help. She makes reassuring statements: "Luisa, it was very wise of you to come in and ask for help. I can see that you understand that these suicidal ideas mean that you need help right away." She tells Luisa what they will be doing in a reassuring manner and communicates to Luisa that the situation is under control: "What I'd like to do is get a better understanding of how you are doing right now so that we can make a plan that will help you as soon as possible. How does that sound to you?"

Even highly experienced therapists can become anxious when they are working with crisis clients. There is nothing wrong with feeling anxious; it shows that you care. Keep in mind how the client is feeling. The client feels that his or her problems are unmanageable and that help is desperately needed. Your calm reassurances will help. The client doesn't feel in control right now, but being with someone else who does know how to manage the situation will be reassuring.

Try to contain your own anxiety during the assessment. You must keep your cool even if you feel nervous. Take a few deep breaths if you need to. Remind yourself that the client is here to get help and will feel better soon. If you are calm though clearly concerned, the client will feel reassured. I can assure you that once you understand the situation and help the client get assistance, the client's emotional distress will be eased, and both of you will feel relieved. Remember that, at any time, you can walk the client to the office of your supervisor or another more experienced colleague and ask for help.

Once the crisis has been resolved, discuss what happened thoroughly with your supervisor. Increasing your understanding and confidence about how to address crisis situations is the best way to reduce the stress and anxiety of coping with them.

ASSESS: THE CURRENT SITUATION

Katherine asks Luisa how long she has been thinking about suicide. Luisa says that she has been thinking about it constantly for the past 5 days. Katherine asks more about Luisa's suicidal ideas. Luisa reveals that she is thinking about jumping off a bridge near her house and that she has walked by the spot several times thinking about jumping. Katherine asks whether Luisa thinks she can control herself and not jump. Luisa is unsure.

Shane asks Robert more about his violent thoughts. Robert says that whenever he sees his brother, he thinks about "jumping him." They have been living in a small apartment together with their mother, and tensions have been running high. When Robert is out of the house, he doesn't think about his brother or their disagreement. He said that he has been trying not to act on the violent impulses since he knows he would regret it later.

Brandi asks Ryan about his thoughts. Ryan says that God has been talking to him and tells him that he needs to spread the Word to the heathens in the neighborhood. (They live in a mostly Hindu Indian neighborhood.)

Whenever you have any concern that a crisis may be developing or anyone may be at physical risk, you must ask about this (Packman, Pennuto, Bongar, & Orthwein, 2004). Not asking may put your client or someone else in danger. Not asking will not protect you legally from not knowing and, in fact, will put you at greater professional risk (Packman, Pennuto et al., 2004). You'll want to thoroughly understand your client's thought process, level of intent, and plans regarding the risky situation (Simon, 2004).

You might want to interview the client individually, or you might want to involve whatever family members came in with the client. If the client is less functional, family members will provide valuable information. In addition, consider that certain cultural groups (such as Ryan's) may have more intergenerational involvement and may conceptualize problems more in the context of the family than the individual (Gonzalez, 1995). Generally, it is helpful to ask the family whether they want to come in to your office together, and take your cue from their response. You can always ask some people to step out briefly later if you think it will be helpful.

ASSESS: HISTORICAL AND DEMOGRAPHIC FACTORS

Katherine knows from Luisa's chart that Luisa has been diagnosed for years with borderline personality disorder and chronic major depression. She also knows that last year, Luisa took an overdose of pills, had her stomach pumped, and was hospitalized for 2 weeks. She knows that Luisa has a history of three other previous attempts of varying lethality. After each attempt, Luisa was hospitalized. Luisa also reports about five other hospitalizations for severe depression and suicidal ideation.

Shane asks Robert if he has been violent before. Robert reveals that he is a recovering alcoholic. He has been abstinent for 15 months. When he used to drink, he was often violent, but he has not been violent since he has been sober. He denied ever getting into any legal trouble because of his violent behavior in the past, and, as far as he knows, no one has ever been in the hospital after a fight with him. With Robert's approval, Shane calls Robert's drug and alcohol counselor, Ms. Patterson, to get her input. She says that Robert has been very compliant with his recovery program and that, to her knowledge, he has not been hostile toward anyone since becoming sober. She feels that he is very motivated to continue to improve and can be trusted to follow through on a crisis intervention plan. She said that she would be happy to see Robert if he could come in for an appointment tomorrow.

Brandi has reviewed the chart and sees that, as far as the clinic knows, Ryan has never done anything to harm himself or others. She asks his parents about this, and they confirm it. He has had several past episodes when he stopped taking his medications, became psychotic, and had to be briefly hospitalized. When Brandi asks the family about his medications, she finds that they have been coping with a medical crisis in a grandchild and have not been monitoring his medications as closely as they often do. Ryan himself insists that he has been taking his medication, but he clearly has a thought disorder and may be too confused to remember his medications; Brandi knows that his insistence is more likely a statement indicating that he has been intending to take his medications rather than an indication that he has actually done so. Ryan wandered off by himself in the middle of the night about 2 years ago, and his family found him in his pajamas wandering about the neighborhood the next morning. They voice their concern that this might happen again.

Has this same crisis situation occurred in the past with this client? If so, that is an indication that the likelihood of its happening again is greater. For example, a history of multiple suicide attempts is the best predictor that a client is at heightened risk of future attempts (Joiner, Walker, Rudd, & Jobes, 1999).

In what situations has the crisis situation occurred? Are these situations the same today or different? For example, if the client has been violent toward family when drunk in the past and has just relapsed on alcohol, the risk is greater. If the client has never been violent when sober and has been reliably sober for several years, the risk is less.

Consider what you know about the client. Ask the client what has or has not worked in past crisis situations. Consider what other professionals have to say verbally and/or in the chart.

PLAN: GIVE AND ELICIT FEEDBACK

Katherine tells Luisa, "I'm concerned about what you're telling me. It was wise of you to come in and talk to me about this. I hear that you can't be sure you'd ask for help if the suicidal feelings get strong again, and you are unsure whether you can control yourself. I suspect you're talking to me about this because you know you'd be safer in the hospital." Luisa responds to Katherine that she does understand that she needs to be in the hospital.

Shane tells Robert, "I see that you are worried about these violent thoughts, and I am as well. But I'm not exactly sure what our plan should be. It sounds to me as if you have been able to control your impulses much better since you have been sober. Is that true? Do you think you and your brother would be safer if you weren't around him right now?" Robert replies to Shane that he feels uncertain about being able to control his violent impulses right now, but he thinks that as long as he avoids his brother, he will be fine. Shane says, "I can think of a few plans that might work for you, and I'd like us to discuss them. One might be to stay with a friend and avoid all contact with your brother for now. We could also consider admitting you to the hospital or to a partial hospitalization program. What do you think?" Robert says that if he can avoid his brother, he knows he won't be violent. Shane feels that Robert is sincere and motivated not to harm his brother, so a less restrictive alternative is appropriate.

Brandi tells Ryan and his parents, "I'm concerned that you will end up in the hospital again. It sounds like, even though you sincerely want to take your medication, you may have been missing some doses lately. [Turning to his parents] It's likely that he will improve soon, if he can regularly get his medication over the next several days. I'm wondering if you feel you can manage him at home or if you are too worried that he might do something unsafe like wander off at night." Ryan's parents worry that he may roam the neighborhood at night again. They think that they can get him to take his medications, but they are worried about what he will do before he stabilizes. Ryan says he thinks he would be okay outside the hospital, then talks again about his intent to convert the heathens. He is observed during this discussion to be looking around the room.

You should give the client feedback—your professional opinion about the situation. Be honest and tactful, if possible. For example, if you believe that the client feels great because she is getting manic, say so. If you are worried about the client's suicidal impulses and think hospitalization would be safer, say so.

Sometimes the situation is fairly cut and dried, such as that of Luisa, and you have specific recommendations. The crisis management plan may be clear to both the therapist and the client. Here, Luisa has been in this situation before and knows what is needed.

Eliciting feedback is important as well. The client's feedback about plans is invaluable. Several possible dispositions might be appropriate, depending on the client's (and family's, if present) interests and motivations. As with Robert and Ryan, in the previous vignettes, you will want to get input from the client (and possibly the family) about the options before a plan is finalized jointly.

Sometimes the input of the family is necessary. In the case of Ryan, the clinician sees that the family has valid worries that he will be unsafe. Since he has a history of wandering about disoriented at night, he has the potential to be a danger to himself. His poor judgment could lead him into dangerous situations, or he could be distracted by hallucinations, wander into the street, and be killed by a vehicle. For his own safety, both the clinician and the family feel that he will be safer in the hospital until he is stable.

PLAN: CONSULT SUPERVISOR

Katherine is uncertain whether she can trust Luisa to wait in the waiting room while she consults her supervisor. They have been working together for only 2 months, and Katherine knows that Luisa is very impulsive. Katherine asks Luisa, "Can you give me a minute to call my supervisor? I need to consult with him briefly." Luisa asks if she should step out, but Katherine assures her that it is fine for her to stay in the office. Katherine calls her supervisor to ask him to come to the office. Her supervisor does not pick up the phone. Katherine then calls a fellow trainee who agrees to go to the supervisor's office and asks him to come to Katherine's office. The supervisor, Ezra Stone, knocks on the door about 5 minutes later. Luisa has met Ezra before. Ezra comes into the office and sits with them while Katherine summarizes Luisa's situation. Ezra agrees with the plan.

Shane feels that Robert can be relied on to wait in the waiting room. He asks Robert to do so, then goes to consult with his supervisor and returns after a few minutes.

Given what Brandi has observed about the family relationships, she feels that Ryan's family can keep him in her office for a few minutes. Brandi asks them if she can step out for a few minutes to consult with her supervisor. She asks, "Can I rely on you to wait here until I get back in about 5 minutes?" They assure her that this is fine.

If you are inexperienced at assessing crises, you will want to consult with a supervisor before giving feedback. Alternatively, if you are more experienced, it may be clear what you need to do, and you will just give your supervisor a quick call to update him or her on the situation at an appropriate point.

If the client has been cooperative and agrees not to leave the facility, you and your supervisor may be able to discuss the case while the client waits in the waiting area or in your office, as with Robert and Ryan in the previous vignettes. However, if you have any concerns about the client's ability to follow through with waiting for 10 to 15 minutes while you consult, as Katherine has concerns about Luisa, your supervisor can join you in the office with the client as you summarize your observations.

If you are afraid that your client will hurt him- or herself, run off, or engage in any risky behavior and you need to step out of the office to find a supervisor, you must ask another staff person to look after the client, or you must take the client to the emergency room if the facility you're working in has one. If your facility has police or security personnel, you may need to call them to escort the client.

PLAN: CONSIDER WHETHER
HOSPITALIZATION IS APPROPRIATE

After discussing her situation with Katherine, Luisa agrees to the plan to go to the inpatient unit.

Brandi tells Ryan and his family that she is worried about his safety and thinks it would be wise for him to be in the hospital. Ryan agrees because he sees that this is what his parents want him to do.

Clients with acute symptoms of psychosis or mania may or may not need to be hospitalized. Each case should be considered on an individual basis. Here are some of the questions you will want to ask yourself regarding the client to determine whether to hospitalize or treat as an outpatient:

- Does the client have insight into own mental illness?
- Can the client be calm and comprehend instructions?
- Does the client verbalize an intention to get and take medications?
- Do you think that the client can be relied on to follow instructions and take medication?
- If psychotic, does the client have sufficient understanding of what is real and what isn't, and can she act appropriately on this knowledge?
- Will the client agree to attend an appointment soon?
- Will the client agree to seek help if worse?
- Can the client or the client's family reliably identify if the client is worse and seek help appropriately?
- Is the family supportive and reliable?
- Is there any risk of harm to self or others?

The client can be managed as an outpatient when the client is engaged well in treatment, has good insight about symptoms, and can be trusted to follow through on appointments and any changes in medication. If there are some deficits in the client's comprehension or follow-though but the client is cooperative and the family is involved, supportive, and reliable, the client may also be able to be treated as an outpatient. If the client can be involved in an intensive partial hospitalization program rather than the more restrictive environment of the inpatient unit, the client and family are more likely to be satisfied with the care (Horvitz-Lennon, Normand, Gaccione, & Frank, 2001).

Sometimes the plan will be to hospitalize the client. Although particular details vary from state to state (Simon, 2004), clients are generally hospitalized when they are a danger to self or others or if they are so mentally ill that they are unable to adequately care for their own needs. In the previous vignette, Ryan cannot keep himself reliably safe because of an exacerbation of his mental illness, so he is considered appropriate for hospitalization.

PLAN: MAKE A CRISIS MANAGEMENT PLAN AND SECURE CLIENT'S VERBAL AGREEMENT

Shane asks Robert if he has a friend he can stay with for a few days. He thinks his friend Tony will let him sleep on his couch.

Finalize a crisis management plan by synthesizing your assessment with the feedback of the client and, if appropriate, the client's family. Get the client's verbal agreement to comply with the plan. (In some settings, there may be a preference for written agreements instead.) Observe the client carefully for signs of insincerity (e.g., hesitancy or sarcastic tone) and reconsider the plan if necessary.

WHEN YOU AND CLIENT DO NOT AGREE ON PLAN

You might have definite ideas about what the plan should be but the client does not like your plan. In this case, carefully explain your concerns and your reasoning to the client and ask for feedback. Then find out what the client's concerns are and do the best you can to address them:

Therapist: "I'm very concerned. You've told me that you can't be sure that you'd call 911 or go to the emergency room if you feel more suicidal. You've come in for help with this, and it's very important to me to take some action to help keep you safe. The only thing I know of that will keep you safe under these circumstances is for you to be in the hospital. Yet you're telling me you don't want to go. What do you suggest that we do under these circumstances?"

Client: "Just let me go. I'll be okay."

Therapist: "Do you have any concerns about being in the hospital?"

Client: "I've seen the movies. I know that psych hospitals are full of dangerous psychos."

Therapist: "Actually, what's in the movies is overly sensationalized. I've visited the unit before, and I can assure you it's a very safe place. The people who are there are seeking help for their problems, just like you are."

Client: "Will you come see me there?"

Therapist: "I can't do that because I need to be here in the intake clinic seeing other people who are in crisis."

Client: "How long will I be there? Can they keep me for weeks?"

Therapist: "They will probably discharge you within a week. And as soon as you aren't suicidal anymore, you can ask to leave at any time, and they can't keep you."

Client: "Okay, I'll go."

When you address the client's concerns, most of the time the client will agree to go to the hospital. In very rare instances, you may have to involuntarily hospitalize a client. Be sure to ask your supervisor what the criteria are for involuntary hospitalization and how this is done in your setting so that you are prepared.

IMPLEMENT PLAN

Luisa expresses some concern about her cats, as she hasn't made any arrangements for them, so Katherine lets her call her mother from the office and ask her to feed the cats while Luisa is in the hospital. Then Katherine escorts Luisa to the emergency room for admission. When in the emergency room, Katherine calls Luisa's psychiatrist to give her an update on the situation. The psychiatrist will need to come to the emergency room to write an admit order.

Robert calls his friend Tony from Shane's office, and Tony tells him that he can stay as long as he needs to. Robert doesn't have any of his clothes or toiletries with him and agrees to ask his mother to bring them over to Tony's. He agrees to stay at Tony's at least until his next appointment with his alcohol counselor, when he can discuss this issue in more detail. Shane suggests that if he does see his brother accidentally before then, he should turn around and leave immediately. Robert readily agrees to do so but thinks this is unlikely. Robert again verbalizes his intent not to hurt his brother despite these impulses. Shane suggests that Robert call his mother as well and update her on these plans. Robert calls his mother from the office, and when he gets off the phone, he says that his mother was relieved and happy to hear that he had taken some steps to get help and resolve this situation. His mother volunteered to bring some of his clothes by his friend's house tonight.

Since the clinic does not have an inpatient unit on-site, Brandi talks to Ryan's parents about where he has been hospitalized before. They have been satisfied with the care he received at St. Joseph's. She recommends that they take him to the emergency room there. She gets a signed release from Ryan to communicate with St. Joseph's. She makes a copy of the release and prints out her progress note about her evaluation of Ryan. She puts these in an envelope and gives them to Ryan's parents with the instructions that they give the envelope to the clinician at the hospital. She puts her supervisor's pager number in the progress note in case hospital staff have any questions. Ryan and his family believe that he will be cooperative in the ride to the hospital, and they agree to take him directly there.

Do whatever you can to implement the plan right then. If you are in a medical center, walk the client from your office to the emergency room for admission. If the client is staying with a friend, have him call the friend from your office and make a plan to get to the friend's house. If the client remains an outpatient, be sure there is an outpatient follow-up appointment made and secure the client's agreement to attend.

DOCUMENT

When documenting a crisis and how it was addressed, it is important to be as thorough as possible. This is the one time when you will want to err on the side of being overly inclusive in your progress note. It is important to do the following (adapted from Rivas-Vasquez, Blais, Rey, & Rivas-Vasquez, 2001):

- Describe the client and chief complaint
- List current symptoms and make appropriate diagnoses
- Summarize relevant historical information, including medical and substance abuse histories as well as prior mental health care
- If time allows, assess and document psychosocial history and family history of mental illness
- Document any consultations you made about the case
- Assess risk and protective factors
- Document client's agreement or disagreement with plan
- Document how the plan was implemented
- Describe, in detail, what your thought process and rationale were in assessing the situation and determining the plan

When you choose a less restrictive plan than hospitalization, be especially detailed about your thought process and rationale. You want the note to be fairly self-contained so that any mental health professional reading it will understand exactly why you made the choices that you did and agree that your choices were consistent with professional standards.

PROGRESS NOTE FOR LUISA

S/O. Luisa Garcia is a 28-year-old Latina female who has been in individual therapy with me for 2 months. Her diagnoses are borderline personality disorder and chronic major depression.

Ms. Garcia presents today with an exacerbation of depressive symptoms: poor eating and sleeping, feeling fatigued, and ruminating constantly about her problems. In addition, she has been thinking seriously about committing suicide and has a plan to jump off a bridge near her home. She states that she has been thinking about this constantly for the past 5 days and has been walking past the site thinking of jumping. She feels uncertain that she can control herself much longer.

Ms. Garcia has a history of suicidal behavior. Last year she took an overdose of her pills and had to have her stomach pumped. Additionally, she had three previous suicide attempts of varying lethality. She has a history of eight previous psychiatric hospitalizations for depression, suicide attempts, and suicidal ideation.

Ms. Garcia does not abuse substances, nor has this ever been an issue for her. She recently lost her mother, on whom she was very dependent, and has been despondent ever since.

A. Ms. Garcia is at significant risk of suicidal behavior given her inability to make a commitment to stay alive and her past history of numerous suicide attempts.

P. Ms. Garcia agreed to inpatient hospitalization at this medical center. She was walked to the emergency room and was medically cleared there, then was admitted to unit 2B.

[Signed]	Katherine Mahoney, B.A.
	Social Work Trainee
[Cosigned]	Ezra Stone, L.C.S.W.

This progress note about Luisa is relatively brief for a crisis note. That is because it is a fairly cut-and-dried situation of acute suicidality in a client with a repeated history of suicidal behavior and because the client was placed in the restrictive environment of the inpatient unit, where they will follow standard procedure and put her on suicide watch.

PROGRESS NOTE FOR ROBERT

S/O. Robert Moore is a 25-year-old White male who presents at the intake clinic stating that he is thinking of killing his brother.

Mr. Moore has a long-standing history of substance abuse and has been treated by the addiction clinic at this facility. With his approval, his substance abuse counselor, Ms. Patterson, was contacted. She said that he has a 15-month history of abstinence, with negative toxicology screens done at random. His compliance with treatment is good, and he has not exhibited any violent or aggressive behavior while in treatment. She stated that she felt he could be counted on to cooperate with any agreed-on crisis management plan.

Mr. Moore admits to having a long history of violent altercations, all of which occurred while he was drunk. However, he states that no one was ever injured seriously, to his knowledge. Mr. Moore denied ever having been charged or convicted of any crimes, which is consistent with all chart documentation.

Mr. Moore stated that he and his brother have been living with their mother in a small one-bedroom apartment. They have been arguing about financial issues and can't get away from each other. He stated that, despite these violent thoughts, he does not want to hurt his brother, which is why he came to the clinic today. Mr. Moore said that as long as his brother is not around, he does not think about hurting him.

A. While Mr. Moore is having homicidal thoughts toward his brother, he showed good judgment coming to the clinic to get assistance in coping with this crisis. He denies any intent to hurt his brother and states that he knows that if he did, he would regret it. He also stated that he wouldn't make his mother suffer like that. He has demonstrated excellent motivation and compliance with treatment over the past 15 months, and his substance abuse counselor has indicated that she trusts him to follow any crisis management plan. Given the above, my assessment is that as long as Robert stays away from his brother and continues to discuss these issues in treatment, he is not at risk of harming his brother.

P. In order to minimize any risk of an altercation, Mr. Moore agreed to call a friend from my office. The friend agreed to let Mr. Moore stay with him as long as he needs to. Mr. Moore agreed to go directly to the friend's house. He called his mother at work, and she agreed to bring some of his clothes and toiletries to his friend's house tonight. This arrangement will prevent him from any interactions with his brother. He agreed to follow up with his substance abuse counselor tomorrow, who will help him further explore these issues and discuss alternative housing options. Will alert Ms. Patterson regarding above.

[Signed]   Shane Abel, M.D.
Psychiatry Resident

As you can see, this note is longer than the previous one. Since Robert will be treated as an outpatient, Shane has very carefully justified his decision-making process. He carefully documents Robert's intent not to harm his brother and Robert's reasons for not doing so. He has ensured that the plan is in place, as much as possible, before Robert leaves his office and documented that he has done so.

Note that there is no mention of Robert's brother being notified of Robert's homicidal thoughts against him—and, in fact, he was not. Why? First, Shane has carefully assessed Robert for homicidal intent and has seen, in fact, that Robert's intent is not to harm his brother. Second, Robert has shown good judgment in seeking help. Robert's reliability in treatment and his agreement to the plan indicate that Robert can be trusted to follow through appropriately. Finally, Shane's professional opinion is that the plan that he and Robert have devised has defused the situation.

PROGRESS NOTE FOR RYAN

S/O. Ryan Fernandes is a 55-year-old East Indian male brought to the clinic by his parents. They are all first-generation immigrants from India, and they are Catholic.

Mr. Fernandes has a long-standing history of schizophrenia. He has been treated for it at this outpatient clinic for 12 years and apparently has had symptoms and treatment since he was 21 years old. His parents report numerous previous hospitalizations, mostly when he stopped taking his medications.

Mr. Fernandes's parents report that he has been pacing all night and talking to himself. His functioning around the house has deteriorated markedly. They admit that they have been distracted lately with the illness of a grandchild and thus haven't been monitoring his medications as closely as they usually do. They also stated that when he has gotten more symptomatic in the past, he has wandered around the neighborhood in his pajamas, talking about "converting the heathens." Today, Mr. Fernandes says that God is telling him that he has been "anointed to convert the heathens." I also observed him looking around the room as if responding to internal stimuli. Mr. Fernandes states that he has been taking his medications, but his report may be unreliable because of current symptoms of thought disorder.

A. Mr. Fernandes is having an exacerbation of long-standing schizophrenia. There is significant risk that he could be a danger to himself by wandering the neighborhood at night when his parents are asleep. He is having auditory hallucinations, probable visual hallucinations, agitation, and delusions that he was anointed by God to convert the heathens. He has almost certainly been missing his medications. His parents do not feel that they can manage him at home at this time.

P. Because of the risk of self-harm through poor judgment, Mr. Fernandes will be taken for hospitalization to St. Joseph's Medical Center. Mr. Fernandes agreed to this plan, and his parents will drive him there. He signed a release of information, and they will bring a copy of this progress note with them for the emergency room staff. I consulted with Dr. Xavier about this plan, and he agreed to the disposition. His pager number is 312-555-0129 if further information is needed.

[Signed]	Brandi Williams, M.A.
	Psychology Practicum Student
[Cosigned]	Thomas Xavier, Ph.D.
	Staff Psychologist

Just because a client with schizophrenia is having an exacerbation of symptoms does not mean that the client needs hospitalization. However, in this case, because of the risk of harm through poor judgment, hospitalization is the wisest choice. Brandi makes this reasoning clear in the previous chart note.

RECOMMENDED READINGS

See chapters 19 to 21 for recommended readings on specific crisis assessment topics.

EXERCISES AND DISCUSSION QUESTIONS

1. What are the procedures for initiating voluntary hospitalization at your facility?

2. What are the procedures for involuntary hospitalization? What are the legal requirements to initiate involuntary hospitalization in your state?

Chapter Nineteen

Suicidality and Self-Harm

Assessing risk of suicide is one of the most important yet terrifying tasks that a beginning clinician can do. It is also professionally risky in terms of practitioner emotional distress and risk for malpractice suits (Packman, Pennuto, Bongar, & Orthwein, 2004). Suicide is the most frequent crisis seen by mental health practitioners (McAdams & Foster, 2000), and almost half the persons who commit suicide are under the care of a mental health practitioner (Institute of Medicine, 2002). Suicide is the 11th most common cause of death in the United States (National Institute of Mental Health, 2004).

Often, beginning therapists work with high-risk populations, such as those in community mental health centers, but suicidal ideation can occur in any population. Thus, you must be prepared to assess and cope with suicidality from your very first day of clinical work.

In this chapter, I focus on performing a thorough suicide risk assessment with adult outpatients. Additional considerations are pertinent to inpatients and emergency settings, and if you are working in those settings, relevant literature should be reviewed (e.g., Simon, 2004). The following steps in assessing, treating, and documenting suicidality are discussed:

- Establish rapport (see chapter 18)
- Assess
  - Screen for suicide risk
  - Current suicidal ideation
  - Past suicide attempts
  - Current and past self-harm
  - Current mental illness and distress
  - Poor judgment, poor self-control, impulsivity, and unpredictability
  - Precipitant and chronic stressors

245

- ○ Demographic and historical factors
- ○ Protective factors
- ○ Other sources of information
- ○ Assess level of risk
- ○ Determine motivation for treatment
- • Plan and implement
  - ○ Determine appropriate intervention level
  - ○ Make a suicide prevention plan and secure client's verbal agreement
  - ○ Implement precautions for outpatients
  - ○ Reduce risk factors and enhance protective factors
  - ○ Hospitalize, if necessary
- • Reduce self-harm and suicidal gestures
- • Document

ASSESS: SCREEN FOR SUICIDE RISK

Tony Sanchez, a mental health trainee, is working in a walk-in intake clinic. He is assigned a new client, Phil Thomas, to interview. Phil has never been to the clinic before, and there is no chart for Tony to review. Phil is a 66-year-old White male who is accompanied by his 64-year-old sister, Susie. Tony speaks with both of them first. Susie says that she has been worried about Phil's mental health since he lost his wife to lung cancer 3 months ago. Lately, she says, Phil has not been taking care of himself, and when she comes by, he has been sitting alone in the dark, with the television on, but doesn't appear to be actually watching it. Tony asks Susie to step outside and wait, then assesses Phil for depressive symptoms. He then screens Phil for suicide risk: "Are you having any thoughts about hurting yourself?" Phil tells him that he sometimes thinks of blowing his head off with his shotgun. Tony asks Phil how long he has had these thoughts. Phil says that he has been thinking of hurting himself ever since his wife's funeral. Tony asks whether Phil has ever had thoughts of hurting himself before his wife died. Phil denies it. Tony asks whether any family members of Phil's have committed suicide. Phil says that his paternal grandfather committed suicide many decades ago. Tony asks Phil whether he has been feeling hopeless. Phil answers, "Yes."

Fred Takahashi is a mental health trainee who has been assigned a new client, Crystal Hughes, a 27-year-old White female. At their first session, Fred notices that Crystal has five parallel superficial scratches on her left forearm and asks her about them. Crystal says that she loves her girlfriend and does not want to leave her, but she is certain that the girlfriend has not been sexually faithful because she snooped last week and found suspicious messages on her e-mail and cell phone. The girlfriend denied this when she accused her last night, and they argued. After their fight, Crystal felt intense distress and anxiety. Fred asks Crystal whether she has been thinking of killing herself. She says that last night, she was thinking of slashing her wrists but ended up cutting herself instead. She locked herself in the bathroom, took out a razor blade, and scratched her arm until it bled. When Fred asks Crystal whether she has been feeling hopeless, she says that she is feeling hopeless and wants to die. Fred asks her if she has any relatives who have committed suicide, and she denies this.

Often, beginning therapists are afraid to ask clients about suicidal thoughts. They fear that asking about suicidal thoughts might implant suicidal ideas in the client's head. However, there is no scientific evidence that this is the case (Moline, Williams, & Austin, 1998). In fact, if you do not ask about suicidality, you may miss an opportunity to intervene to prevent a suicide, and you may put your professional career at risk.

Every time you meet a new client, it is wise to do a suicide assessment (Moline et al., 1998). Your client may have been prescreened for you by your supervisor and/or the clinic, but life circumstances can change quickly, so you also should assess for suicidality. Determining an accurate diagnosis of mental illness (if one is present) and asking the following four screening questions should be an adequate screening for suicidality:

"Are you having any thoughts about hurting yourself? [If yes] Tell me about that."
"Has that ever been a problem for you?"
"Have you been feeling hopeless?"
"Have you had any family members who have committed suicide?"

Most clients will answer no to all these questions, and you are done in just a couple minutes. Simon (2004) suggests that if the answer to any of these questions is positive, a thorough suicide risk assessment should be done. The rest of this chapter describes the procedure for doing a suicide risk assessment.

If the client hesitates when you've asked about suicide, then answers no, remark on that: "Are you sure? I noticed that you were hesitant." In addition, if the client has significant depressive symptomatology, further probing about suicidality may be indicated, even if denied (Jacobs & Brewer, 2006). Note that studies have found that many clients who have suicidal ideation will deny it when asked, so if the client has other significant risk factors, you may want to talk to family members or significant others and/or ask again when there is a stronger therapeutic alliance.

Note that assessing for suicide risk is an ongoing process with many clients. Suicide risk varies from minute to minute, hour to hour, and day to day because suicidal behaviors are impulsive and transient (Simon, 2006). Clients with a recent suicidal crisis should have their suicidal ideation reevaluated every time they are seen until they are stable and the suicidal ideation is consistently over. Clients with chronic suicidal ideation may need to be assessed at every session as long as the suicidal ideation lasts.

ASSESS: CURRENT SUICIDAL IDEATION

Tony asks Phil more questions about his current suicidal ideation: "Phil, tell me some more about your thoughts about hurting yourself." Phil says, "I think about taking out my rifle, putting it in my mouth, and pulling the trigger." Tony ascertains that there is a gun in the house, along with ammunition, and that it is kept in a locked cabinet in the basement. Tony asks Phil, "Do you think you would ever actually pull the trigger?" Phil says that he doesn't know. Tony asks Phil how often he thinks about hurting himself. Phil says that he thinks about it off and on every day.

Fred asks Crystal more about her suicidal ideation. Crystal says that she has been thinking about taking all her Prozac, but at other times she thinks about slitting her wrists. She says that it would serve her girlfriend right to come in and find her bleeding to death in the tub. Fred asks her whether she thinks she would act on these thoughts. Crystal says that she thinks she might. Fred asks how often she is thinking about killing herself. Crystal says that she has had these thoughts off and on for years but that she has been thinking about this more since she found the messages last week.

The presence of current suicidal ideation is the most important predictor of suicide risk. Here are some of the questions you could ask to assess suicidal ideation (informed by Jacobs & Brewer, 2006):

> "When did the suicidal ideas start? Are the thoughts every day? How often throughout the day? When was the last suicidal thought. Today? Yesterday? Last week?"
> "Have you made a specific plan to hurt yourself?"
> "Do you think you would ever act on those thoughts? Why or why not?"
> "Are these passing thoughts, or are you serious about them?"
> "Do you have any ideas about how you might kill yourself?"
> "How often have these thoughts occurred?"
> "What is the closest you've come to hurting yourself?"
> "Have you ever started to hurt yourself but stopped before doing anything?"
> "How would you hurt yourself?"
> "Do you have any guns or weapons available to you?"
> "Have you made any preparations to hurt yourself?"
> "If you begin to have thoughts about hurting yourself again, what would you do?"

You do not need to ask every one of these questions to every client—these are just to give you an idea what you may need to ask to get the full picture. Once you have this information, you need to consider the likelihood that the client will act on the ideation (this discussion is informed by Joiner, Walker, Rudd, & Jobes, 1999). The most important predictors of acting on suicidal ideation are having a plan and having the intent to act on it. In assessing the plan, consider the following:

- Presence of a specific plan
- The client has the means and the opportunity to enact this plan (e.g., a gun is readily available)
- The client has been preparing to enact this plan (e.g., the client wants to overdose and has stockpiled medications)

In assessing intent, consider the following:

- Whether the client has determination and courage to follow through on suicide attempt
- Whether the client feels competent to kill self
- Whether suicidal ideas have been persistent and intense

Clients who have suicidal thoughts but neither a suicidal plan nor suicidal intent have *passive suicidal ideation*. They will talk about their suicidal ideation in this way:

"I wish I were dead."
"Everyone would be better off if I were gone."
"I wish I had never been born."
"I don't care about my life anymore."

These clients, unless they have other significant suicidal risk factors (as discussed in the rest of this chapter), are considered to be either not at risk (Joiner et al., 1999) or at low risk of suicide. However, even if the suicidal ideation is passive, you should continue to perform and document a full suicide risk assessment (Simon, 2004).

Clients with a suicide plan and/or suicidal intent have *active suicidal ideation*. Even if the suicidal ideation has been fleeting and brief, consider the client to be at risk if there are suicide plans (Joiner et al., 1999). If clients have active suicidal ideation, they will talk about suicidal ideation like this:

"Whenever I go over that bridge, I think that if I was really brave, I would crash off with the car into the water."

"I've got a gun, and I often think I should kill myself."

"Sometimes I think of hanging myself off the rafters in the garage. No one would find me until I were dead."

"I think about taking an overdose of my pills, but I know that my children would be devastated."

"If I had the guts, I'd kill myself."

"If I killed myself, then my boyfriend would understand how he hurt me."

In conclusion, here are some initial determinations about levels of suicide risk that you could make from assessing current suicidal ideation:

- The client has passive suicidal ideation but no other significant risk factors (as described in the rest of the chapter). Risk level: none to low.
- The client has passive suicidal ideation and has other risk factors of significance. Risk level: low to high, depending on what the other risk factors are.
- The client has active suicidal ideation. Risk level: moderate to high on the basis of this risk factor alone. Note that as the interview progresses, the client may become interested in following through with the treatment plan and that intent may lessen, decreasing risk.

ASSESS: PAST SUICIDE ATTEMPTS

When asked by Tony, Phil denies any history of past suicidal ideation, behavior, or self-harm prior to his wife's death.

When asked, Crystal says that she has been hospitalized twice in the past after making suicide attempts. She points out very faint scars on her wrists that Fred had not noticed before and said that she cut her wrists when she was 16 years old after being rejected by a boyfriend. She said that the second hospitalization was last year and that she had taken a half bottle of Xanax but then got scared and called 911.

Past suicide attempts are the second most important predictor of current suicide risk after the presence of active suicidal ideation. Persons who have made past suicide attempts are at a much higher risk than any other group for completed suicide. Past attempters have risk of completed suicide that is 38 times (in an aggregate of many studies; E. C. Harris & Barraclough, 1997) to over 100 times (in a review of international studies; Owens, Horrocks, & House, 2002) greater than the general population. Persons who have attempted suicide at least twice, known as *multiple attempters*, are the group at greatest risk of future suicide and suicide attempts (Joiner et al., 1999). Thus, past suicide attempts must be thoroughly evaluated, and clients with past attempts, especially those with more than one attempt, must be very carefully monitored and treated. *Note that past suicidal ideation, without any history of suicidal behavior, is so common that it is a poor predictor of risk*, although it can still be informative to assess.

To assess past suicide attempts, ask the following:

"Have you had any thoughts of hurting yourself in the past?"
"Have you ever done anything to hurt yourself in the past?"

If the client appears to be confused or you suspect forgetfulness or minimizing, ask further specific questions, such as "Have you ever been hospitalized for an emotional problem?" or "What was going on when you went to the hospital?"

When the client reveals a past episode of suicide attempts, gather as much information about that episode as possible:

"How old were you?" (or "When was that?")
"What was going on with you at the time?"
"Were you using drugs or alcohol then?"
"How did you hurt yourself? What happened then?"
"Did you get any help? Did you go to the hospital?"
Then ask the client, "Other than that, were there any other times in the past when you felt like hurting yourself?"

Keep asking this question and then asking about the specific episodes until the client denies that there are any other previous episodes of suicidal thoughts or behavior.

You should always review any mental health records that are immediately available regarding past suicidality. If ongoing treatment is anticipated, send releases to get records from past treatment facilities for any client with any level of suicide risk (Packman, Pennuto et al., 2004). If the family is available, consider getting a written or oral (crisis situation) agreement from the client to talk to them (and document that agreement in the chart), then ask them for their perspectives on the client's past suicidal behavior (Simon, 1988).

The clients who tell you about past suicidal ideation, attempts, and self-harm will fall into several (possibly overlapping) categories:

- More than one previous suicide attempt with intent to die
- One suicide attempt with intent to die
- Past suicidal gesture(s) without intent to die (e.g., scratches wrist with razor just before boyfriend is due home because she is angry at him)
- Self-harm behavior without intent to die (e.g., superficially scratches self with knife on leg or gives self an ugly homemade tattoo on arm with ink from a pen)
- Past suicidal ideation but no attempts or self-harm
- No previous history of suicide attempts, self-harm, or ideation

These groups are listed from most to least risk of suicide (Joiner et al., 1999; Nock & Kessler, 2006). Again, be very cautious with any client who has more than one previous suicide attempt; these clients should be considered to be at moderate to high risk if additional significant suicidal risk factors are present (Joiner et al., 1999). The risk level of the other groups is significantly lower and must be assessed in the context of other risk factors that are present. Note, however, that a suicidal gesture can be fatal, even if not intended to be, and thus past suicidal gestures should be considered to be indicative of significantly higher risk.

ASSESS: CURRENT AND PAST SELF-HARM

Crystal reports that after she cut herself yesterday, she felt relief and could "float above my problems." She said that she didn't feel any pain at all from the scratches. Fred asks her if she has hurt herself before. "Many times," Crystal replies.

"Have you ever done anything to hurt yourself?" will usually elicit self-harm behavior as well as suicidal behavior. However, initially the client may deny this but volunteer it later, or you may see suspicious injuries and ask about them, as Fred did earlier in the chapter.

It is not always possible to know whether a client meant a past episode of self-harm to be fatal. However, whenever possible, ascertain whether the self-injurious behavior was meant as an actual suicide attempt: "Did you actually mean to kill yourself?"

There is a lack of definitional clarity regarding self-harm and suicide; however, Nock and Kessler (2006) argue that a distinction can and should be made between genuine suicide attempts and suicidal gestures in which there is not any intent to die but rather a cry for help. Self-harm is a sign of acute distress. Current and past self-harm is often seen in multiple suicide attempters. Additionally, self-harm is associated with other risk factors for suicidal behavior: substance abuse (Nock & Kessler, 2006), antisocial personality disorder (Nock & Kessler, 2006), borderline personality disorder (Linehan et al., 2006), comorbidity (three or more diagnoses; Nock & Kessler, 2006), and histories of childhood sexual abuse (Gratz, 2003). Note that self-harm is more common in women (McAndrew & Warne, 2005).

Self-inflicted injuries are often burns or scratches on the skin; they are often on the arms but may also be on the legs, abdomen, or other areas of the body. Clients may wear clothing that covers the area when in public. Self-harm can also include self-poisoning by overdosing on medications, alcohol, or street drugs.

If the client admits to injuring self, ask where the injuries are. If there are cuts or other injuries in an area that you can observe, without the client inappropriately disrobing, you might ask if you can see them. Even if you are not a physician, it is likely that you will be able to see whether the cuts are superficial or whether it would be wise to have a medical evaluation. If your have any doubt whether the client significantly damaged self, a physician or nurse should be consulted. If the self-inflicted injury is in a more private location, such as the inner thigh, you should get a nurse, psychiatrist, or another physician to examine the injuries. If none of these health professionals is on-site, you may need to obtain a release of information to talk to the client's physician.

ASSESS: CURRENT MENTAL ILLNESS AND DISTRESS

Tony assesses Phil for symptoms of depression. Phil has poor appetite and has lost 15 pounds in the past 2 months. He is not sleeping well. He is feeling either numb or depressed most of the time and cries uncontrollably when thinking about how much he misses his wife. He feels guilty that he did not appreciate her enough when she was alive. Tony screens Phil for bipolar disorder, post-traumatic stress disorder (PTSD), and psychotic symptoms, but these are denied.

Fred assesses Crystal for mental illness. She had a history of bulimia in high school but denied any problems with that in recent years. She has many symptoms of major depression. When asked about manic symptoms, she describes an episode in the past that might have been hypomanic, but Fred is not sure. Clearly, Crystal is in great distress.

After active suicidal ideation and past suicidal behavior, the presence of certain mental illnesses is the third-strongest predictor of suicide. All other factors are less significant predictors in research studies than these three. Almost all mental illnesses have been associated with increased mortality from suicide (E. C. Harris & Barraclough, 1997; Institute of Medicine, 2002).

E. C. Harris and Barraclough (1997) reviewed the research and derived combined risks of suicide for a number of mental illnesses (based on criteria from the *Diagnostic and Statistical Manual of Mental Disorders* [3rd ed., revised]; *DSM-III-R*) by aggregating numbers across studies. These numbers indicate the degree of increased risk compared to the general population. Here are the findings of this study:

- Eating disorders, 23 times (23 times the rate of suicide in the general population)
- Major depression, 20 times

- Bipolar I disorder, 15 times (since the diagnostic criteria of the studies that were aggregated were based on *DSM-III-R*, bipolar II was not included)
- Dysthymia, 12 times
- Obsessive-compulsive disorder, 10 times (the authors suspect that number should be higher)
- Panic disorder, 10 times
- Schizophrenia, 8.5 times
- Brief reactive psychosis, 15 times
- Personality disorders, 7 times
- Adjustment disorder, 14 times

Note that E. C. Harris and Barraclough (1997) did not include PTSD in this study, and comparable rates are unavailable. However, it is known that PTSD does increase risk of suicide (Hudenko, n.d.).

A review of risk factors in depression (Institute of Medicine, 2002) indicated that certain depressive symptoms are more predictive of suicide: suicidal ideation, hopelessness, guilt, loss of interest in usual activities, low self-esteem, cognitive distortions, and few perceived reasons for living. Hopelessness, especially, may be a particularly significant risk factor for suicide (Packman, Marlitt, Bongar, & Pennuto, 2004).

Emotional distress is likely to be an important factor mediating the relationship between a diagnosis of mental illness and suicidality. Thus, in addition to noting the client's diagnosis, carefully attend to the client's distress about current symptoms. In particular, such factors as comorbidity of diagnoses and symptom severity can increase suicide risk (Simon, 2004). The reality of having a mental illness is often highly distressing for high-functioning clients; this may put them at greater suicide risk (Simon, 2004). The combination of severe depression along with anxiety and/or panic attacks can be especially distressing and predictive of suicide risk (Simon, 2004). Since clients are discharged so quickly from inpatient units, they are rarely completely stable. The week after discharge is an especially high-risk period for suicide, and the 3 months after discharge continue to be high-risk time for suicide (Appleby et al., 1999).

ASSESS: POOR JUDGMENT, POOR SELF-CONTROL, IMPULSIVITY, AND UNPREDICTABILITY

Tony assesses Phil for substance abuse. Phil admits that he has often been drinking a six-pack of beer every day, sometimes followed by hard liquor. Phil says that the alcohol dulls the pain of his loss. At this point, Phil admits that when he is very drunk, he will sometimes take out the shotgun and cradle it on his lap, thinking of killing himself. However, he states that lately his sister Susie has been bringing him to her Alcoholics Anonymous (AA) meetings with her, as Susie is a recovering alcoholic herself. He stated that he has been trying to cut down on the alcohol, and that he had 2 days last week when he did not drink.

Crystal admits that she occasionally uses cocaine and marijuana. She said that she was drunk when she made the two previous suicide attempts. She stated that she drinks alcohol on the weekend when out with friends. When screened for psychotic symptoms, Crystal says that she sometimes hears a voice telling her to kill herself.

Client characteristics that are indicative of greater impulsivity or less self-control are generally linked to greater suicidality (Joiner et al., 1999). Those who are incarcerated and those with antisocial personality disorder are at increased risk (Verona, Sachs-Ericsson, & Joiner, 2004). Clients with a history of poor follow-through in treatment are at greater risk (Joiner et al., 1999). Certain symptoms may also contribute to lack of self-control; the client may not be getting much sleep or may have reduced concentration. Clients with a history of head trauma are at greater risk of suicide (Krakowski & Czobor, 2004).

The presence of command hallucinations to commit suicide should be evaluated (Simon, 2004), so ascertain whether clients with psychotic symptoms are having auditory hallucinations telling them to kill themselves. If so, find out if the client feels that the commands can be resisted, if the client wants to resist the command, how often the voices are occurring, and if there is a known voice (client may be more likely to act if the voice seems to be that of a known person).

Alcohol or drug abuse significantly increases the risk of suicide (and other impulsive behaviors as well; all risks from E. C. Harris & Barraclough, 1997):

- Sedative dependence and abuse, 20 times (20 times the rate of suicide in the general population)
- Multiple dependence and drug abuse, 20 times
- Opioid dependence and abuse, 14 times
- Alcohol dependence and abuse, 6 times
- Cannabis heavy use, 4 times

ASSESS: PRECIPITANT AND CHRONIC STRESSORS

Tony asks Phil about his stress. Phil talks about how he has had to learn how to do his own laundry and cooking since his wife died. His wife managed all the finances as well, and he has been ignoring the bills. Phil has arthritis in both hips, which has been very painful lately. He has been putting off getting the hip replacements that his doctors recommended. He is uncertain if he can afford to keep his current condo, given the loss of his wife's pension and Social Security.

Crystal tells Fred that she has been under a lot of stress. Her younger sister has been staying with her and would otherwise be homeless, but they argue all the time. Crystal is distressed about the recent argument with her girlfriend and fears that they will break up. She hasn't gone to her job for the last 3 days and fears that she will be fired.

Ask the client about recent stressors: "Has anything stressful been going on in your life lately?" Both Phil and Crystal have experienced significant stressors lately that have contributed to emotional instability and suicidal ideation.

A wide variety of stressors have been linked to suicide attempts. These include losing a job, poverty, sickness-related absence from work, and chronic illness or disability (K. L. Knox, Conwell, & Caine, 2004). The presence of shame, possibly associated with important recent losses, can also increase risk of suicide (Simon, 2004). Serious medical problems such as AIDS, seizure disorder, spinal cord injury, brain injury, Huntington's chorea, and multiple sclerosis have been found to increase the risk of suicide two to seven times (E. C. Harris & Barraclough, 1997), so it would be wise to consider any chronic serious medical problem a suicide risk factor. Interpersonal trauma, whether recent (e.g., domestic violence) or remote (e.g., childhood physical or sexual abuse), increases risk of suicidality (Packman, Marlitt et al., 2004). Social isolation increases risk of suicide in general (Packman, Marlitt et al., 2004)—those who are single or live alone are at greater risk of suicide (Institute of Medicine, 2002)—and the loss of a spouse is a particularly salient stressor that can precipitate suicidality (Louma & Pearson, 2002), especially among men under 35 years old.

ASSESS: DEMOGRAPHIC AND HISTORICAL FACTORS

Tony considers Phil's demographic risk factors. Phil is a White male, over the age of 65, and thus is in a very high-risk group. He has recently become a widower, increasing his risk. He also has a family member who committed suicide, which again increases his risk.

A number of demographic factors are associated with suicidality. Men are three to four times more likely to commit suicide then women, although women make three to four times as many attempts (Simon, 2004). Whites and Native Americans are more likely to commit suicide than Asian Americans or African Americans. Historically, older people were at greater risk for suicide, although that may be changing (Packman, Marlitt et al., 2004). However, White males over the age of 65 are at particularly high risk, and White males over 85 are at even greater risk (Simon, 2004). People who live in more rural areas are at increased risk (Singh & Siahpush, 2002). People who are divorced are at greater risk than those who are married (Institute of Medicine, 2002).

Some historical factors that are associated with suicide risk include suicide in a parent, which is estimated to increase risk in the client six times (Brent et al., 2002). Suicide in other family members increases risk of suicide in the client as well (Simon, 2004). Strangely, women who have breast implants have about two to three times the rate of suicide as comparable women in the general population (McLaughlin, Wise, & Lipworth, 2004).

ASSESS: PROTECTIVE FACTORS

Tony asks Phil what has kept him alive until now. Phil talks about how much he loves his two grandsons, who live nearby. They used to get together every week and play catch and board games. Phil learned to play their favorite video games, "although I always lose," he says with a smile. He says, "I know what it is like to lose a grandfather to suicide and don't know if I can do that to them. But maybe they'd be better off without me." He says that he has been avoiding his grandsons "because they shouldn't see me like this." Tony tells Phil that he is sure that his grandsons would not be better off without him and that, in fact, if he committed suicide, that would put them at greater risk of suicide later in life. Phil says that he would not want that to happen. Tony suggests that Phil and his grandsons can be a comfort to each other, and Phil agrees that this might be true. Tony asks Phil about his relationship with his sister. They have always been close and raised their children and grandchildren together. Susie has been looking in on Phil and making him eat and go out to AA meetings every day. Phil says that he feels that she has helped keep him alive. Tony asks Phil, "Would you be willing to come for treatment regularly, for your family, if not for yourself?" Phil says that he would.

Fred asks Crystal what has been keeping her alive. She says that she has a close relationship with her younger sister and has been trying to help her out since her sister lost her job last month. Both of their parents have died, and she feels responsible for her sister. She says, "I think about killing myself, then I think about how my little sister would then be all alone."

Each client has unique protective factors. Ask whether client has any reasons to live:

"What has kept you alive so far?"
"What made you decide to come in and talk to me today?"
"Why do you say that you couldn't commit suicide?"

Carefully note what these reasons are. These are probably protective factors. Clients who have more coping skills, greater self-control, greater self-efficacy, and more adaptive coping skills are at less risk (Institute of Medicine, 2002).

Protective factors often involve social and family functioning. Having young dependent children, being pregnant, or having a caring partner can be protective (Institute of Medicine, 2002). Thinking about the pain that suicide would cause to one's close family members can be protective. A close circle of friends or any other supportive group can be protective. Being actively involved in organized religion can be protective (Institute of Medicine, 2002), and some religions have explicit prohibitions against suicide that clients may take very seriously.

Engagement in treatment can be considered a protective factor. Being in a low-risk suicide group (e.g., young African American women) can be considered a protective factor. A sense of efficacy to cope with the crisis can be protective. If the client feels hopeful and has plans for the future or events to look forward to, this can be protective. Even being afraid of the pain of committing suicide can be considered a protective factor (for a longer list of empirically generated reasons for living, see Linehan, Goodstein, Nielsen, & Chiles, 1983).

ASSESS: OTHER SOURCES OF INFORMATION

Tony feels that Phil is not at immediate risk to hurt himself or leave the clinic, as Phil has verbalized his willingness to get help. He asks Phil to wait in the waiting room and asks if it is okay for him to talk to Susie for a few minutes. Phil gives his verbal agreement. Tony then asks Susie some questions. He briefly verifies Phil's report that he has not been suicidal in the past and has never gotten any mental health treatment. Susie says that Phil was not bathing regularly after the funeral until she started stopping by each day. She said that he seems to be recognizing more that he needs to get professional help and stop drinking. However, she worries about him a great deal. He has been refusing to go anywhere with her but to the grocery store and AA meetings until today.

When possible, talking to the client's family and significant others, as Tony does in the previous vignette, will sometimes reveal significant information that the client did not volunteer. Collateral information from the family can be especially useful when no other historical documentation is available, as in the case of Phil.

Whenever you are working with a client, you should be aware of information that is in the client's chart. This is even more important with any potentially suicidal client. You must thoroughly review the chart, document that you did so, and be aware of any relevant information from the chart that is pertinent to the suicide risk assessment. You should also be in regular contact with other mental health professionals at your facility who have regular sessions with the client and be aware of what they have learned regarding the client's suicide risk. Keep up to date with current chart notes from other clinicians as treatment progresses.

If the client was treated in private practice, chart records can sometimes be unavailable or insufficient. In those cases, obtain a signed release, call the practitioner and discuss any suicidal behavior or ideation during the previous episode of treatment, and then document the call thoroughly in the client's current chart. If the client was treated at other facilities, you should obtain copies of those records and review that information as well. Often, phone contact with a prior treating mental health practitioner and/or review of a faxed discharge summary can and should be done in a timely manner (Simon, 2004). Again, document this clinical activity in the chart.

ASSESS: LEVEL OF RISK

Tony's initial assessment is that Phil is at moderate risk. Phil has significant risk factors, specifically, that he is a recently bereaved older White male. Phil also has a suicide plan; specifically, he been thinking of using a gun, a very lethal method of suicide. Phil has also been drinking, which puts him at greater risk. However, Tony sees that Phil has expressed and demonstrated some willingness for treatment and that he has remaining family members who care about him and have good relationships with him. Phil also has no previous history of suicidal ideation or behavior. Tony suspects that if he can engage Phil in treatment, that will lower his risk quickly, but Tony is willing to revise his risk assessment to high risk if Phil does not readily agree with all his recommendations and the suicide prevention plan.

Fred's initial assessment is that Crystal is at high risk. Crystal has significant risk factors, including two previous suicide attempts, substance use, recent self-harm, and acute distress. Crystal has two suicide plans that she has been contemplating. Fred thinks that Crystal should be hospitalized.

Each client is a unique individual and has unique risks and protective factors. Thus, no one risk factor can be used in isolation, and a thorough evaluation is needed in every case. Keep in mind that no particular suicide can be predicted with accuracy. Suicide is a *low-base-rate* event (Institute of Medicine, 2002), meaning that it happens so infrequently that accurate prediction is impossible. Literally thousands of research studies have evaluated various aspects of suicidality, yet still, with any single client, it is impossible to accurately predict suicide. We can only ascertain whether the client is at risk and the level of risk.

When comparing the current situation to past suicide attempts, consider the following signs of high risk:

- In the past, the client was involuntarily committed for being a danger to self and others. In this case, you'd be more concerned about the client's ability to follow through appropriately.
- Risk factors have worsened. For example, the client has a new boyfriend who has introduced her to crack cocaine.
- The client's suicidal behaviors have progressively worsened over the years (Yufit, 2005). Again, be very concerned if this is the case; the client is probably high risk.

Here are some signs of lower risk in the case of past suicide attempts:

- Risk factors have improved. For example, the client is now abstinent from alcohol.
- Demographic risk factors have improved. For example, a client might have cut her wrists when she was 16 years old and had a breakup with a boyfriend. You meet the client when she is 32 years old, and she has passive suicidal ideation and a young child. The client's demographic risk factors have changed for the better (she is no longer an adolescent, and she is the mother of a young child), so she is probably at much less risk now than in the past.
- In recent crisis situations, the client has asked for help from professionals, thus refraining from any suicidal behavior.

When we think about Crystal, we see that her risk level is probably about the same as in the past circumstances in which she made suicide attempts (e.g., when using substances or under stress). Therefore, hospitalization is a prudent choice.

Many articles and books talk about the importance of assessing risk level, but few give guidelines for labeling the level of risk for a particular client. However, several references (Jacobs & Brewer, 2006; Joiner et al., 1999; Simon, 1988) are useful in this regard. Although no description can be comprehensive, I have provided some case vignettes and descriptions in appendix 20 to help you learn how to assess and label your clients' risk levels. I recommend that you use these to supplement what you have learned in this chapter so that you understand how to make a risk-level determination.

ASSESS: MOTIVATION FOR TREATMENT

Tony sees that Phil has shown good engagement and motivation for treatment. It is a good sign that he has been willing to follow his sister's recommendations and go to AA as well as come to the clinic today. Tony is concerned, but he also sees positive signs regarding Phil's engagement and motivation for treatment. As the interview progresses, Phil appears relieved and more willing to get help. Phil even smiled when talking earlier about his grandsons.

As you discuss a suicide prevention plan and attempt to work with the client to reduce risk factors and enhance protective factors, you will notice the emotions and responses of the client. Ask yourself these questions:

- Is the affect of the client becoming brighter as the session progresses?
- Does the client readily agree to treatment recommendations?
- Does the client readily agree to the suicide prevention plan?
- Is the client open to your reframing of the situation (e.g., that coming in for evaluation and treatment was wise and courageous)?

All these would indicate that the client is becoming more hopeful as the evaluation session progresses and thus will now be at significantly lower risk. This means that outpatient treatment could be considered for this client if careful consideration of other risk factors does not contraindicate it.

Be concerned if you notice signs that the client is unlikely to engage in continued treatment, including these:

- The client seems unconnected to you.
- The client seems uninterested in treatment recommendations and uninvolved in the treatment process.
- The client repeatedly talks about barriers to mental health treatment (e.g., "I can't come in because I have to take care of my elderly mother").
- The client indicates that only weak people need treatment.

- The client has a history of stopping treatment immediately after past crises resolved.

As Simon (1988) states, "The presence of a therapeutic alliance is a bedrock indicator of the patient's willingness to seek help and sustenance through personal relationships during emotional crisis, and is one of the most important nonverbal statements of a desire to live" (pp. 92–93). So be aware of any signs that your client is not engaging in treatment or has been unable to in the past because a suicidal client who is unwilling to engage in continuing treatment is at greater risk (Joiner et al., 1999).

PLAN: DETERMINE THE APPROPRIATE INTERVENTION LEVEL

Tony asks both Phil and Susie back into his office since he sees that they are close, and he realizes that involving Susie in the treatment will enhance the likelihood of success. He says to Phil, "I see that you have been suffering a lot lately. Unfortunately, your grief has been so severe that it has turned into ongoing depression. Depression is very treatable. I can see that we need to take what is going on with you very seriously. I'd like to ask you to attend an intensive daily program that we have here at this facility. You would come every weekday for intensive treatment, but you'd get to stay in the comfort of your own home at night. Would you be willing to do that?" Phil agrees to this plan.

You will need to choose between three levels of intervention for your clients who have suicidal ideation. Here are the levels:

- Individual weekly psychotherapy as usual: suitable only for no-risk or low-risk clients.
- More intensive outpatient treatment, tailored to the client's needs: suitable for clients with moderate risk who readily and believably agree to suicide prevention plan and attend treatment. Tailor the more intensive treatment to the client's individualized needs. Consider the following:
  - Partial hospitalization program
  - Substance abuse treatment
  - Dialectical behavior therapy or other psychotherapy group
  - More individual therapy sessions per week
  - Community support groups (such as AA)
- Hospitalization: suitable for a high-risk client.

PLAN: MAKE A SUICIDE PREVENTION PLAN
AND SECURE CLIENT'S VERBAL AGREEMENT

Tony says to Phil, "I'm still concerned about your suicidal thoughts. We can't help you if you aren't alive to be helped. I know that it has been painful to lose your wife, but I also know that you have a lot of family members who love you and want you to be around for them." Phil nods his agreement. Tony continues, "I'd like to ask you to make a suicide prevention plan with me. I'd like you to agree to give up the gun and let Susie dispose of it or keep it in a safe place for you to have later when you are feeling better. Would you be okay with that?" Phil indicates his agreement. Tony continues, "I'd also like you to agree to call 911 or go to the nearest emergency room if you are having these ideas of hurting yourself and you think that you might be at risk of actually doing something to hurt yourself. Can I count on you to do that?" Phil readily agrees.

Should you suggest that the outpatient client call you when feeling more suicidal? I do not recommend it. You cannot be available 24/7, so if the client is depending on you and you are not available by your phone, then what should the client do? This uncertainty may confuse someone who is feeling acute distress. Do not take responsibility for saving your client's life; this is a clinical mistake (Simon & Gutheil, 2004), and it is not realistic. If you can't trust the client with that responsibility, the client should be hospitalized.

An appropriate suicide prevention plan is one that is available to the client 24/7 and is not dependent on your constant availability (McWilliams, 2004). If the client will be treated as an outpatient, the client must agree to a suicide prevention plan. Give the client two alternatives if the suicidal ideation worsens: either call 911 or go to the nearest emergency room. The 911 operators can dispatch appropriate personnel to the client's home to take the client for evaluation. Any emergency room will be able to evaluate the client and hospitalize as needed. Obtain and document the client's verbal agreement to adhere to this plan. If the client has any hesitation, ask what the concerns are and address them thoroughly until the client can accept the plan. If the client cannot accept the plan, there may be more ambivalence about continuing to live than the client initially revealed. This should be further evaluated and addressed as you decide whether to treat the client as an inpatient or an outpatient.

A possible alternative suicide prevention plan would be to have the client call you first, but if you are not available, then to seek help from 911 or the nearest emergency room (Simon, 2004). However, that plan can be problematic with certain borderline clients who might decide to call you, tell you that they are going to commit suicide, and then expect that you will exert all efforts to rescue them by phone while they are actively resisting your efforts. The client needs to work out ambivalence about the suicide plan in the psychotherapy session, not act it out when in a crisis. So if you sense that the client may act out ambivalence about suicide in this way, *do not* tell the client to call you when suicidal; instead, use the 911/emergency room suicide prevention plan and address ambivalence about living at every psychotherapy session until it is resolved (or hospitalize if at risk).

Whether to make a written or verbal no-suicide contract with the client is a controversial topic. I tend to agree with Simon (1988, 2004), who feels that the primary purpose of a suicide contract is to alleviate the anxiety of the therapist. He goes on to caution that making a suicide contract "may falsely relieve the therapist's concern and lower vigilance without having any appreciable effect on the patient's suicidal intent" (Simon, 1988, p. 93). There is no evidence that written contracts reduce suicidal behavior, and repeated studies show that many clients will commit suicide even with a written contract (Simon, 2004). *Always do a thorough suicide risk assessment whether or not the client signs a written contract.*

Be concerned if you notice any signs of continued suicidal intent. These signs could include the following:

- The client has tunnel vision and is unable to accept therapist's input or reframe.
- The client seems reluctant, sarcastic, or hopeless about treatment recommendations.
- The client's affect or verbalizations suggest reluctance to comply with suicide prevention plan.

If you notice any of these signs, reconsider hospitalization.

IMPLEMENT: PRECAUTIONS FOR OUTPATIENTS

Tony turns to Susie: "Susie, can I count on you to go to Phil's house right after we meet today and take the gun and the ammunition away with you?" Susie indicates her agreement. Tony cautions, "Could you be sure that the gun is secured in a locked area and that Phil has no access to it?" Susie agrees to do so. Tony asks if there are any other guns available to Phil, but both of them indicate that there aren't.

Sometimes, when weighing the risks, benefits, and protective factors, you will decide that a client with suicidal ideation can be effectively treated as an outpatient. This will probably be a client who has passive suicidal ideation and a good treatment alliance. However, clients like Phil, with occasional active suicidal ideation, who can be trusted to seek help if their urges to hurt themselves worsen, can be effectively treated as outpatients.

Safety precautions must be considered when treating clients with suicidal ideation as outpatients (Simon, 2004). Sixty percent of suicides are by firearms, the most frequently used method of suicide for both men and women (National Institute of Mental Health, 1999), so if there are any guns in the home, they should be removed, disarmed, and secured in a location outside the home by a responsible adult (not the client). Too many medications in the home can be a suicide risk, so others in the home should secure their personal medications, and the psychiatrist may wish to limit the client's medications to a week's supply. If the client has been having thoughts of suicide by car, it would be wise to take public transportation or have others do the driving for now. To achieve these goals, you may need to meet with a responsible friend, relative, or significant other of the client and obtain that person's assistance.

Note, however, that no home environment can be truly made safe for someone who is intent on committing suicide; all that can be done is to remove some potential means that could be used impulsively, allowing the client more time to think clearly and obtain professional help. If you find yourself obsessing over how to make the client's home safer, that might be a sign that you don't trust the client to seek help if needed; in that case, the client should be hospitalized instead.

IMPLEMENT: REDUCE RISK FACTORS AND
ENHANCE PROTECTIVE FACTORS

Tony talks to Phil about other interventions. Tony says, "As I mentioned before, depression is very treatable, and I think that there is an excellent chance that you can feel much better within the next few weeks. In order for this to happen, I'd suggest several things. First, it's very important that you attend regular weekly psychotherapy sessions. Can I count on you to do that? Let's schedule a regular session time for you [takes a few minutes to schedule session]. Second, I see that your sleep is not good at all. I would like you to talk to a psychiatrist today and get some medication so you can sleep better. Usually, getting better sleep makes a significant impact on how a person is feeling. How does that sound?" Phil indicates that he is willing to see the psychiatrist. Tony then says, "I think it is great that you have been going to AA with Susie. Can I count on you to continue to do that every day for the next few weeks?" Phil says that he will do so. Tony then says, "One last thing that

I think is crucially important is for you to start seeing your grandsons again.
I suspect that they miss you a lot and would like to see you. How soon can you
go over and see them?" Susie jumps in and says that she can drive him over
to see the grandsons this evening. Phil agrees to go even though he seems
somewhat reluctant.

Don't stop planning after you make a suicide prevention plan. In order to
deescalate the client's suicidality, you must begin to reduce risk factors and
enhance protective factors as soon as possible. Identify any risk factors that
can be modified (e.g., recent relapse on alcohol or a lack of sleep that contributes to feelings of desperation) and address them immediately. Identify
any possible protective factors that can be reinforced (e.g., involve family
and friends or return to regular social events) as soon as possible (Simon,
2006).

Working with the client to develop a plan to reduce suicidality over the
short term can help your client reduce feelings of hopelessness that have been
linked strongly to suicidality (A. T. Beck, Brown, & Steer, 1989; Joiner et al.,
2005). The following paragraphs address three key intervention points.

First, you will want to assess the social support of the client and work with
the client to make a plan to increase social support over the short term. If
there are any supportive family members, discuss with the client how to en-
list their emotional support (Packman, Pennuto et al., 2004). In the previous
vignette, Tony enlists Susie to help Phil make it to AA and to see his grandchildren. If the client has a history of being interested in religion and has a religious group that he has found uplifting in the past, reengaging with that
group can be helpful. However, note that certain religious involvements
might add to the client's distress (e.g., the client is gay, and church preaches
against it) and should not be encouraged early in treatment.

Cultural considerations can be important in determining social support. If
the client belongs to an ethnic group where there is strong family interde-
pendence and/or extended family support, this can help support the client
(unless there is significant conflict). Of concern, White clients may be the
most socially isolated since they probably are not embedded in an actively
involved extended family and may not be highly engaged with a faith community.

Second, you will want to help the client realize that the problems are treatable. Tony has mobilized resources within the mental health system to improve Phil's emotional functioning as soon as possible. He is clarifying that
treatment is possible, available, and likely to help. In addition, note that Tony
emphasizes the likelihood of improvement without actually making any con-
crete promises since each client is different and improvement cannot be predicted with certainty.

Third, use psychotropic medications to quickly reduce symptoms and acute distress (Simon, 2004). Symptoms that can be treated quickly with medications include insomnia, agitation, anxiety, panic attacks, and psychotic symptoms. Educate the client about how these medications should help within days.

IMPLEMENT: HOSPITALIZE IF NECESSARY

Fred suggests to Crystal that hospitalization would be most appropriate given how distressed she has been feeling. Crystal agrees but says she feels discouraged that she needs hospitalization again. Fred takes steps to initiate hospitalization.

When starting at a new mental health facility, you should always be familiar with how clients are hospitalized in that setting before starting to see any clients. Paperwork and procedures for psychiatric hospitalization vary from facility to facility and from state to state. In some states, outpatient commitment is also possible. Be aware of the laws regarding involuntary inpatient and outpatient treatment in your state. Talk to your supervisor about how involuntary hospitalization is initiated at your facility. Your supervisor should orient you to both the voluntary and the involuntary hospitalization protocols.

Voluntary hospitalization is when your client agrees to be hospitalized. An *involuntary hospitalization* is the hospitalization of a client who refuses to be hospitalized but whom clinicians believe is a danger to self or others. Involuntary hospitalization generally requires considerable paperwork and a secure location to keep client and may require the agreement of two mental health professionals.

In the process of hospitalization, do not leave the client alone and unattended unless you have a very good reason to assume that the client will not leave or engage in self-harm in your absence. If you work in a facility that has an emergency room and an inpatient facility, you or another staff member should walk the voluntary client down to the emergency room and ensure that the client is under observation. If the facility does not have these services, a reliable individual, such as a family member or friend, should escort the client directly to the agreed-on hospital. Personal items can be brought to the client later; the top priority is for the client to be taken to the hospital immediately and directly.

IMPLEMENT: REDUCE RISK OF SELF-HARM

Self-harm behaviors are often used to cope with distressing feelings. In a study of 93 clients with self-injurious behavior, clients were asked their reasons for engaging in the behavior (Briere & Gil, 1998). At least a third of the clients endorsed each of these reasons: feel body is real (43%), distraction from memories (58%), distraction from painful feelings (80%), feel inside body (43%), mark to show pain inside (60%), stop guilt (38%), stop flashbacks (39%), self-punishment (83%), feel alive (38%), feel self-control (71%), get attention or ask for help (40%), make body unattractive (37%), manage stress (77%), stop hurt by others (45%), reduction of tension (75%), feel something (57%), and release pent-up feelings (77%). As you can see, many of these reasons involve affect regulation, specifically trying to cope with distressing feelings, flashbacks, and dissociation. After engaging in self-harm, the subjects felt less anger at self, less anger at others, and less fear, emptiness, hurt, loneliness, and sadness. After self-harm, they had more feelings of relief and shame (Briere & Gil, 1998).

The findings of this study clearly indicate that individuals who use self-harm to cope are in need of alternative coping methods. And, in fact, research has found that individuals who engage in self-harm have deficits in their problem-solving abilities (J. Evans, 2000). Until the client learns alternatives and is motivated to use them, the self-harm will likely continue.

Given these findings about coping deficits, here are some early interventions you can consider using to deescalate self-harm behavior:

- Maintain your empathy to the client throughout and gently emphasize the importance of addressing self-injurious behavior consistently in therapy.
- Ask the client how the self-injurious behavior helps:

  "How were you feeling before you burned yourself with the cigarette?"
  "What was happening that led you to have that feeling?"
  "How did you feel after you burned yourself?"

- Agree that the client needs effective ways to ease distress and acknowledge the client's feeling that self-injurious behavior has helped:

  "I certainly agree that you need something effective to do when you feel fearful or when you are having flashbacks. I can see that you feel that biting yourself has really helped you when you felt like that."

- Educate the client about the dangers of the self-injurious behavior:

  "I'm concerned because you could end up getting a serious infection or permanent scarring, or you could cut too deep and injure a blood vessel or a nerve."

- If appropriate, reframe the relationship between the client's trauma history and the self-injurious behavior:

"You've already suffered more than enough hurt in your life. I don't think you deserve to suffer any more injuries."

- Suggest that alternative ways of coping can be used when the client is feeling in distress:

  "I'm hoping that we can work together and help you figure out healthier ways to cope when you are upset. I understand how important it is to have something you can do to feel better."

- Recognize that the self-injurious behavior may not stop immediately. Discuss how to reduce its dangerousness—perhaps by substituting holding an ice cube in the hand or snapping a rubber band on the wrist (Linehan, 1993).
- Tell the client in a nonjudgmental way that you'd like to discuss the self-injurious behavior every week that it occurs and help the client think about other ways to cope in those situations.
- Enroll client in a dialectical behavior therapy (DBT) group or teach DBT skills on an individualized basis.

The DBT approach has the greatest research evidence of effectiveness in treating self-harm (Burns, Dudley, Hazell, & Patton, 2005). Specifically, it is effective in reducing self-harm episodes among clients with borderline personality disorder and multiple self-harm episodes (Linehan et al., 2006), probably because it is a structured approach that directly addresses coping effectively with distress.

DOCUMENT

Thorough documentation of suicidal ideation and risk factors is an essential portion of the suicide risk assessment (Moline et al., 1998). In the future, you or other clinicians may need this information when assessing another suicidal crisis in the same client. In addition, you will want to be sure to delineate all the risk factors so that you and other clinicians can work to reduce the client's risk.

You must document completely so that in case of legal action sufficient information is available to prove that your evaluation and actions were up to your profession's "standard of care" (Packman, Pennuto et al., 2004). Remember that, in a legal context, "if it wasn't written down, it didn't happen" (Gutheil, 1980, p. 479). As Moline et al. (1998) assert, "Clear, specific and objective written documentation of treatment and preventative actions taken by you are a good safeguard against liability" (p. 74).

Your thought processes in clinical decision making must be documented. If you did not hospitalize, make your reasons for this perfectly clear in the chart (Packman, Pennuto et al., 2004). *If you do not hospitalize, the client's risk level should be no more than moderate.* Document clearly why you made that risk determination. *Never* state that a client is high risk unless you plan to hospitalize the client.

Document all suicide risk assessments contemporaneously for your professional protection against lawsuits since there remains a risk that the client will commit suicide anyway. *Documentation of a suicide risk assessment must be completed (and cosigned if necessary) before you leave the facility for the day.* If you work in a medical center, your client may later present for treatment at the emergency room when you are not available. Your notes will help the clinician on duty make an appropriate determination. In addition, if your client commits suicide and you haven't written a note documenting your earlier suicide assessment, you are in a highly problematic legal position.

For a suicide risk assessment, the following is an outline of what to address in the progress note. This outline is for a client who will be treated as an outpatient:

- Ms. A's current suicidal ideation is . . . [active, passive, intent, plans, means]
- Current behavior relevant to suicide risk assessment is . . .
- Ms. A reported the following past suicidal behavior and ideation . . . [discuss incidents in sufficient detail]
- The suicide risk factors for Ms. A are . . .
- The suicide protective factors for Ms. A are . . . She verbalizes that she does not intend to act on her suicidal ideation because . . .
- Ms. A's past compliance with treatment is . . .
- Ms. A's current engagement in treatment is . . .
- I consulted with [other professionals] regarding Ms. A and [their agreement/input regarding plan]
- Ms. A verbalizes her intent not to commit suicide, and if she feels that she is at greater risk of doing so, she agrees to come to the emergency room or call 911 for assistance.
- Given the above, Ms. A is at [low, moderate] risk for suicide at the present time.
- I did not hospitalize Ms. A because . . .
- Ms. A has agreed to participate in the following treatment and activities to reduce her risk of suicide . . . [include what interventions you chose, why you chose them, time frames for interventions, and why you didn't choose alternative interventions (Simon, 2004)]
- During the session . . . [detail other actions or plans undertaken during session; e.g., sister agreed to remove gun from home]

• Ms. A will be next seen by [insert person] at [insert date].

If you feel that you cannot make a persuasive argument using this outline for managing the client as an outpatient, then the client should be hospitalized.

If a client with significant suicide risk drops out of treatment, make a good-faith effort to reengage the client in treatment. In consultation with your supervisor, consider sending appointments by mail, contacting the client on the phone, and/or contacting family members for assistance in getting the client to attend. Document all these efforts carefully before you close the case.

COPING IF A CLIENT COMMITS SUICIDE

Leah Perry, a psychology intern, completed an intake interview with a new client in a medical center yesterday. As part of her interview, Leah had assessed depressive symptoms and suicidal ideation. Although apparently moderately depressed, the client denied any suicidal ideation and intent, and he denied any history of suicidal ideation or behavior. Today, she gets a message on her voice mail from the client's wife stating that the client committed suicide late last night.

Research suggests that the suicide of a client is one of the most stressful professional events possible (Horn, 1994). Trainees and early career professionals may be especially vulnerable to more intense emotional reactions and stress after a client suicide (Horn, 1994).

Experiencing a client's suicide is unfortunately all too common. Therapists who work with inpatients and/or those with more severe mental illness are more likely to have a client who commits suicide (Kleespies, 1993). Mental health practitioners have a 25% to 50% risk of having at least one client commit suicide in their careers, and of those, psychiatrists have the most risk (Chemtob, Bauer, Hamada, Pelowski, & Muraoka, 1989; McAdams & Foster, 2000). Three studies found that during psychology training alone, the risk for client suicide was 10% to 17% (Kleespies, 1993; Kleespies, Penk, & Forsyth, 1993; Kleespies, Smith, & Becker, 1990), and a sample of psychology trainees found that about 30% had a client attempt suicide during their training years (Kleespies, 1993).

If your client has committed suicide, there are several practical matters you must address (for a thorough treatment of these issues, see Simon, 2004). Tell your clinical supervisor and your administrative supervisor. The malpractice insurer who covers your training site should be contacted by the appropriate person within 30 days. You need to understand that confidentiality does not expire with the client, and you need to consider how you will relate to the family through this difficult time. Risk management, unfortunately, needs to be considered carefully. Read more about these complex issues *immediately* if a client commits suicide.

The suicide of a client impacts your emotional functioning in two ways (this entire paragraph is informed by Horn, 1994). You have the feelings that go along with losing a significant person to suicide, and you experience the suicide as a critical event in your professional development. Ordinary emotional reactions to suicide may begin with shock, disbelief, and denial and then progress to guilt, shame, sadness, and blame. On a professional level, you may worry about professional competence and experience self-doubt. You may fear that fellow professionals are being silently critical. You may be preoccupied with intrusive thoughts about the client and worry about legal issues as well. You may also have some avoidance symptoms (McAdams & Foster, 2000).

Do not share all your feelings with the grieving family; they have enough emotional distress already. Any doubts are probably your emotional reaction and not based on the realities of the treatment you provided; talking about your doubts with the client's family will sow inaccurate concerns that your poor management contributed to the suicide—*don't do it.* Saying the words "I'm sorry" to the family could be problematic as well (Simon, 2004).

Instead, proactively address the emotional and professional impact by discussing feelings and concerns with trusted colleagues, including supervisors and consultants, especially those who have also lost a client to suicide (Kleespies, 1993). The emotional support of your family, friends, and peers can be helpful as well (S. Knox, Burkard, Jackson, Shaack, & Hess, 2006) as long as you are careful to not violate the deceased client's confidentiality.

If your supervisor approves, you can consider attending the client's funeral if the family feels it is appropriate, or you might write a note of condolence to the family. When ready, you may want to review the case in detail with a supervisor or with a consultation group in order to gain more understanding of what transpired.

Later, you will regain emotional equilibrium and reach acceptance and understanding of the event. As a result of the suicide, you may be more attuned to clients' emotional pain and may learn more about effectively managing high-risk clients (S. Knox et al., 2006). You may be more careful with clinical record keeping and more aware of legal liabilities, and you may be more willing to seek consultation regarding high-risk cases (McAdams & Foster, 2000). These reactions can lead to improved sensitivity and quality of care.

However, negative emotional effects are possible as well, as you could develop feelings of fear and helplessness when treating suicidal clients and become overly protective of high-risk clients (Horn, 1994). If you have these reactions, you should seek personal therapy and consultation for assistance.

CONCLUSION

No one chapter can be considered anything more than an introduction to the complex subject of assessing and managing suicidality in clients. It is essential that you continue to learn more about this subject through reading, consultation, and lectures. The following list of recommended readings will help you get started on this process.

RECOMMENDED READING

Jacobs, D. G., & Brewer, M. L. (2006). Application of the APA Practice Guidelines on Suicide to clinical practice. *CNS Spectrums, 11*, 447–454. Retrieved October 21, 2006, from http://www.cnsspectrums.com/aspx/articledetail.aspx?articleid=471.
This article has two particularly helpful tables: Table 2, "Questions About Suicidal Feelings and Behavior"; and Table 3, "Guidelines for Selecting a Treatment Setting for Patients at Risk of Suicide or Suicidal Behaviors."
Packman, W. L., Pennuto, T. O., Bongar, B., & Orthwein, J. (2004). Legal issues of professional negligence in suicide cases. *Behavioral Sciences and the Law, 22*, 697–713.
Packman and colleagues provide a thorough discussion of legal malpractice issues relevant to client suicide and how the clinician can practice to minimize risk.
Simon, R. I. (2004). *Assessing and managing suicide risk: Guidelines for clinically based risk management.* Washington, DC: American Psychiatric Publishing.
Although targeted to fellow psychiatrists, Simon's volume is essential reading for any clinician who wants to be well informed and confident in the clinical management of suicide risk. Chapters on inpatient management of suicidality and suicide aftermath are helpful in those situations. I recommend that you have a copy on hand so that, in the unfortunate event that a client commits suicide, you have an appropriate reference to help you.

EXERCISES AND DISCUSSION QUESTIONS

1. Does your facility use suicide contracts with clients? Do you think this is a good idea with these particular clients? Why or why not?
2. Do you know any clinicians who have lost a client to suicide? Has your supervisor or any of your coworkers lost a client to suicide? Ask these colleagues how they dealt with it.
3. If a client were to commit suicide, what would you need to do from a procedural standpoint at the facility? What do you think would help you cope personally and professionally with this tragedy?
4. Write a progress note documenting Tony's assessment of Phil.
5. Write a progress note documenting Fred's assessment of Crystal.

Chapter Twenty

Violence Risk Management

When a client is suicidal, only one person is at risk: the client himself. However, when a client may be violent, others are at risk. The risk of violence depends on three types of factors: those concerning the client, factors concerning the potential victim, and the specific aspects of the situation. The violence could be either psychological (such as threats or insults) or an actual physical assault. While psychological violence is also of concern clinically, this chapter focuses on prevention and management of potentially physically violent situations toward other persons.

This chapter focuses on the assessment, prevention, and management of potentially violent or actually violent clients in the adult outpatient mental health setting. In other settings, different risk factors are significant. If you plan to work in another setting (e.g., corrections, schools, or with children or adolescents), review the literature regarding violence in that setting for the most accurate information on risk and management.

Three specific situations are discussed in this chapter: (a) assessing and treating a client who has a general risk of being violent in the future, (b) assessing and treating a client who has a risk of being violent to a specific person or persons, and (c) coping with violent and potentially violent situations in the mental health workplace. Different approaches must be taken from a clinical and legal perspective with clients who have *nonspecific risk* of future violence toward no particular identifiable individual versus a client who makes threats or appears dangerous to a *specific* person or persons. The topics covered are as follows:

- Rapport and informed consent
- Assess

- ○ Violence risk screening
- ○ Violence risk level
- ○ Violence protective factors
- ○ Nonspecific risk: situations with high risk for violence
- ○ Nonspecific risk: potential victims at greatest risk
- ○ Specific risk against an individual
- ○ Specific risk: the *Tarasoff* case
- • Plan and implement
- ○ Specific risk: duty to warn
- ○ Specific risk: considerations regarding making a report
- ○ Containing the danger of violence
- ○ Treat effectively to reduce future risk
- ○ Deescalating the angry, agitated client
- ○ Implementing: if violence is occurring or imminent
- ○ Planning to reduce the risk of violence toward the clinician
- • Documentation

RAPPORT AND INFORMED CONSENT

At the outset of treatment and as part of the informed consent process, address limits to confidentiality regarding violence. In a population that is at low risk for violence, a brief mention of these limitations in written informed consent documents that the client signs at the outset of treatment would be sufficient. However, in a higher-risk population for violence (e.g., community mental health or substance abuse treatment), a written document, followed by a brief oral review, may be helpful to ensure that the client understands. When your client has been informed, it will not be a surprise if you need to take steps to ensure anyone's safety. Proper informed consent will help maintain the therapeutic alliance if you need to take any precautions, as the client had been informed from the outset.

ASSESS: VIOLENCE RISK SCREENING

All clients should have an initial screening for current and historical violent behavior and ideation in the first session. As suggested earlier, you can precede difficult questions by stating, "Now, I am going to ask you a few standard questions that I ask everyone." Here are suggested screening questions:

"Are you having any thoughts of hurting anyone?" [Ask follow-up questions as needed to ascertain exactly what violent or threatening behavior, if any, has transpired recently.]

"Have you ever been violent in the past? When? Can you tell me more about what happened?"
"Have you ever had any legal or criminal problems?" If so, ask the following questions: "Have you ever been arrested? Have you ever been in jail or prison? What were the charges?"

If the client answers no to all these questions, you can assume that the client is not at risk for violence. If the client answers yes to any of these questions (or if there were legal problems and the charges involved accusations of violence), you should do a full assessment of violence risk. You should also assess whether the client has any weapons and knows how to use them (Kumar & Simpson, 2005).

For past violence, you will want to know how many times the client has been violent and when this occurred. For each incident, you will want to understand how the client assaulted the victim (e.g., with fists or a weapon), the relationship the client had with the victim (e.g., girlfriend or "a guy" who angered client at a bar), and how injured the victim was after the assault (Flannery, 2005). You will also want to ask the how client feels about having been violent in the past and what the client thinks has triggered past violent behavior (Kumar & Simpson, 2005).

If the client denies a history of violence but you still have some suspicions or concerns, ask the following:

"What is the most violent thing you have ever done?"
"What is the closest you have ever come to being violent?"
"Do you ever worry that you might physically hurt someone?" (Monahan, 1993)
"Have you ever been hospitalized for having thoughts about hurting someone else?"

If significant others are available for interview, you can question them as well, such as "Are you concerned that [client name] might hurt someone?" (Monahan, 1993, p. 244). You will also want to review past chart records at your facility and send for chart records at other facilities.

ASSESS: VIOLENCE RISK LEVEL

Which clients are most likely to be violent? Be especially concerned if a client has violent intent (e.g., the client verbalizes intent to hurt others or admits to making threats of violence to others). A history of violent behavior is the risk factor that is most strongly associated with violence risk (Barlow, Grenyer, & Ilkiw-Lavalle, 2000).

The following is a summary list of violence risk factors (adapted from T. R. Anderson, Bell, Powell, Williamson, & Blount, 2004, and informed by

Barlow et al., 2000; Flannery, 2005; Flannery, Schuler, Farley, & Walker, 2002; Krakowski & Czobor, 2004; Swanson et al., 2002):

- Younger age: Persons in their late teens and early 20s are at greatest risk; however, even clients up to their early 30s can still be at increased risk. Note, however, that the mean age of assailants in one study was 35 years old (Flannery et al., 2002).
- Older age: Geriatric patients with dementia can also be at risk of violent behavior.
- Socioeconomic status (SES): Persons with lower SES are at greatest risk.
- Race: When SES is controlled for, race is not a risk factor.
- Victim status: Individuals with a childhood history of physical abuse or observing domestic violence are at greater risk of violence.
- Childhood behavior problems: Clients with a history of truancy or conduct problems are at a greater risk of violent behavior. Clients with a younger age of first violent behavior are at a greater risk.
- Childhood instability and family dysfunction: Greater parental psychopathology and a history of being placed in foster care are indicative of greater risk of violence.
- Client's perception of stress: The greater the perception of being under stress (e.g., unemployment, relationship or family problems, homelessness, or health problems), the greater the risk of violence.
- Adult exposure to violence: The greater the exposure to violence in the client's current environment, the greater the likelihood of violent behavior.
- Ready access to guns: Greater access to guns is indicative of greater violence risk.
- Neurological status: Clients with neurological abnormalities or a history of head trauma can be at greater risk.
- Substance use or abuse is indicative of greater violence risk, as is current intoxication.
- Bipolar clients in a manic phase are at greater risk of behaving violently, especially when agitated and irritable.
- Schizophrenic clients who have paranoid ideas that they are in danger or who have command hallucinations telling them to be violent are at greater risk of being violent. One study (McNiel, Eisner, & Binder, 2000) found that two-thirds of clients with command hallucinations to be violent had been violent in the past 2 months.
- Posttraumatic stress disorder (PTSD) can be predictive of greater risk of violence.
- Antisocial/psychopathic personality traits indicate a greater risk of violence, although recent research suggests that being antagonistic (or low in the agreeableness personality factor; Skeem, Miller, Mulvey, Tiemann, & Monahan, 2005) is the antisocial trait that is most related to violence proneness.

- Borderline personality–disordered clients can be at greater risk of violence.
- Admission status: Patients admitted involuntarily are at greater violence risk on the inpatient unit.

Note that while males are at more risk for violence in the general population, in mental health settings, males and female clients are at equal risk for behaving violently (T. R. Anderson et al., 2004). Mental illness, in general, may not be related to greater violence risk, but clients with certain specific symptoms are at greater risk. Schizophrenic clients who do not abuse substances and take their medications (and thus, do not have acute psychotic symptoms) may not be at any greater risk for violence than the average person.

Ask about weapons, their availability, and the client's history with using these weapons (T. R. Anderson et al., 2004). For example, a combat veteran who has guns in the home is at much greater risk than an office worker who has no access to weapons and does not know how to use them.

ASSESS: VIOLENCE PROTECTIVE FACTORS

If the individual has good treatment engagement and good treatment adherence, the likelihood for violence is lessened. Even individuals with psychopathic traits (antisocial personality traits) can have lessened risk for violence with suitably intensive treatment; they have (wrongly) historically been thought to not benefit much from treatment (Skeem, Monahan, & Mulvey, 2002). If the client has a history of following treatment recommendations appropriately, this would be a protective factor as well.

If the individual believes that violent behavior would be wrong, this is a protective factor. If the individual understands the negative consequences of behaving violently and wants to avoid these consequences by controlling his behavior, this is a protective factor. Perhaps the client's family, cultural, or religious values support nonviolence; if so, this is a protective factor. In addition, the client may be able to have some empathy for the potential victim (Kumar & Simpson, 2005), which can be a protective factor as well.

ASSESS NONSPECIFIC RISK: SITUATIONS WITH HIGH RISK FOR VIOLENCE

In what situations are clients most likely to be violent? Little appears to be known about dangerous situations outside mental health facilities. However, dangerous situations on inpatient psychiatric units have been studied. When on an inpatient unit, patients may be at greater risk of danger during times of change: admission, change of shifts, mealtimes, visiting hours, and any period of change when nursing staff are busy with unit tasks (Barlow et al., 2000). Aggression is more common during morning and afternoon shifts and is infrequent at night (Barlow et al., 2000). Patients are likely to be violent if they are being denied something that they want on an inpatient unit, such as increased privileges or cigarettes. They may be violent when rules are being enforced (Flannery, 2005).

ASSESS NONSPECIFIC RISK: POTENTIAL VICTIMS AT GREATEST RISK

Who are the potential victims of violence? If the client is at general risk of violence, the client is most likely to be violent toward family and significant others (T. R. Anderson et al., 2004) or mental health practitioners (Barlow et al., 2000). Mental health practitioners who work in inpatient settings or in the emergency room are generally at the greatest risk (Petit, 2005). Practitioners who work in the nonprofit sector and those who work for community mental health, corrections, or drug/alcohol treatment programs are at greater risk, while attacks in private practice are rare (Jayaratne, Croxton, & Mattison, 2004). Practitioners who are younger than 45 years old or male are more likely to be threatened or assaulted (Jayaratne et al., 2004). Practitioners who are less experienced are more likely to be assaulted; one study found that one-third of psychiatric residents had been physically assaulted by a patient (Schwartz & Park, 1999). On inpatient units, nurses are at greater risk of assault than psychiatrists (Lawoko, Soares, & Nolan, 2004). There is no evidence that the race or ethnicity of the therapist influences the likelihood of being assaulted (Jayaratne et al., 2004).

ASSESS SPECIFIC RISK: AGAINST AN INDIVIDUAL

The standard violence risk questions as described previously were developed in the context of exploring which clients were at general violence risk in the community. As Borum and Reddy (2001) point out, considering these actuarial risk factors is unlikely to be a sufficient clinical assessment if a client makes violent threats toward another person or otherwise appears significantly dangerous toward a specific person.

Here are the six factors Borum and Reddy (2001) suggest using to evaluate a client's immediate threat toward a specific person as well as questions to ask oneself about the client for each factor:

- A—Attitudes that support or facilitate violence: Does the client believe that the use of violence is justified under the circumstances? Does the client believe that there have been intentional provocations by others? Does the client think that being violent will be successful in accomplishing his or her stated goals? Does the client have personal attitudes (such as antisocial, patriarchal, misogynistic, or prejudicial) consistent with violent behavior? Does the client feel that there are no other options or that there is nothing to lose?
- C—Capacity: Does the client have the physical and intellectual capacity to carry out the threat? Does the client have access to means, access to the target individual, and the opportunity to commit the act? How well does the client know the target's routines and whereabouts?
- T—Thresholds crossed: Has the client already engaged in behaviors to further the plan of attack? Have any of these behaviors broken any laws already (showing a willingness to engage in antisocial behavior)?
- I—Intent: Weighing this information and other statements made by the client, does there appear to be actual intent to engage in the violent act?
- O—Others' reactions: Does the client report that significant others are encouraging or discouraging of the violent plan? Are significant others immediately available to provide input about the client's behavior and likelihood to act? Are they fearful that the client will act on violent statements?
- N—Noncompliance versus compliance with risk-reduction interventions: Is the client willing to participate in interventions to reduce or mitigate risk? Is the client motivated to prevent this violent act? Does the client feel that treatment will be effective? Does the client have a good treatment alliance? Has the client adhered to treatment recommendations in the past? Does the client have insight into the need for treatment and potential for violence?

Note that these six factors form an acronym to assist memory: ACTION.

ASSESS SPECIFIC RISK: THE TARASOFF CASE

Prosenjit Poddar, raised in rural India, arrived in Berkeley, California, in September 1967 to study graduate electronics and naval architecture. Beginning in the fall of 1968, Poddar began romantically pursuing Tatiana Tarasoff, a community-college student who lived with her parents nearby. Tarasoff was never really interested, but cultural differences produced much misunderstanding. In March 1969, Poddar blurted out a marriage proposal, which was promptly rejected. Angry and humiliated, he returned home and voiced to his roommate thoughts of killing Tarasoff. Over the next few months, Poddar's behavior was plainly paranoid: taping telephone conversations with Tarasoff, then staying in his room for days on end listening to them, and telling coworkers that he would like to blow up Tarasoff's house.

Finally, in June 1969, Poddar's roommate persuaded him to see a university health service psychiatrist. At the initial interview, Poddar told the psychiatrist of his thoughts of killing an unnamed young woman with whom he was obsessed. Antipsychotic and sleep medication were prescribed and weekly therapy appointments with a psychologist were scheduled. Poddar kept these appointments for eight weeks, repeatedly confessing his homicidal ideas toward the unidentified woman. In August 1969, the therapist told Poddar that he would take steps to restrain him if he continued such talk. Poddar immediately stopped coming to therapy. The therapist conferred with the treating psychiatrist (and with another university psychiatrist) and then wrote a letter to university police stating that Poddar [should be committed for observation in a mental hospital].

The campus police tracked Poddar down at his new apartment (very near Tarasoff's house) and interviewed him in front of his new roommate, Tarasoff's brother, about the death threats. Poddar acknowledged a troubled relationship with an unidentified young woman but denied any death threats. The brother knew that the alleged threats were against his sister but did not take them seriously. The officers, "satisfied that Poddar was rational, released him on his promise to stay away from Tatiana."

The university health service's chief of psychiatry, astonishingly, "then asked the police to return [the psychotherapist's] letter, directed that all copies of the letter and notes that [he] had taken as therapist be destroyed, and 'ordered no action to place . . . Poddar in [a] 72-hour treatment and evaluation facility.'"

Poddar purchased a gun and began to stalk Tarasoff. One evening just before Halloween 1969, he found her at home alone and killed her, called the police, and waited to be arrested.

Tarasoff's parents sued the university health service's chief of psychiatry; the psychiatrist who initially interviewed Poddar; the psychologist who saw him for the eight sessions, along with one other campus psychiatrist who had the misfortune to have taken part in one discussion about what to do at the time Poddar broke off treatment; and the campus police. Their complaint alleged that "defendant therapists did in fact predict that Poddar would kill and were negligent in failing to warn." (Herbert, 2002, pp. 417–418; reference notes removed for clarity)

In the 1970s, this legal case in California established the following case law precedent in that state: If the therapist's client makes violent threats against a specific individual, the therapist must warn that intended victim. This case is generally referred to by one name, *Tarasoff*, the last name of the woman who was killed and her parents, who sued. The events leading up to the case are described in detail in the previous quote.

Note that Poddar's psychologist and psychiatrist clinically managed Poddar's violent threats appropriately. They were concerned about his potential for violence. The psychiatrist prescribed antipsychotic medications to attempt to reduce delusional thoughts. They conferred appropriately about the case and even consulted with an additional clinician as needed. When Poddar dropped out and still appeared to be a violence risk, they directed the police to detain him and hospitalize him involuntarily (although the police did neither). Also note that Poddar didn't kill Tarasoff until weeks after this and after terminating therapy.

At least one of Tarasoff's family members knew about the threats since Tarasoff's brother was Poddar's roommate and heard the interview with the police. It also should be noted that Tatiana Tarasoff was not even in the United States at the time of the psychologist's request for Poddar's hospitalization (Gutheil, 2001). What was being alleged in the case was that the treating mental health professionals should have, nonetheless, contacted Tatiana Tarasoff directly and warned her personally of the threat against her. This was an unprecedented demand of the clinician and not consistent with confidentiality laws of the time.

PLAN AND IMPLEMENT WITH
SPECIFIC RISK: DUTY TO WARN

Be aware that state laws regarding *Tarasoff*-type situations vary dramatically (Herbert & Young, 2002). In most states there is statute law, while in other states there is case law, and in other states there may still be no law at all. In some states, law even contradicts the *Tarasoff* ruling (Herbert & Young, 2002; Walcott, Cerundolo, & Beck, 2001). Which mental health professionals are covered by *Tarasoff* statutes varies as well (Herbert & Young, 2002).

Statute law is law that is passed by legislators, such as state senators and representatives, and is codified by the state or federal legal system. *Case law* is a body of law based on judicial decisions of legal cases; new law can be made or existing law interpreted and clarified. Thus, the original *Tarasoff* ruling in California was Californian case law. However, it has since been supplanted by statute law in California (Herbert, 2002). Case law in one state is not technically law in another state, but it may be cited in rulings in the other states nonetheless (see example of Florida case law citing *Tarasoff* in Walcott et al., 2001).

A *duty to warn* is written into some state statutes (this paragraph is informed by Herbert & Young, 2002). These states indicate that when a client makes a specific threat against one or more individuals, the clinician makes a warning. Whether the warning goes to the intended victim, the police, or both varies by state. In addition, whether the clinician can exercise professional judgment and expertise to decide whether the threat is credible and then decide *not* to make a warning—if the client has no intent or ability to carry out the threat—depends on the state as well.

Thus, no general guidelines can be given for making a report to an intended victim or victims, the police, or both since state statutes vary so much. Read the statute for your state (if there is one). Unfortunately, experts conclude that in states where there is no law, "the clinician is continuously in jeopardy: warn, and face breach-of-confidentiality exposure; keep silent, and risk a *Tarasoff* suit" (Herbert & Young, 2002, p. 280).

The term *duty to protect* is often used in statutes rather than *duty to warn*. However, when this term is used in a state statute, the laws of most states indicate that the clinician's duty is discharged solely by warning the intended victim and/or law enforcement (Herbert & Young, 2002) and that direct actions to actually protect the victim from the client (such as civil commitment) are not mandated, although these actions are sometimes suggested. In other words, even though clinicians may interpret the terms *duty to warn* and *duty to protect* differently, they are used essentially interchangeably in state laws. Herbert and Young (2002) conclude, "Much has been made of this [difference in terminology]. In fact, the earlier phrase [duty to warn] was accurate, the later one [duty to protect] rhetorical and misleading" (p. 275).

Think again about the actual case where Poddar murdered Tarasoff. In this case, the clinicians took many steps to protect Tarasoff from Poddar. In most clinical situations, the steps they took would have contained Poddar and, through effective treatment, would have kept him from murdering anyone. Herbert and Young (2002) conclude, "If anything, *Tarasoff* thus weakens the case for a duty to protect by providing a potential defense (if a warning was given) against a suit for negligent noncommitment" (p. 275). This leaves clinicians in a peculiar state of affairs: In many states, a warning to the intended victim and/or law enforcement is required, but actual clinical steps to contain the potential perpetrator of murder or violence are not.

In conclusion, when deciding an appropriate course of action after a client makes a threat of violence against another individual, ethically we do not want our clients murdering anyone. Therefore, we cannot rely solely on state law for guidance about appropriate case management; we must also consider ethics *and* our clinical expertise to manage the situation effectively.

PLAN AND IMPLEMENT WITH SPECIFIC RISK: CONSIDERATIONS REGARDING MAKING A REPORT

Efram Rosenberg is a mental health trainee working with a substance-abusing Iraq War veteran, Casey Simmons. The veteran has lived with his family since returning from the war. Casey is having a difficult time getting a job. He has long-standing conflicts with his father, who had been physically abusive when he was a child. Casey tells Efram, "I just want to hit him sometimes, I get so mad," but denies ever having been violent toward his father or having any actual intent to do so. Casey says, "I know how much Dad's violence messed me up, so I'd never do that to anyone, not even him." While Efram believes that Casey has no violent intent, he is concerned because he has performed a violence risk assessment and has determined that Casey has some risk factors, namely, his high level of stress, his history of childhood physical abuse, continued family discord, and substance abuse. Efram makes it a priority to help Casey obtain alternative housing that supports his abstinence. No report of a violent threat is made, although Efram is practicing in a state with a statute mandating duty to warn.

A hospitalized client, Maria Barnes, is angry because her student therapist is on vacation. She rages to Allison Wolinski, a mental health trainee on the unit, "I'm going to kill him." Allison is concerned and tells the rest of the unit staff. Allison then calls the therapist's supervisor at the outpatient clinic at the same medical center. They practice in a state with a duty-to-warn statute that indicates that a warning must be made to the intended victim if the clinician assesses a threat is serious. Allison and the supervisor agree that they trust the judgment of the unit staff, and they know that the staff will not release Maria while she still verbalizes threats. Thus, they consider the risk very low. Nonetheless, they agree to call the therapist, thinking that he would want to know what transpired. Allison called the therapist on his cell phone and told him about the threat. The therapist was unconcerned since he knows that Maria is very labile and that this is just her way of expressing anger. When the therapist returns, therapy resumes as before, including discussions of separation, abandonment, and anger management.

Samantha Jenkins is a 24-year-old psychotherapy client. She comes in for her regular psychotherapy session with her student therapist, DeShawn Taylor. Samantha is angry and loud. She curses when talking about her live-in boyfriend, whom she suspects of being unfaithful. DeShawn knows that Samantha has been violent toward her boyfriend in the past when they were having arguments. Samantha says, "I've decided now. I've got to shoot him. There's nothing you can do to stop me." She then abruptly leaves the office before DeShawn can further assess her intent, whether she actually has a gun, or anything else. DeShawn practices in a state with no statute or case law about duty to warn. He goes to his supervisor's office right away and appropriately interrupts his supervisor's session with another client ("I'm very sorry, but I have to talk to you about a crisis immediately") to consult. Since both agree that Samantha poses a serious threat toward her boyfriend, DeShawn calls the home and warns the boyfriend of Samantha's threat. Although not required by

law, DeShawn provides the boyfriend with specific advice: "I believe that this
is a sincere threat against your life. I recommend that you leave your apartment
immediately and go to a location that Samantha will not associate with you.
This location could be a motel or a friend's house or, even better, go out of town
for a few days until she has been found and detained. I want to be sure you are
safe until a mental health clinician determines that you are no longer at risk of
being harmed." He then contacts the police, tells them of the threat, and asks
them to pick up Samantha and take her to the state hospital for commitment.

The previous vignettes illustrate some important points regarding making a
report. In the first vignette, the client expresses some thoughts about hurting
his father. Gellerman and Suddath (2005) carefully review the relevant research and case law regarding violent fantasies versus threats of violence.
They conclude, "The research suggests that violent fantasies are present in a
large number of 'normal' individuals who presumably have not acted crimi-
nally based on these fantasies. There is insufficient scientific evidence that violent fantasies should be considered absolutely predictive of future dangerousness" (p. 293). Therefore, violent ideation, without any violent intent,
should not necessarily be considered a threat triggering *Tarasoff* reporting (if
required by your state). Instead, violent ideation is one piece of evidence that
must be considered in making a well-balanced assessment of violence risk.
Gellerman and Suddath (2005) suggest that when a client reveals a violent
"fantasy," the clinician should evaluate further, including assessing the nature
and quality of the ideas, the degree to which a person is preoccupied with
them, whether foreseeable victims can be identified, and what the client's potential is of acting on the violent ideas.

In the first vignette, the client is not threatening his father but instead is revealing violent ideation. Efram has done a violence risk assessment and determined that the client may have some violence risk factors but that he has
no history of violence, nor does he have any intent to be violent. Taking appropriate clinical steps to reduce the client's overall risk is thus the most appropriate step. In conclusion, *having violent ideation (or fantasies) does not*
constitute making a threat. Violent ideation must be evaluated within the context of a full violence risk assessment to determine whether anyone is actually in any danger.

In the second vignette, Allison contacts the therapist, who the client made
threats against, even though she felt that the risk was very low. In this case,
she felt that the therapist would want to be informed, and she cannot be sure
that the therapist will check the chart notes before going to see the client on
the unit. Since they all practiced at the same facility, no breach-of-confidentiality issues were involved, so there is no downside to reporting the threat.
Allison is also aware that mental health professionals are at significant risk of

violence from clients, in general, so she wisely wanted to be extra cautious. In conclusion, it is wise to maintain good communication between professionals by keeping fellow health care practitioners aware of all changes in violence risk factors for mutual clients (Kumar & Simpson, 2005).

In the third vignette, DeShawn and his supervisor must make an appropriate decision about how to manage this emergency. No law guides them. However, they believe that Samantha's threat could have been sincere, so they feel ethically compelled to protect her boyfriend's life, even if this means violating Samantha's confidentiality. Samantha is clearly unable to control her own behavior appropriately since she made threats in the session. They agree that she needs to be hospitalized to protect others. Our ethical concerns for the safety and well-being of others and the client dictate this action because, clearly, an involuntary hospitalization would be better for the client than a conviction of murder. As Mossman (2004) states, "The existence of a moral obligation to save others, and the absence of clear standards to define the obligation does not mean that there are never clear cases where we know another person is in danger and should do something reasonably simple to avert the danger" (p. 363). In addition, as Gutheil (2001) states, "Because the clinician works, not for the patient, but for the healthy side of the patient, the use of a *Tarasoff* warning may be seen to take place in service to that side of the patient that wishes not to harm another person" (p. 349).

PLAN AND IMPLEMENT: CONTAINING THE DANGER OF VIOLENCE

Ashley Evans is a mental health trainee working with Richard Walker, a client who has chronic schizophrenia. Richard has been incarcerated for burglary. He also has paranoid schizophrenia, and his medications do not fully control his symptoms despite the best efforts of the psychiatrist. Richard continues to be paranoid and thinks that others are out to get him. He says that he feels angry and that he thinks about attacking others at times. However, he verbalizes his understanding that this is wrong and would lead to incarceration, which he wants to avoid. He states that he therefore does not want to be violent to anyone.

Since your client is seeing you in a mental health facility, the client has demonstrated some degree of cooperation and insight so far. Try to build on that, using whatever rapport you can establish when you ask the client to collaborate with you to make a plan to avoid violent behavior.

Determine, with the client, who is at greatest risk for being victimized. Assess whether the client has any actual intent to hurt the individual(s) or whether the client is wrestling with violent thoughts but intends to continue to refrain from violent behavior. Assess how the client has been able to refrain from acting violent up to now. If the client feels unable to control him- or herself from being violent, the client needs to be in the hospital.

Make a plan for more intensive treatment that is appropriate to the client's needs and risk level; some options are inpatient, partial hospitalization, substance abuse treatment, or more frequent sessions. Refer the client to community programs and resources to reduce environmental stressors as much as possible. For example, a bipolar client who abuses substances and is at risk of being violent to elderly parents should be referred to a residential program that supports substance abuse recovery. This plan would reduce the risk factor of substance abuse while getting more distance between the client and the parents, who were at risk of being victimized.

Talk to the client about making an outpatient safety plan. If the client feels at risk of becoming violent, he or she should leave the provoking situation and call 911 or go to the nearest emergency room. If the client readily agrees to do so and verbalizes a sincere motivation to avoid violent behavior, this is a positive sign that it may be possible to treat the client as an outpatient.

If weapons are available, help the client obtain the assistance of a reliable family member or friend to remove the weapons from the house and secure them in another location. In addition, ask if the client has any weapons with him right now and, if so, ask the client to give them to you and secure them in a locked desk or filing cabinet. Later, you can follow your facility's policies for disposal of weapons obtained from clients. Obtain the client's sincere promise not to obtain any more weapons until both of you agree that it is safe to do so.

Sometimes you will need to consider hospitalization. Here are some of the questions you should ask yourself when making that decision:

- Does the client have a history of previous violence? If so, the client is at greater risk.
- Is the client impulsive or abusing substances? If so, the client is at greater risk.
- Will client agree to attend the more intensive treatment that you have recommended, and do you trust the client to attend? If so, you may be able to manage as an outpatient.
- Will the client agree to seek help if violent thoughts worsen? If the client readily agrees to the outpatient safety plan, the client might be managed as an outpatient.
- Can the client articulate intent not to hurt anyone? If so, this is a good sign. If not, hospitalization is probably warranted.
- Can the client articulate why it would be poor judgment to hurt anyone? If so, consider outpatient treatment. Hospitalize if the client says something like this: "It would be worth it to hit him, even if I were locked up because of it."

IMPLEMENT: TREAT EFFECTIVELY TO REDUCE FUTURE RISK

Treatment for the potentially violent client should emphasize reducing risk (Flannery, 2005). Maintain good communication about current level of risk between all mental health care practitioners involved with the client (Kumar & Simpson, 2005). As allowed by the client, involve the client's family in encouraging and supporting the client in treatment.

The client should be engaged in substance abuse treatment as needed. If the client has PTSD, this should be treated with individual therapy and psychotropic medication as needed. Anger management group therapy may be appropriate, or anger management and assertiveness skills can be addressed in individual therapy.

Since certain symptoms may increase risk, effective treatment may reduce a client's violence risk to match that of the general population (Friedman, 2006). Thus, if your client has been violent in the past when experiencing paranoia and/or command hallucinations or when manic, the best way to prevent violence is to control these symptoms effectively with medications. Schedule the client frequently and work with the client and the client's family to improve medication compliance (see chapter 15 for adherence strategies). Work closely with the psychiatrist to change the medication as needed to control symptoms better. Consider antipsychotics that can be given as a shot every 2 to 4 weeks.

If a potentially violent client is dropping out of treatment and has not attended one or more psychotherapy sessions, it is wise to make a good-faith effort to reengage the client in treatment (Monahan, 1993) for the safety of society and for your own risk management. In consultation with your supervisor, consider sending the client additional appointments by mail, contacting the client on the phone, and/or contacting family members for assistance. Document all these efforts carefully in the days or weeks before you close the case.

PLAN AND IMPLEMENT: DEESCALATING
THE ANGRY, AGITATED CLIENT

[Physical signs of imminent violence include] . . . a clenched jaw, flared nostrils, flushed face and clenched or gripping hands. . . . Demanding immediate attention, pacing, restlessness, pushing or slamming things, yelling, profanity, physical aggressiveness and verbal threats can all be early indicators of pending violence. Bell (2000) further elaborates warning signs of imminent violence including eye movement and appearance (such as dilation of the pupil or darting eye movements), proximity (such as a patient invading the clinician's personal space), inability to comply with reasonable limit setting and patient's perception of fear in the clinician. (T. R. Anderson et al., 2004, p. 387)

The previous description is a helpful summary of verbal and nonverbal signs that a client is at risk of imminent violence. In many situations, clients can be deescalated. Never respond to yelling or angry statements with sharp, angry statements of your own; this will probably escalate the situation. When talking with an agitated, angry client, always use a quiet, soothing tone of voice. Reflect the client's feelings: "I can see that you are feeling very upset and angry right now." Reassure the client that he or she has done the right thing and that you plan to help: "You did the right thing coming in to the clinic to ask for help. I'd really like to get a better understanding of what is going on with you and see if we can make a plan together that will help you." Ask the client to calm down and behave appropriately: "Calm down. Sit down, please. It's difficult for me to get an understanding of what's wrong when you are yelling and pounding on the desk. Can I ask you to take a few deep breaths and then try to tell me what's wrong in a quieter voice? I can help you better if I can understand what's going on more." Consider offering medication empathetically (T. R. Anderson et al., 2004): "I can see that you are very distressed. Perhaps our psychiatrist can help you with some medication that will help you calm down. Would you like me to help you look into that?"

IMPLEMENT: IF VIOLENCE IS OCCURRING OR IMMINENT

Monique Brown is a mental health trainee who is in her office writing some progress notes. Suddenly, she hears thumping from the next office and hears her colleague cry for help.

In rare occasions, violence could be happening nearby, or you could believe that violence is imminent. If you hear a violent situation, call the police or security immediately. Do not hesitate because of uncertainty; it would be much worse to hesitate in a dangerous situation than to make a mistake and call the police unnecessarily. Your facility may have security staff; if so, call them, as they can arrive quickly. If not, call 911 for help. You might be trained to assist appropriately in a violent situation, or you might not. Discuss with your supervisor what you should do in those cases.

You might also hear an ambiguous situation, such as a client is yelling in an angry manner in the next office. In that situation, you may wish to assess the situation first. Knock on the door (even if there is a do-not-disturb sign) and look at the situation. If the clinician appears calm and in control, you may simply ask the clinician if everything is okay. You may also wish to politely ask the client to be quiet:

> "I'm not sure if you realize it, but everyone can hear you in the hall. Could I ask you to talk more quietly, so as not to disturb other clients and staff?"

If the situation looks tense, you may wish to ask the clinician to step out for a minute before you ask if everything is okay. If it is not okay, ask what you can do to help.

If you feel that a client is becoming threatening toward you in a session, use your judgment as to whether you think you can talk the client down or whether you need help. It is not okay for the client to yell, make threats, or make prejudicial or harassing remarks toward you. Politely, calmly, and firmly ask the client to behave in an appropriate manner:

> "Mr. Thomas, I'll have to ask you not to hit your hand on the desk like that or talk so loudly. Do you think you can calm yourself down?"

A client who is too agitated and angry to calm down should probably be hospitalized. If this is an intake client, you do not have to frustrate yourself and the client by fully assessing all the history and symptoms at this point because it is clear that hospitalization is needed right now. Inpatient staff can assess the client more fully later when calm and able to participate appropriately. If you think the client will cooperate, say something like this:

> "Mr. Thomas, I can see that you are very upset right now. It was very wise of you to come here and ask for help. Given what you've told me so far, I think that the safest place for you would be the hospital. Could you come to [location] with me so I can get that started for you?"

Ask another staff person to go with you to escort the client to the emergency room or a quiet, secure location so that arrangements can be made for hospitalization. It might be helpful for the client to be sedated.

Ask your supervisor what to do in your setting if you have a client who is agitated and at immediate risk of being violent, yet refuses to agree to hospitalization. In general, you would want to move away from the client and be sure that assistance is available. If possible, the area should be cleared of other patients and staff who are not needed for the crisis. Appropriately trained staff, security personnel, or police should be the ones to restrain the client if that is necessary. It might be helpful for the client to be sedated while arrangements are made for involuntary hospitalization.

IMPLEMENT: REDUCE THE RISK OF VIOLENCE TOWARD THE CLINICIAN

[After considering extended hospitalization] the patient told me that she had seen the hospital and decided that she would like to live on a houseboat while in treatment. The request was not one that I had expected, so I was a bit taken aback.

Topeka, after all, is a landlocked city. I explained to her that it wouldn't be possible to accommodate her request. She then looked at me in a menacing way and asked, "Are you proposing marriage to me?" Although the situation was filled with uncertainties, I was clearheaded about one thing: I was not proposing marriage to her. I told her so, and she came at me with several swift karate kicks, one of which hit me in the right thumb [and broke it]. (Gabbard, 2004b, p. 427)

In the hour before he was killed, on Sunday, Sept. 3, Dr. Wayne S. Fenton, a prominent schizophrenia specialist, was helping his wife clear the gutters of their suburban Washington house. He was steadying the ladder, asking her to please stop showering debris on his clean shirt; he had just made an appointment to see a patient and wanted to look presentable. . . . At 4:52 p.m. that Sunday, the Montgomery County police found the 53-year-old psychiatrist dead in his small office, a few minutes' drive from his house. They soon tracked down the patient he had agreed to meet that afternoon, Vitali A. Davydov, 19, of North Potomac, who admitted he had beaten the doctor with his fists, according to charging documents. (Carey, 2006)

BLS [Bureau of Labor Statistics] rates measure the number of events per 10,000 full-time workers—in this case, assaults resulting in injury. In 2000, health service workers overall had an incidence rate of 9.3 for injuries resulting from assaults and violent acts. The rate for social service workers was 15, and for nursing and personal care facility workers, 25. This compares to an overall private sector injury rate of 2. . . . The average annual rate for non-fatal violent crime for all occupations is 12.6 per 1,000 workers. The average annual rate for physicians is 16.2; for nurses, 21.9; for mental health professionals, 68.2. (Occupational Safety and Health Administration, 2004, p. 5)

The previous quotes illustrate the fact that mental health care professionals are at greater risk for workplace violence than most other professions. While this risk cannot be eliminated, certain steps can be taken to increase the safety of the clinician's work environment. The clinician needs to consider the safety of the office (Berg, Bell, & Tupin, 2000). Chairs should be arranged in the office so that the clinician can exit the office without being blocked by the client. Sharp objects, such as scissors and letter openers, should not be left out. Heavy decorative objects, such as sculptures, should not be accessible.

When working with high-risk populations, panic buttons should be installed, among other safety measures (Berg et al., 2000). Do not work in a secluded area alone with a client at high risk for violence. At least one other clinician should always be within earshot.

Because of the level of risk on inpatient units, all mental health practitioners working on the unit should have specialized training in self-defense. Inpatient professionals should also be trained in how to "take down" a violent patient and know how to use physical restraints. For a detailed review of how to alter the environment to reduce physical violence risks within an inpatient psychiatric unit, see Yeager et al. (2005).

DOCUMENTATION

Good documentation is essential in violence risk situations for two reasons. First, your documented assessment of violence risk at this particular time is essential clinical information that must be preserved in writing to help you and other clinicians who work with the client in the future. If the client is at risk of behaving violently again, studying the information that you have provided can help other clinicians evaluate that future risk more knowledgably. Second, lawsuits regarding harm could be brought against you in the future. A good contemporaneous violence risk assessment is the best defense (Elbogen, Tomkins, Pothuloori, & Scalora, 2003). As opposed to general progress notes, where being brief is a virtue, progress notes that discuss violence risk factors should include every relevant detail that you are aware of and may be quite lengthy.

As mentioned previously, a violence risk assessment is generally done at intake. One should also be done at discharge from inpatient or intensive outpatient programs if indicated and whenever there are significant changes in risk factors or violent ideation emerges. For a general violence risk assessment, the assessment for an outpatient can be outlined as follows:

* The violence risk factors for Mr. X are . . .
* Current behavior relevant to violence risk assessment is . . .
* Mr. X reported the following past violent incidents . . . [discuss incidents in detail]
* Mr. X's current violent ideation is . . .
* The violence protective factors for Mr. X are . . . He verbalizes that he does not intend to act on his violent ideation because . . .
* Mr. X's past compliance with treatment is . . .
* Mr. X's current engagement in treatment is . . .
* Mr. X verbalizes his intent not to engage in violent behavior, and if he feels that he is at greater risk of doing so, he agrees to come to the emergency room or call 911 for assistance.
* Given the above, Mr. X is at [no, low, moderate] risk for violent behavior at the present time.
* Mr. X has agreed to participate in the following treatment and activities to reduce his risk of violent behavior . . . [include what interventions you chose, why you chose them, and why you didn't chose alternative interventions].
* Mr. X will be next seen by [insert person] at [insert date].

Note that this outline pertains to a client who will be managed as an outpatient. If risk for violence is high, the client should probably be hospitalized instead. If you feel that you cannot make a persuasive argument, using this outline, for managing the client as an outpatient, then the client should be hospitalized.

In a situation where there is specific risk against an individual, all the factors assessed (remember the ACTION acronym) should be carefully documented, as should the reasoning for any clinical decision making and ensuing treatment plans. Relevant issues from the previous outline should be documented as well. If you make a *Tarasoff* warning to anyone, document whom you warned (the intended target, the police, or both), when you made the warning and why, and your clinical efforts to reduce risk to that individual.

If you have been involved in a violent or potentially violent situation with a client, document what the circumstances were, what you did, and what happened as soon as possible after the incident. If a colleague was injured by a client, the colleague might not be able to document in a timely manner; someone may need to get the information and document instead. This timely documentation is essential for the safety of other clinicians who may work with the client in the future.

Be certain that all these types of documentation are completed contemporaneously; do not go back and add further details to the assessment weeks or months later. You must do it at the time you saw the client. In addition, complete this documentation before you go home for the day; if you were concerned enough to assess violence risk, you should be concerned enough to document it the same day. This is essential because other clinicians may need this information after hours and will not have it unless you've written it up. In addition, in the worst-case scenario, if you do not document immediately and the client is subsequently violent, you are in an untenable legal situation.

COPING IF YOUR CLIENT KILLS

In my capacity as expert witness for the defense, I reviewed the discharge summary. It was a superb document, including a carefully justified risk-management plan and detailed recommendations to the patient and family members regarding adherence to the plan. . . . Then I noticed the secretarial inscription at the bottom of the last page. . . . The summary had obviously been written on the day after the killing and back-dated to appear as if it had been written before the patient had been discharged. . . . When I informed the defense counsel of the ruse, she immediately decided to settle the case—which she had previously thought was eminently winnable—for the amount the plaintiff was asking, rather than risk a trial at which the tainted discharge summary would be placed before the jury. (Monahan, 1993, p. 248)

I was retained on a case in which the patient discharged from a community mental health center later killed a stranger. On the day after the killing made the front page of the local newspaper, the director of the facility wrote numerous comments, in black ink, across the only copy of the discharge summary. These are some of them: "How could we have missed this!" "Somebody should have gotten his records," "Really shoddy work on our part." One can imagine the dollar signs glistening in the plaintiff's attorney's eyes when she saw this subpoenaed document. The case, needless to say, was settled on very generous terms. While unburdening one's conscience and self-flagellation may do wonders for the psyche, they are very hard on the net worth. Indeed after this case, the mental health center in question was no longer able to buy liability insurance. No one would sell it to them. (Monahan, 1993, p. 249)

The worst-case scenario may happen: Your client may have murdered someone, and there is a lawsuit. Monahan (1993) also advises that you not make any written or verbal statements of guilt or responsibility for what happened.

If your client kills, there are some things you should never do. Never go back and alter or add chart documents to include more information, even if they were incomplete. "It is, in short, much better to admit that you didn't keep good records and hope that the jury believes you when you tell them what happened than to manufacture good records after the fact at the cost of your own integrity and credibility" (Monahan, 1993, p. 248). All risk assessments and risk management plans must have been written in sufficient detail contemporaneously.

Do discuss the case thoroughly with your supervisor. You will undoubtedly feel quite distressed. You are likely to have many feelings about your inability to foresee and prevent the crime. You are likely to be preoccupied by thoughts and even dreams of the crime. This is normal. To regain your personal and professional functioning, seek professional support through supervision and personal therapy.

RECOMMENDED READING

Borum, R., & Reddy, M. (2001). Assessing violence risk in *Tarasoff* situations: A fact-based model of inquiry. *Behavioral Sciences and the Law, 18*, 375–385.
Borum and Reddy discuss the process of evaluating an individual for immediate violence risk toward a specific individual. Careful review and consideration of the assessment process discussed in this article is recommended for all clinicians.
Petit, J. (2005). Management of the acutely violent patient. *Psychiatric Clinics of North America, 28*, 701–711.
Petit thoroughly discusses the management of a client with acute risk of being immediately violent in the clinical setting.

EXERCISES AND DISCUSSION QUESTIONS

1. Find and review your state laws for *Tarasoff*-type situations. You may need to contact your state professional association if only case law exists or to verify if there is no law.
2. Given the laws in your state, how would you proceed with the vignette situations in this chapter? Would you do anything differently? Why?
3. Write progress notes for the three vignettes on pages 284–286.

Chapter Twenty-One

Child and Elder Maltreatment, Intimate Partner Violence, and Rape Crises

All psychotherapists need to know how to address situations of abuse and maltreatment. This chapter addresses your responsibilities in several different situations: child and elder maltreatment, intimate partner violence, and rape. These crises involve legal, ethical, and clinical considerations.

As legal considerations may vary from one state to another, I have attempted to highlight the greatest variations. Note that there are two types of law that might apply: statutes, which are laws that are passed by the state legislature, and case law, which is law that is established through judicial rulings on particular cases. Some sources for legal information by state are highlighted at the end of this chapter; your supervisor and your state professional organization can also assist you.

BEING A MANDATED REPORTER AND LEGALLY REQUIRED BREACHES OF CONFIDENTIALITY

When the client has been apprised of limits to confidentiality at the start of treatment and then reveals a problematic situation, your obligations regarding mandated reporting of abuse and legal requirements to report potential violence will not be a surprise. In fact, Steinberg, Levine, and Doueck (1997) found that when the informed consent process had been clear and explicit about limits to confidentiality, clients reacted significantly more positively to the therapist making a report of child abuse, and there was a trend toward these clients being more likely to remain in treatment.

As a mandated reporter, you have the individual responsibility to ensure that a report was made to the state authorities. Sometimes institutional policies require that one individual in the institution make all the reports to the appropriate state authority. But be aware that you, the mandated reporter, remain legally responsible for ensuring that the report was made and that it was made in a timely fashion (Alvarez, Donahue, Kenny, Cavanaugh, & Romero, 2004).

CHILD MALTREATMENT: OVERVIEW

Determining whether to make a report of child maltreatment can be a very difficult decision. As a beginning psychotherapist, you may feel particularly confused. In this section, I review some reporting recommendations based on current literature. However, be aware that this is a basic overview and that further professional education is essential. Psychotherapists who work extensively with children or families need to be especially well informed.

Child maltreatment comes in many different forms. The four types of child maltreatment are sexual abuse, physical abuse, emotional abuse, and neglect (this paragraph is informed by Alvarez, Kenny, Donahue, & Carpin, 2004; Lambie, 2005). Note that if one sibling is being maltreated, in over half the cases, others are as well (Hamilton-Giachritsis & Browne, 2005).

- *Sexual abuse* includes contact (fondling, intercourse, or inappropriate touching of genitalia) and noncontact (exposure to pornography or sexual acts).
- *Physical abuse* that results in injury is reportable, and other acts that have the potential for injury, such as shaking, striking, or kicking, are reportable in most cases.
- *Emotional abuse* is a "pattern of behavior that impairs a child's emotional development or sense of self-worth, including constant criticism, threats, or rejection, as well as withholding love, support, or guidance" (Lambie, 2005, p. 254); note that some states do not require that emotional abuse be reported (Lambie, 2005).
- *Neglect* is when the child's basic needs for food, clothing, health care, supervision, education, emotional care, and so on are not being met.

Note that these are general definitions, and you need to be familiar with how child abuse and neglect are defined legally in your state. Because research has shown that many students do not recognize certain acts of child abuse and neglect as reportable (Smith, 2006), appendix 21 provides examples and signs of maltreatment.

Be proactive and be ready to address the issue of child maltreatment as it arises. Know the exact wording of your state law regarding reporting of child maltreatment since state laws can vary considerably (Kalichman, 1999). Be sure that all clients have given written informed consent at the beginning of therapy and that the informed consent process directly addresses mandated reporting of child abuse and neglect (Kalichman, 1999). Have the hotline number for your state's child protective services readily available. It is likely that your state will require a follow-up written report (Alvarez, Donohue, et al., 2004). If so, keep blank copies of the form on hand. Finally, ensure that you have done sufficient professional reading and/or attended continuing education on child maltreatment.

CHILD MALTREATMENT: MAKING A DECISION TO REPORT

Matthew Gray is a mental health trainee who is seeing a client who is a single mother. His client talks about her son's misbehavior with frustration. She states, "Then I smacked him upside the head."

Yasmin Chopra is a mental health trainee who is working with a substance-abusing single father. She has been encouraging him to take his teenage daughter to mental health treatment for weeks. The daughter has a known history of severe depression and suicidal threats, although Yasmin's client has denied that the daughter has verbalized any problems lately. Yasmin's client is attending sessions irregularly and voices little concern about his daughter while getting more involved in substance use. He has not taken the daughter for treatment as recommended. Yasmin is very concerned.

> During the child interview, Brenda [a child] is nervous and shy. You ask Brenda about what is worrying her, and she tells you, "I can't tell you." You ask her if she can show you in a drawing. She proceeds to draw two naked people. You ask Brenda to tell you about the picture and she says, "He's peeing on her." You ask her to identify the characters in the picture and she states, "That's my daddy and that's me and sometimes my daddy pees on me." She proceeds to cry and is unwilling to talk anymore. (Finlayson & Koocher, 1991, p. 466)

In assessing the child abuse situation, you need not be certain that abuse took place; you need to have only a "reasonable suspicion." Note that under the law, it is not your job to further assess the situation and make a determination whether abuse actually took place; that is the job of child protective services (Renninger, Veach, & Bagdade, 2002). Once you develop a reasonable suspicion, you must make an oral report within 24 hours (although some states allow more time; Lambie, 2005).

Be certain to make a report of child maltreatment whenever you hear a first- or secondhand report of abuse because this surpasses the criteria of "reasonable suspicion" (Kalichman, 1999). Here are some examples of situations in which you need to make a report of child abuse:

- A child reports abuse or maltreatment, even in vague terms.
- An adult client talks about behavior suggestive of abuse, such as Matthew's client in the previous vignette.
- A client's behavior demonstrates neglect of a minor, such as Yasmin's client in the previous vignette.
- A client or a child's peer reports that a child has been abused.
- You observe physical signs of maltreatment; this also surpasses the criteria of "reasonable suspicion" (Kalichman, 1999).
- You observe an episode of emotional abuse.
- You observe that a child appears undernourished.

Do not go beyond your professional competence to be certain whether a child has been maltreated (Kalichman, 1999); certainty is unnecessary to make a mandated report. If you are not a medical professional, do not undertake any physical examinations. If you do not have extensive forensic training in validating abuse, do not attempt to do so; your untrained efforts will contaminate the investigation process. If you work primarily with adults, do not have the child come in and attempt to interview him or her. When a professional feels compelled to gather more information in these ways, it is a sign that a reasonable suspicion exists, and a report should be made instead (Kalichman, 1999).

There is a gray but important area between spankings and beatings that are administered with an object (e.g., a hairbrush or a belt) or fists. Generally, spankings are not considered child abuse (Renninger et al., 2002). If your client talks about administering or receiving "whoopings," you may need to ask what this consists of. However, some experts suggest that it is wiser to report any corporal punishment anyway and let the appropriate authorities make a determination about whether abuse has taken place (Kalichman, 1999).

If the information you have received from the client falls in this gray area or you are otherwise uncertain about whether to make a report, consult with your supervisor or another trusted licensed professional. *Be sure that you consult on the very same day that you obtained the information from the client.* You can also call child protective services in your state and discuss the concerns with a worker who will help you decide whether a report is warranted. These discussions will help clarify whether to make a report. If you decide in consultation with a colleague or with a worker at child protective services not to make a report, document that you consulted and what the reasoning was behind your decision not to report, with specific reference to your state's laws.

Be careful not to underreport. If you have been informed that maltreatment has occurred but you find that another professional already reported it, you still have a legal liability to initiate a report yourself (M. A. Small, Lyons, & Guy, 2002). Insist that the phone worker document your call to make a report; some workers may not fully understand that you are legally required to report, even if a report has been made already. In addition, receiving more than one report provides child welfare workers an indication of the seriousness of the situation. In some states, there is no requirement to report unless you have actually seen the maltreated child yourself; however, professional ethics dictate that you make a report nonetheless if you have a reasonable suspicion (Kalichman, 1999). Sometimes underreporting is due to lack of awareness of different types of child maltreatment. Be aware that child physical or sexual abuse can come from siblings or peers as well as adults. Moreover, children can sometimes be maltreated while in foster care (Gelles, 2006) or in an institution (Kalichman, 1999). An adolescent can ostensibly agree to have sex with an adult, but this may actually be statutory rape and thus reportable, depending on their ages and state law. Psychotherapists must also be aware that in rare events, caregivers can intentionally produce illness in a child or other dependent person; this is called Munchausen syndrome by proxy (Pasqualone & Fitzgerald, 1999).

On the other hand, be careful not to overreport. Overreporting will contribute to overtaxing your state's already overburdened child protective system. An example where a report is not warranted is a child who has emotional symptoms that could possibly be suggestive of abuse (e.g., is withdrawn or fearful) but there are no other signs of abuse (Besharov & Laumann, 1996). These emotional symptoms could be due to childhood mental illness or to a chaotic but not abusive family situation, and your report would likely be unsubstantiated; however, continue to be alert to possible indicators of abuse in these cases.

Research shows that many suspected cases of abuse are never reported (Alvarez, Kenny et al., 2004). Psychotherapists are often reluctant to make reports because they are unsure whether abuse actually occurred. In addition, there appear to be some cultural factors that may result in White therapists and those born in the United States being more likely to make reports than non-White therapists and immigrant therapists (Ashton, 2004). Remember that it is not your job, legally, to determine the full facts in the case; that is the job of child protective services. You need to have only a "reasonable suspicion" of maltreatment.

Some therapists fear that that reporting will hurt the therapeutic relationship. However, Steinberg et al. (1997) found that only one-quarter of clients drop out subsequent to a report, whereas in three-quarters of cases, the therapy relationship is unchanged or improved. Psychotherapists may worry that they will be sued for making a report, but all states provide legal immunity for reports made in good faith (Alvarez, Kenny et al., 2004). On the other hand, depending on state law, psychotherapists can risk facing charges, jail time, or loss of license for failure to report, or a psychotherapist might also be sued by a victim or the victim's family for failure to report (Alvarez, Kenny et al., 2004). Finally and by far most important, failure to report will result in the child experiencing continued maltreatment and emotional distress.

CHILD MALTREATMENT: MAKING A REPORT

When a mandated report must be made, there are two goals. First, we are motivated compassionately, ethically, and legally to be sure that children are safe. Second, we want to maintain the therapeutic relationship so that we can help alleviate the family situation that led to the maltreatment.

Prepare to call by gathering together all the relevant contact information that you have regarding the child and the child's family (this paragraph is informed by Kalichman, 1999). This information could include the name of the child, the child's age, sex, address, and current whereabouts. Other helpful information would include ages and names of other children in the home, names and addresses of the child's parents, information of the circumstances and nature of the maltreatment, and the identity of the suspected perpetrator. Of course, you may not have all this information. If not, that is okay; simply supply as much information as you have. Do not provide confidential information about the client that is not directly relevant to the episode of maltreatment (e.g., adult client's own history of abuse).

Your client may be the child, the perpetrator, or another family member. When deciding how to proceed, first ask yourself whether the child will be at more risk if the family is aware that a report is being made (Kalichman, 1999). If so, do not tell the family that you will be making a report before you do so. However, if the risk to the child will not increase if the family is aware of the report, involving them in the reporting process can help maintain trust in the therapeutic relationship.

When you involve your adult client in the reporting process, first explain the necessity of making a report. Positive therapeutic outcomes were associated with this reporting strategy: Inform the client yourself that you need to make a report and explain why in terms of your own clinical assessment rather than as a requirement imposed by state law (Weinstein, Levine, Kogan, Harkavy-Friedman, & Miller, 2001). If you have appropriately informed the client of limits to confidentiality at the beginning of treatment, the need to make this report will probably not be a surprise. You should also explain what is likely to happen when a report is made.

Second, several alternatives can be offered to the client to participate in or observe the process of reporting. The client could make the call to report the abuse in the office with you observing (do not rely on the client to report the abuse later). Or the client could observe you making the call so that the client knows exactly what you said during the call. If the client does not want to participate in either of these options, you should make the report immediately when the session ends.

When you or the client make the call, be sure to obtain the name, position, and contact information for the worker who takes the call. If the client calls, follow this up with a call of your own or talk to the worker yourself with the client there so that it is documented by child protective services that you have made the mandated call.

CHILD MALTREATMENT: DOCUMENTATION AND FOLLOW-UP

Make a note in the chart of any other professional you consulted with prior to making the call. Document the circumstances of the call: Had you informed the client that you were making the call? Did the client participate in making the call? Note the time of the call and the name or employee number of the person you talked to (Kalichman, 1999). Document exactly what information you provided to the worker. *Document that you made the call on the day that you made it.*

If your state requires a written form, keep a copy of that. Document any follow-up calls you made to child protective services or that they made to you. Document any activities related to the case as they happen.

ELDER MALTREATMENT

Margaret, an 82-year-old retired musician, lives with her 65-year-old son, Maurice. Maurice is a pathological gambler who spends all of his time at the racetrack. Margaret suffers from congestive heart failure and mild dementia. She is unable to dress, wash, or feed herself without assistance. Margaret's physicians have advised Maurice that she should not be left alone at home. Maurice ignores their advice, frequently fails to feed or bathe his mother, and uses the money she gives him to refill her prescriptions to bet on the horses. Consequently, Margaret is not able to obtain needed medication and her heart condition has worsened significantly. Her nutrition is poor, and she is mildly dehydrated. Margaret has also burned herself several times while trying to prepare her own meals. (Welfel, Danzinger, & Santoro, 2000, p. 285)

In a caregiver support group for elderly people, group members were discussing stressful caregiving situations. Mr. Smith began talking about how he sometimes became frustrated with his wife, a victim of Alzheimer's disease. "When you say you're frustrated, what do you mean exactly," the facilitator asked him. "Well," he answered, "I guess I mean I have to do things I would rather not have to do." "Such as what?" the facilitator probed. "Well sometimes she won't get dressed, just real stubborn she is. I'll try showing her what I mean by taking off my clothes, but it doesn't register. So then I'll try to take off her blouse, gently, but she'll back away from me. I'll try talking to her, but nothing. So I'll slap her a few times, I'll say 'You have to listen to me' then she cooperates. It's real frustrating." (Bergeron & Gray, 2003, p. 96)

Evidence suggests that elder abuse is significantly underreported and underidentified. Neglect is the most common form of elder abuse and is defined as "withholding of necessary food, clothing, and medical care to meet the physical and mental needs of an elderly person" (Jayawardena & Liao, 2006, p. 128). Caretakers may neglect elders intentionally or unintentionally. Caretakers may be unable to provide adequate care. Physical, emotional, and financial abuse are also common, and different forms of abuse often co-occur:

- *Physical abuse* includes "pushing, striking, or causing bodily injury, force-feeding, or improper use of physical restraints" (Jayawardena & Liao, 2006, p. 128).
- *Emotional abuse* involves threats, humiliation, or insults.
- *Financial abuse* entails misappropriating the elder's funds or property for the caretaker's own financial gain. Perpetrators of elder financial abuse can also be individuals "outside the family, such as contractors, salesmen, attorneys, caregivers, insurance agents, clergy, accountants, bookkeepers, and friends" (Kemp & Mosqueda, 2005, p. 1123).
- *Sexual abuse* of the elderly is rare, although it may be more underreported than other types of elder maltreatment (Loue, 2001); it is any unwanted sexual contact, perhaps with an elder who is too cognitively impaired to consent.

Elders can also be neglected or abandoned by caregivers. See appendix 22 for detailed signs and examples of elder maltreatment.

Abusers of the elderly in the home can be spouses, adult children, spouses of adult children, and other relatives (Jayawardena & Liao, 2006; Rudolph

& Hughes, 2001). Abuse by the spouse is sometimes a continuation of long-standing domestic violence (Loue, 2001). Abuse can also take place in an institutional setting (Loue, 2001). The elderly who are most at risk have dementia, short-term memory problems, mental illness, or alcohol abuse (Shugarman, Fries, Wolf, & Morris, 2003) or are dependent or aggressive (Loue, 2001). Maltreatment risk factors associated with the caregivers are "advanced age, alcoholism, intellectual deficits, inadequate communication skills, substance abuse, depression, poor physical health, stress, social isolation, financial difficulties, and dependence on the elderly individual" (Loue, 2001, p. 167).

Probably even more than with child maltreatment, laws for defining and reporting of elder abuse vary considerably from state to state (Jogerst et al., 2003); however, elder maltreatment is mandated to be reported in all 50 states (Loue, 2001). Elders are generally defined as being 60 years old or older (except for California, Maryland, and Nebraska, where the age is 65, and Alabama, where the age is 55; Jogerst et al., 2003). However, many of the same reporting principles apply (certain individuals are designated as mandated reporters; a reasonable suspicion, not certainty, is needed for the report; reports in good faith are immune from prosecution; and mandated reporters can be prosecuted for failure to report).

Be aware of the requirements of your state laws and keep the number for reporting elder abuse handy. Consider and document the same issues as you would in the case of child maltreatment: obtaining proper informed consent, effectively using consultation, and involving the client in making the report. For a detailed review of the recommended procedure for mandated reporting in elder abuse, see Welfel et al., (2000).

ELDER SELF-NEGLECT

[Self-neglecting elders in the United Kingdom lived in homes with] conditions of extreme disrepair with buildings in a state of collapse, holes in the roof, ceilings, walls and broken windows. Interiors were often sparsely furnished with bare floorboards and makeshift stoves/cooking facilities including open fires on the floor. In many cases there was no electricity, running water, or proper sanitation. . . . [Elders lived with] blocked toilets, offensive household odours, and infestations of fleas, flies, rats, and maggots. There were reports of large numbers of pets, particularly cats, within dwellings. A commonly reported feature involved houses being crammed full of belongings, which spilled over into the garden area. Such clients hoarded rubbish, clothes, newspapers, family belongings and miscellaneous items. (Lauder, Anderson, & Barclay, 2005, p. 320)

Elder self-neglect appears to occur at much greater frequency than elder maltreatment from others (Lauder et al., 2005). *Self-neglect* is defined as "not engaging in those self-care actions that are required to produce socially acceptable levels of personal and household cleanliness and personal health and well-being" (Lauder et al., 2005, p. 317). The elderly person's home is likely to be "dirty, full of rubbish and in a general state of disrepair" (Lauder et al., 2005, p. 320). Self-neglecting clients may be socially isolated, and they may be difficult to treat because they may not attend appointments or open their mail. Self-neglect is more common in women and the very old (Thompson & Priest, 2005).

About half the states require that self-neglect be reported to adult protective services as well (Loue, 2001). But often the issue of the elder's competency to make his own decisions, in the context of self-neglect, is not adequately addressed in state reporting laws (Loue, 2001).

MALTREATMENT OF VULNERABLE ADULTS

Some adults who are not elderly are nonetheless considered *vulnerable adults* because of their disability status (Teaster, 2000). Most adult protective services programs serve both elderly and other vulnerable adults, but Louisiana, Massachusetts, and Oregon have separate divisions or agencies (National Committee for the Prevention of Elder Abuse & National Adult Protective Services Association, 2007). The vulnerable adults' disabilities can be physical, mental, or emotional. Self-neglect, physical abuse, and caregiver abandonment or neglect were the most common categories of investigated reports, each encompassing about 20% of the total (National Committee for the Prevention of Elder Abuse & National Adult Protective Services Association, 2007).

If you feel that it may be appropriate to make a report regarding a vulnerable adult, talk to your supervisor. Further information can be obtained from the link to your state on http://www.elderabusecenter.org or by calling your state elder abuse hotline (since this hotline is likely to handle cases with vulnerable adults as well).

INTIMATE PARTNER VIOLENCE

Pannee Raksuwan is a mental health trainee working in an emergency intake clinic. Her intake client, Sandra Johnson, states that her husband tried to strangle her. She has prominent bruises and is feeling dizzy, perhaps from a mild concussion. Sandra tells Pannee about her history of chronic depression with multiple suicide attempts. Sandra states that she plans to leave; she is upset and crying. She admits to a history of returning to her husband a week or two after the abuse.

Shoshanna Rosenberg is a mental health trainee working with a gay client, Frank. The client repeatedly describes arguments with his partner. Shoshanna asks whether these arguments have been physical at times. With some reluctance, Frank admits that he and his partner hit each other when they are angry. Frank had to go to the emergency room for a dislocated finger once after his partner pushed him against a wall.

Intimate partner violence (IPV) is a common phenomenon worldwide and within every American cultural group, although there is some international variation in rates (Loue, 2000). One multiracial study of heterosexual couples found that men were most commonly the primary perpetrator of violence (54%), but mutual violent perpetration (35%) is common as well, and female primary perpetration (11%) is not unusual (Weston, Temple, & Marshall, 2005). Another study found that mutual violence in heterosexual couples is the most common pattern (Williams & Frieze, 2005). However, the negative emotional and physical impact of IPV may be stronger on women (K. L. Anderson, 2002; Weston et al., 2005). Intimate partner violence can also occur in gay and lesbian couples (McKenry, Serovich, Mason, & Mosack, 2006).

Perpetrators of domestic violence have a high incidence of childhood trauma, adult mental illness and substance abuse (Stuart, Moore, Gordon, Ramsey, & Kahler, 2006). The victims of IPV suffer disproportionately from post-traumatic stress disorder (PTSD), substance abuse, depression, and other anxiety disorders (Robertiello, 2006) as well as brain injuries (Valera & Berenbaum, 2003) and physical health problems (Dutton et al., 2006).

Evidence suggests that IPV is underdetected by health care professionals. A chart review of women's emergency visits found that fewer than 30% of charts documented that the woman was screened for IPV (Richter, Surprenant, Schmelzle, & Mayo, 2003). A survey of licensed psychologists found that less than 20% of psychologists screened routinely for IPV (Samuelson & Campbell, 2005). If the clinician does not ask about IPV, the clinician will probably miss it.

Intimate partner violence and child abuse often co-occur (Knickerbocker, Heyman, Slep, Jouriles, & McDonald, 2007), so the presence of one type of abuse should trigger a full assessment of violence, abuse, and neglect within the family. Observing IPV as a child leads to a higher rate of childhood problems (Kitzmann, Gaylord, Holt, & Kenny, 2003), adult psychopathology (Diamond & Muller, 2004), and adult perpetration of partner violence (Ehrensaft et al., 2003).

Often victims present to mental health clinicians with depression or anxiety symptoms. One simple screening procedure for domestic violence is the Partner Violence Screen, which consists of the following three questions:

> "Have you been hit, kicked, punched, or otherwise hurt by someone within the past year? If so, by whom?"
> "Do you feel safe in your current relationship?"
> "Is there a partner from a previous relationship who is making you feel unsafe now?" (Feldhaus et al., 1997, p. 1358).

If the client has experienced IPV, Samuelson and Clark (2005) recommend that safety be assessed through these types of questions:

> "What threats have been made?"
> "Do you and [name of abuser] live together? How often do you see each other? Does he/she have a key to your apartment?" (and other questions to assess accessibility of client to abuser)
> "Do you want immediate protection by law enforcement or the safety of a shelter?"
> "Do you have a plan to protect yourself [and your children] if the danger escalates?"
> "Do you know how to access community resources if you feel unsafe?"

In our society, it is common knowledge that resources are available for victims of domestic violence. Often, those who are ready to leave the perpetrator have already taken steps to contact law enforcement, leave the partner, or go to a domestic violence shelter. So clients who are seen in therapy and who are experiencing ongoing domestic violence may be ambivalent about leaving the partner or do not intend to leave. In those cases, sometimes all the clinician can do is provide support, concern, education, and information to the client.

The client may not realize that physical attacks are a crime and might not understand the negative impact of IPV on one's own mental health and that of the children. Samuelson and Clark (2005) recommend having the following information ready to provide to victims of interpersonal violence: hotline numbers, local shelters, domestic violence therapy groups, law enforcement, legal aid, advocacy groups, educational and financial services, and food and housing assistance.

In some states, IPV is mandated to be reported to the state. In other jurisdictions, there may be requirements that certain types of injuries (e.g., gunshot wounds) be reported (Loue, 2000). However, in other states, there is no mandate for reporting IPV at all. Talk to your supervisor about what the laws are in your state.

RAPE

Dante Rogers, a mental health trainee, is getting into his office early in the morning at the college counseling center. He checks his voice mail to find a distraught and not entirely coherent message from his client Michelle Barnes. He listens to the message several times, and it becomes clear that Michelle was calling in the early morning hours stating that she had experienced date rape. He calls Michelle's cell phone right away. She is still distressed, but her roommate is with her. He tells Michelle to come in to the office right away, and she agrees to do so. He then calls his first two scheduled clients to reschedule them.

Angelica Willis, a mental health trainee, is working in a state prison for men. An inmate whom she does not know requests to speak with her. She meets with him, and he starts crying, stating that he has been raped. He asks her not to tell anyone since he is fearful of being killed by the rapist and his gang.

The mental health practitioner can encounter a rape crisis in any clinical setting. The client may seek mental health treatment first rather than medical treatment. Most communities have rape crisis centers that can send a volunteer or paraprofessional to assist the rape victim throughout the emergency medical assessment and treatment process.

Rape is underrecognized and undertreated in men; a recent survey found that 5% of rape victims were male (Azikiwe, Wright, Cheng, & D'Angelo, 2005). Men appear to be most at risk of rape in prison (Wiwanitkit, 2005). Male survivors of sexual assault were raped by men in over 85% of cases, and in almost all cases there was forced anal penetration (Wiwanitkit, 2005).

As a health care practitioner, you need to be informed about all the issues that a sexually assaulted client will need to address: emotional, medical, and legal. Cybulska and Forster (2005) delineate the tasks that should ideally be accomplished in the immediate aftermath of rape:

- Treating severe injuries (e.g., the client may need antibiotics or a tetanus shot for bite wounds)
- Assessment of safety
- Forensic medical examination
- Emergency contraception with testing to rule out preexisting pregnancy as needed
- Prophylaxis against sexually transmitted diseases, including HIV
- Screening for sexually transmitted diseases, including HIV
- Counseling and psychological support
- Support for the victim's partner and family if appropriate

To this list, I would add making a report of the crime. Clearly not all rape victims will be willing to participate immediately—or sometimes ever—in all aspects of this process.

As you probably know, emergency departments have trained professionals available to gather forensic medical evidence in rape cases. After the rape occurs, the client has a limited time in which there is any chance that valid evidence can be gathered. The passage of time, defecating, showering, and changing clothes all reduce the chances of obtaining evidence (A. Anderson, 1999; Cybulska & Forster, 2005). Sperm survives in the vagina for 7 days and in the rectum for 3 days (Cybulska & Forster, 2005). After 7 days, no forensic evidence can be gathered; however, any injuries that are healing can still be documented medically (Cybulska & Forster, 2005). A rape victim advocate from the local rape crisis center can knowledgably help support the client throughout this process.

Whether or not forensic evidence has been gathered, the client needs to be evaluated for pregnancy (if a fertile female), for sexually transmitted diseases, and for injury. The emergency room staff should offer emergency contraception. Emergency contraception can be administered in the emergency room, reducing the chances that the distressed rape victim misses filling her prescription (Azikiwe et al., 2005). Medications can be administered to reduce the chance that HIV and other sexually transmitted diseases will infect the client. It is important that you know about these treatments because you may need to educate the client to ask for them; in many cases, medical care for rape victims is incomplete, especially with regard to emergency contraception (R. Campbell, Wasco, Ahrens, Sefl, & Barnes, 2001).

If the client wishes to make a police report and press charges, it is helpful to obtain the assistance of a rape victim advocate. Unfortunately, many negative outcomes can occur for the rape victim in the legal arena. The case may be dismissed against the client's wishes, and if the client succeeds in prosecuting, the legal process of doing so can sometimes be retraumatizing (R. Campbell et al., 2001).

In counseling the client, the first goal is to reduce the client's immediate level of distress (for simplicity, I refer to the client as female in this discussion). Let the client talk to you at her own pace. Listen nonjudgmentally and provide validation and support; this will help calm her. Assist the client in calling the rape crisis center from your office for assistance if she hasn't already. Educate the client about her medical and legal options and help her decide how to pursue these if she is willing to do so. Help the client activate her social support network if she hasn't done so already (e.g., the client may want to call her sibling, parent, best friend, or other individual to support her through the legal and medical aftermath). Help the client figure out how to reestablish a feeling of safety; perhaps she would like to stay with a close friend or her family for a few days. She may need prescriptions for medications to manage anxiety, agitation, or sleeplessness. Before she leaves, make a plan for follow-up treatment no later than 1 week from now. You also may wish to have the client check in by phone between sessions in the first week or two.

Whatever the client decides to do from a medical or legal perspective, clear and careful records should be made of the client's statements about assault since the client might need these records to press charges later (Cybulska & Forster, 2005). Some of the information you would want to document might include the following:

• Date and time of the assault
• Circumstances of the assault
• Location
• Type of assault (physical and/or sexual)
• Orifices involved, condom use, and whether ejaculation occurred
• Client's actions after the assault (Cybulska & Forster, 2005)

Inform your client that, for her legal benefit, you plan to completely document whatever she says to you about the assault. Remind her of relevant confidentiality issues as needed. However, use great care in asking about details of the trauma because it may be overly distressing for the client to repeatedly discuss it or to discuss it in detail. Any medical professionals who treat her must ask her most of these questions in order to provide effective medical care based on her specific situation.

Rape causes a higher rate of PTSD than most other traumas, and your supervisor can help you figure out how to assist your client further after this initial crisis and stabilization phase.

COPING WITH MALTREATMENT, VIOLENCE, AND NEGLECT

Addressing these traumatic experiences with clients is distressing. Thoroughly discuss what has transpired with your supervisor and seek support from trusted colleagues and in personal therapy as needed. In addition, read about vicarious traumatization in chapter 23 and about therapist self-care in chapter 24.

RECOMMENDED READING: CHILD MALTREATMENT

Alvarez, K. M., Donohue, B., Kenny, M. C., Cavanagh, N., & Romero, V. (2004). The process and consequences of reporting child maltreatment: A brief overview for professionals in the mental health field. *Aggression and Violent Behavior, 10*, 311–331.

Alvarez and colleagues provide a detailed portrayal of the nuts and bolts of child protective services reporting and investigation process. This article should be essential reading for all mental health professionals.

Kalichman, S. C. (1999). *Mandated reporting of suspected child abuse: Ethics, law, and policy.* Washington, DC: American Psychological Association.

Kalichman provides an in-depth discussion of mandated reporting of child maltreatment, including helpful case discussions and reports of legal cases. Read this book if you anticipate working with families or children or if you will be working with a high-risk population.

RECOMMENDED READING: ELDER MALTREATMENT

Loue, S. (2001). Elder abuse and neglect in medicine and law: The need for reform. *Journal of Legal Medicine, 22,* 159–209.

Provides a detailed review of the area of elder abuse, including current legal complexities.

Thompson, H., & Priest, R. (2005). Elder abuse and neglect: Considerations for mental health practitioners. *Adultspan Journal, 4,* 116–128.

Thompson and Priest provide helpful information for psychotherapists who will be working with the elderly, including how to assess the home situation, cultural considerations, and suggestions for intervention.

Welfel, E. R., Danzinger, P. R., & Santoro, S. (2000). Mandated reporting of abuse/maltreatment of older adults: A primer for counselors. *Journal of Counseling and Development, 78,* 284–292.

Provides a detailed overview of the process of mandated reporting for elder abuse and neglect.

RECOMMENDED READING: INTIMATE PARTNER VIOLENCE

Samuelson, S. L., & Campbell, C. D. (2005). Screening for domestic violence: Recommendations based on a practice survey. *Professional Psychology: Research and Practice, 36,* 276–282.

Samuelson and Campbell current practices and give helpful recommendations for screening and intervention.

RECOMMENDED READING: RAPE

Campbell, R., Wasco, S. M., Ahrens, C. E., Sefl, T., & Barnes, H. E. (2001). Preventing the "second rape": Rape survivors' experiences with community service providers. *Journal of Interpersonal Violence, 16,* 1239–1259.

Campbell and colleagues research and discuss the actual experiences of rape survivors in the mental health, medical, and legal arenas.

Cybulska, B., & Forster, G. (2005). Sexual assault: Examination of the victim. *Medicine, 33*, 23–28.
Cybulska and Forster describe in detail the process of medical examination of the female sexual assault victim.

WEB RESOURCES

http://www.childwelfare.gov
This website provides a comprehensive review of all state-mandated reporting laws for child abuse and neglect as well as other information about child welfare. The website is a project of the U.S. Department of Health and Human Services.
http://www.elderabusecenter.org
Website for the National Center on Elder Abuse. Provides guidance in finding state statutes regarding elder abuse reporting and more information about elder abuse.

EXERCISES AND QUESTIONS

1. Find and review your state laws for child and elder maltreatment. Are there situations in your state where you might become aware of abuse, yet not be required to report it? What would you do then? Are written reports required? What is the statute of limitations? How soon do you need to call after you have a reasonable suspicion of abuse? Does the statute specify any differences between information learned as part of your professional duties and personally obtained information?
2. How is statutory rape defined in your state?
3. Does your state mandate reporting of elder self-neglect? How is that defined?
4. Does your state mandate reporting of domestic violence? Under what circumstances?

Section V

CARING FOR YOURSELF AND YOUR CLIENTS

Chapter Twenty-Two

Challenging Relationships and Emotions

Emotional reactions from the client and your own feelings about the client often arise even during the very first session. These emotions are often the first clue that key relationship patterns are occurring within the session. Relationship patterns are expressed through thinking, emotions, behavior, and physiological reactions (J. S. Beck, 2005). The aim of this chapter is to give you an introduction to conceptualizing these emotional reactions when they occur.

As we all know, psychotherapy can be an emotional experience for a client. Often strong emotions are related to persistent relationship patterns. In addition, occasionally the client will implicitly or explicitly express emotions toward you, potentially leading to confusion or distress on your part.

Of course, you have feelings in therapy as well. Often these feelings will be positive (e.g., you like the client, you empathize with the client, or you are pleased with the client's effort in therapy). At other times, these feelings may be perplexing or troubling (e.g., the client is boring you, or the client makes you feel anxious). Sometimes therapists are even ashamed about some of the feelings that they have in therapy (e.g., feeling disgust toward the client or feeling attracted to the client).

Different schools of psychotherapy have different ways to conceptualize these emotions and relationships. In this chapter, as in the rest of this book, I attempt to frame clinical issues in a theoretically integrative manner. However, in this chapter, my terminology—although, it is hoped, not my conceptualization—departs from this ideal. Psychodynamic psychotherapists have a long history, dating back to Freud, of giving names to the clients' emotional reactions and relationships patterns in therapy (transference) and therapists' emotional reactions and relationships patterns in therapy (countertransference). I am not aware of any similarly useful terms in other traditions.

COGNITIVE-BEHAVIORAL CONCEPTUALIZATION OF RELATIONSHIPS IN PSYCHOTHERAPY

A great deal of evidence exists that some of Freud's (1965) theories of transference and countertransference, though somewhat exaggerated and distorted, often exist in practically all forms of psychotherapy. For example, we can in all likelihood endorse these clinical findings: (a) Clients and therapists bring influences of their personal history to the therapeutic encounter; (b) they consciously, and especially unconsciously, project their feelings and wishes onto each other; (c) consequently, clients and therapists often have a biased or prejudiced view of each other's personality and effectiveness; and (d) they both can use their transference and countertransference thoughts, feelings, and behaviors to help and/or hinder the therapeutic process. . . . Therapists often are obsessively and compulsively convinced that their particular theory and practice of therapy is the only one capable of helping their clients. Therefore, they rigidly and inefficiently stick to its narrow ways and refuse to use other methods that would be more helpful. (A. Ellis, 2001, pp. 1000–1001)

They [patients] usually have very negative ideas about themselves, others, and their worlds—views that they developed and have maintained since childhood or adolescence. When these beliefs dominate their perceptions, patients then tend to perceive, feel and behave in highly dysfunctional ways, across time and across situations—including in the therapy session itself. (J. S. Beck, 2005, p. 4)

When noticing their own discomfort or maladaptive behavior (for example, avoiding important topics, overcontrolling or undercontrolling patients, speaking sharply or without empathy), therapists should identify their dysfunctional thoughts and beliefs and conceptualize their area of vulnerability. . . . Because therapists are human, it is inevitable, and sometimes even helpful, that they occasionally have a dysfunctional reaction toward their patients. As professionals, therapists need to conceptualize why the problem arose so they can take stock of their contribution to the problem and solve it. (J. S. Beck, 2005, pp. 114, 127)

As Albert Ellis stated in the first quote, transference and countertransference are well-recognized phenomena in psychotherapy. As far as I know, however, he never integrated his recognition of them into his theoretical perspective.

The second quote from Judith Beck emphasizes the importance of examining the client's ideas about relationships with others during therapy. This second quote could even be interpreted as a description of transference from a cognitive-behavioral perspective. The third quote, also from Beck, describes a phenomenon very much like countertransference from a cognitive behavioral perspective. Clearly, she is describing similar phenomena, although she does not use the same terms.

RESEARCH EVIDENCE OF TRANSFERENCE

> Classically, transference has been considered an unconscious process in which the patient displaces or "transfers" onto the therapist feelings and thoughts originally directed toward the important people of childhood. (Goldstein, 2000, p. 167)

> [Transference occurs when] a perceiver's mental representation of a significant other is activated in an encounter with a new person, leading the perceiver to interpret the person in ways derived from the representation and also to respond emotionally, motivationally, and behaviorally to the person in ways that reflect the self–other relationship. (Andersen & Chen, 2002, p. 620)

Transference was first recognized by Sigmund Freud back in the 19th century. Research and clinical practice has supported the idea of transference since then. The previous two quotes indicate that *transference* entails transferring feelings, thoughts, and behaviors from a past significant relationship to a current relationship. And, as Andersen and colleagues have shown (e.g., Andersen & Chen, 2002), transference can happen in an individual's personal life as well as within the therapy relationship.

A growing body of research scientifically demonstrates the presence of transference in the therapeutic relationship. Andersen and Berk (1998) have found that "mental representations of significant others serve as storehouses of information about given individuals from one's life, and can be activated (made ready for use) and applied to (used to interpret) other individuals, and that this is especially likely when the new individual in some way resembles a significant other" (p. 81).

Research by Beach and Power (1996) demonstrated that transference occurs in all types of psychotherapy. They transcribed psychotherapy sessions from psychotherapists of varying theoretical orientations and discovered comments indicative of transference in each. Interestingly, fewer transference statements were voiced by clients in the cognitive and cognitive-behavioral groups. They also found that psychoanalytic therapists made more detailed comments in response to client transference statements.

A different research approach toward transference was taken by Bradley, Heim, and Westen (2005). They used standardized instruments to survey psychologists and psychiatrists regarding the thoughts, feelings, motives, conflicts, and behaviors expressed by the clients toward the therapists. They then subjected the resulting data to factor analysis, which is a statistical method of identifying categories in the data. Five groups of transference feelings emerged:

- Angry/entitled: The client makes excessive demands on the therapist while also being angry and dismissive, generally found with borderline and narcissistic clients.

- Anxious/preoccupied: The client fears the therapist's disapproval and rejection and may be overly compliant or dependent.
- Avoidant: The client seems to want to avoid connecting with the therapist emotionally.
- Sexualized: The client appears to have sexual feelings toward the therapist and may behave in a seductive manner.
- Secure/engaged: The client feels comfortable with the therapist, and they have a positive and secure working alliance.

Interestingly, the researchers were concerned that these findings might be an artifact of the significant number of psychodynamically oriented therapists in the sample, so they reanalyzed the data excluding those therapists and found basically the same results. Note that there are many possible emotional reactions that are not categorized by this research; probably only the most common transference patterns showed up in the factor analysis.

These different research projects have one commonality: that transference exists and that it is a normal event that occurs during therapy and in the client's personal life. Thus, as psychotherapists, we must be prepared to recognize it and use it therapeutically to help the client understand his or her relationships more deeply. Then the client can choose to change long-standing relationship patterns if he or she feels that they are unhealthy.

USING TRANSFERENCE IN THERAPY

It is the establishment and working through of the transference that is thought to be crucial to the attainment of insight in psychoanalysis and psychoanalytic psychotherapy. Traditionally, the therapist strove to serve as a "blank screen," in an atmosphere of neutrality, abstinence, and anonymity, thus providing a setting most conducive to the displacement of feelings. . . . [Now therapy is considered] a process that is more interactional, interpersonal, and subjective in nature, characterized by a mingling of transference and countertransference between patient and therapist. The therapist, like the patient, is viewed as a unique individual with his own theory of how therapy works, his own idiosyncrasies, his own conflicts and his own past, all of which contribute to the unfolding of the transference. (Goldstein, 2000, p. 168)

The research cited in the previous section shows that clients frequently display challenging emotional reactions and relationship patterns, otherwise known as transference, in therapy. These emotions may be toward you or toward important others in the client's life.

Beginning therapists can take their clients' emotional reactions toward them very personally. Therapists are concerned about their clients and want to help.

To have their clients feel fearful, angry, or distant in response can be confusing and frustrating. The key to addressing these reactions is to reconceptualize them and use them to gain greater insight into the client's life problems.

Although transference can occur toward anyone and is not simply a phenomenon of therapy, it is more likely to occur when there is some resemblance to an individual who was very influential to the client (Andersen & Chen, 1998). By virtue of your professional authority and your caretaking for the client, your role already has some resemblance to that of the client's parent (or other significant childhood caretaker). This role will contribute to transference arising during the psychotherapy session. In addition, the client may have rigid, inflexible ways of dealing with interpersonal situations and thus act out a typical manner of relating to others in the session (J. S. Beck, 2005).

Historically, in psychodynamic approaches, as indicated in the previous quote, the therapist uses insights about the client's transference to make *transference interpretations*. When you make a transference interpretation, you are trying to describe explicitly some aspect of the relationship between you and the client that is occurring implicitly (Hobson & Kapur, 2005). Another definition of transference interpretations is "an explicit reference to the patient's ongoing relationship with the therapist" (Hoglend, 2004, p. 280). Here are some examples of transference interpretations:

- "I'm noticing that you are hesitant to talk to me about your difficulties with your classes. I'm wondering how you are expecting me to react if we discuss that?"
- "[H]ow did you feel when I suggested that you might have some influence [on your husband]? (pause) Did you feel a little anxious? . . . What did it mean to you when I said it?" (J. S. Beck, 2005, p. 71).
- "You seem a little different this week. I wonder, are you feeling less connected to therapy and to me? . . . Are you also thinking that I feel less connected to you?" (J. S. Beck, 2005, p. 82).

Note that these transference interpretations are more like questions than statements. You may not even know what the answers would be; you need only identify that a reaction arose in the client that signifies transference and begin the process of inquiring about it. While there are many ways to make transference interpretations, these interpretations are phrased as "inviting a mutual exploration of possibilities rather than . . . talking 'at' the patient or prescribing the truth" (Hobson & Kapur, 2005, p. 277).

Hoglend (2004) notes that transference issues can also be explored in therapy without making transference interpretations directly. Instead, you might "interpret conflicts and/or interpersonal patterns in the patient's contemporary relationships or search for memories of past relationships, without including a reference to the patient-therapist interaction" (p. 281). Hoglend terms these therapeutic interventions *extratransference interpretations.* Some examples of this kind of intervention would be the following:

- "I've noticed that you often do not talk about your difficulties with your friends. Are you worried that they would react negatively if you did so? [After client reacts to that point] How do you think you developed these expectations of other people?"
- "What were you thinking when you talked to your mother on the phone?" (J. S. Beck, 2005, p. 211).
- "So you were trying to e-mail your sister and you began to feel bad. What was going through your mind?" (J. S. Beck, 2005, p. 213).

Note that the therapist is actually helping to guide the client in constructing her own extratransference interpretations. The client's views about others can then be examined using cognitive therapy techniques if you choose (J. S. Beck, 2005).

You don't need to present a transference interpretation that dazzles your client with your insight and therapeutic brilliance ("You treat me as if I were your mother, expecting me to be harsh and controlling"). I suspect that it was this type of comment that Hoglend (2004) examined when he found that there is a significant risk that clients will not take transference interpretations well. Clients may be defensive or anxious in response to transference interpretations or find them intrusive and unpleasant. They can see the therapist as critical, hostile, or dominant. And they can feel that the therapist is focusing too much on the therapy relationship and ignoring the client's very real current interpersonal problems, symptoms, and difficulties in coping. All these reactions pose some threat to the continuation of therapy, the strength of the therapeutic alliance, and hence the therapy outcome.

In his review of the research on transference, Hoglend (2004) concluded that research suggested that a high level of transference interpretations (five or more per session) is poorly tolerated by clients, often resulting in dropout and/or lack of improvement. Extratransference interpretations were much more readily tolerated by the clients. Interestingly, a Norwegian research study found (contrary to theoretical expectations) that clients with more interpersonal problems and more symptoms responded better to therapy that included transference interpretations and that clients who were higher functioning responded better to therapy without any transference interpretations (Hoglend, Johansson, Marble, Bogwald, & Amlo, 2007).

Clearly, transference interpretations are powerful interventions that are not fully understood in the current research paradigm. So how can the beginning therapist use transference interpretations when starting to see a new client? In summary, here are some suggestions:

- Be gentle when making either transference or extratransference interpretations. Ask questions or wonder what is happening rather than making statements.
- Since transference interpretations can be challenging to the client (Hoglend, 2004), you may wish to avoid them until you feel that rapport is sufficient that the client can tolerate them. Then provide no more than one transference interpretation per session until you feel confident that the client can handle more (a low level of interpretation as defined by Hoglend, 2004).
- Take your time before you make any interpretations. Let several instances accrue before suggesting a specific interpretation and "postpone the interpretation of transference until it is close to the patient's awareness. If it is prematurely interpreted, the patient may be totally unable to relate to what the therapist is saying and might feel misunderstood. One useful adage suggests that one should formulate the interpretation and think about it four times before verbalizing it" (Gabbard, 2000a, p. 64).
- If the client does not tolerate transference interpretations, it is okay to avoid them; still, you can use your conceptualization to inform therapy because the client will report the same challenges with significant others that you observe in the therapy relationship.
- Use extratransference interpretations as frequently as needed and tolerated.
- Clients with borderline personality disorder may find transference interpretations especially beneficial (Levy et al., 2006). Other clients with significantly disturbed interpersonal relations can benefit significantly as well.
- Subsequent work on the issues that emerge from these interpretations can be done from different theoretical perspectives. For references, see the list of recommended readings at the end of this chapter.
- Even if no transference or extratransference interpretations are ever made in therapy, the client's habitual ways of reacting to others can be transformed over time. The therapeutic relationship itself can be a powerful vehicle for learning about interpersonal relationships (Gabbard, 2000a). If the therapist is nurturing, understanding, kind, and helpful toward the client, the client can internalize new ideas about significant relationships, helping to have more healthy relationships in other spheres of life.

WHAT IS COUNTERTRANSFERENCE?

Therapists working with borderline clients are likely to discover that, from time to time, interactions with clients elicit in themselves strong emotional reactions ranging from empathetic feelings of depression to strong anger, hopelessness, or attraction. It is important for the therapist to be aware of these reactions and to look at them critically so that they do not unduly bias his or her responses. However, far from being an impediment, these feelings can be quite useful if the therapist is able to understand his or her emotional responses to the client. Emotional responses do not occur randomly. If a therapist experiences an unusually strong response to a client, this is likely to be a response to some aspect of the client's behavior, and it may provide valuable information if it can be understood. It is not unusual for a therapist to respond emotionally to a pattern in the client's behavior long before that pattern has been recognized intellectually. (Freeman, Pretzer, Fleming, & Simon, 1990, p. 194)

The therapist whose reactions are countertransference-based is faced with the task of deciphering which of his or her personal issues is being stimulated and how. . . . I propose that countertransference be conceptualized as therapist reactions that stem from areas of personal conflict within the therapist. . . . [This definition] does not require that therapist conflicts be unresolved. Rather, it allows for the possibility that countertransference might also arise from therapist issues or conflicts that are partially resolved (I do not believe that one's issues are ever completely resolved). (Hayes, 2004, pp. 23, 31)

Therapists of all theoretical stripes recognize that it is normal to have emotional reactions to clients. Having feelings about your clients is a very complex matter. Sometimes these feelings will be helpful in therapy, and at other times they will confuse you; this is also normal. One of the most challenging tasks before you as a therapist is to learn to interpret the messages that your feelings about the client are giving you. There are many ways to conceptualize countertransference (Dalenberg, 2000), so I have selected just one for simplicity's sake.

The first major type of countertransference is your emotional reactions to the client that are based on the client's presentation: the client's behavior, what the client says, how it is said, and so on. This is the type of countertransference being described by Freeman et al. in the first of the previous quotes. Generally, these are emotional reactions that anyone might have to the client. These emotions give you important clues to the client's interpersonal world outside the session. As Judith Beck (2005) states, "It is useful for therapists to use their own negative reactions to patients as a cue to assess the degree to which patients' behavior and attitudes in the session are representative of their behavior and attitudes outside of the session" (p. 84). This type of countertransference is sometimes called *objective countertransference* (Kiesler, 2001).

The second major type of countertransference is based on your personal issues. In other words, something about the therapy is stimulating you to have a personal emotional reaction to the situation. Fauth (2006) defines this type of countertransference thusly: "therapists' idiosyncratic reactions (broadly defined as sensory, affective, cognitive, and behavioral) to clients that are based primarily in therapists' own personal conflicts, biases, or difficulties (for example, cognitive biases, personal narratives, or maladaptive interpersonal patterns)" (p. 17). This type of countertransference is sometimes called *subjective countertransference* (Kiesler, 2001). (Note: If you read more about countertransference in the literature, you will see that some researchers and theorists [e.g., Fauth, 2006; Hayes, 2004] define the term *countertransference* as *only* this second type of emotional reaction to the client—explicitly excluding the therapist's emotional reactions that are based on the client's presentation.)

Since countertransference can be in response to the client's presentation or can be based on your own personal idiosyncratic reactions, having the insight to tell the difference is an essential therapeutic skill. In addition, keep in mind that it is something of an arbitrary distinction to divide countertransference into these two major categories because, as Gabbard (2001a), states, "countertransference is a jointly created phenomenon that involves contributions from both patient and clinician. The patient draws the therapist into playing a role that reflects the patient's internal world, but the specific dimensions of that role are colored by the therapist's own personality" (p. 984).

COUNTERTRANSFERENCE BASED ON THE CLIENT'S PRESENTATION

Anita Cook is a mental health trainee who is working with Laura Ward, a woman who is living with her husband. Laura is battered by her husband about once a month. Laura has shared all her abusive experiences with Anita. She also says that she is afraid to leave him because he might kill her. Anita feels sympathy for Laura's fear and pain. Anita then starts to suggest how Laura can effectively leave her husband. Laura says, "But I love him, and the children need their father." They repeatedly take these two opposing stands for several sessions. Anita tells her supervisor that Laura is "stubborn and resistant."

Aaron Webb is a mental health trainee who is working with Eugene Turner, a recovering alcoholic and addict. Eugene has been convicted for selling crack, and he is on parole. Aaron likes Eugene and sympathizes with his struggles. Eugene grew up in poverty, and he has post-traumatic stress disorder from being physically abused by a stepfather in his youth. Eugene lives in a halfway house under very strict rules. He is supposed to be in every night at a certain time. Eugene has an ambivalent and conflictual relationship with his mother, who is his primary emotional and financial support. Eugene tells Aaron that he has been sticking to all the halfway house rules. Then Eugene urges Aaron to call the halfway house. Aaron gets a release of information and does so. After faxing the release over, Aaron talks to a staff member who informs him that Eugene has been coming in late for several nights and is at risk of having his parole violated. Aaron feels intense rage when he hears that Eugene has been lying to him but is also confused because this is not a typical feeling for him. Aaron is well aware that addicts can struggle with telling the truth. Since Aaron recognizes that this rage is unusual for him, he understands that it is probably a countertransference reaction. Aaron does not know exactly how he came to experience the rage; however, he uses the feeling as a guide for the next session without acting it out. Aaron says to Eugene, "I've been somewhat confused after our last session. You told me that you were sticking to all the house rules, but you also encouraged me to call the house, where you knew I would learn otherwise. I'm wondering what was going on with you when you decided to do that? How have others reacted to you when you've told them things that aren't true in the past?" Aaron discovers that Eugene is fearful of trusting others out of concern that they will be angry and then lies to avoid their rage, increasing the chances that they will be angry later. This pattern apparently first developed between Eugene and his stepfather.

Countertransference must be attended to carefully, as unexamined feelings on your part will lead the therapy astray. For example, you may begin to react to the client like everyone else does instead of offering the client an opportunity to think about how his or her behavior affects others and how the behavior can be changed. Or you may fall into the trap of reenacting the client's important relationships from the past rather than exploring the client's current interpersonal challenges that stem from those relationships.

As I noted before, there are many different definitions of countertransference. For simplicity, I describe three types of countertransference that are based on the client's issues.

The first type of countertransference based on the client's issues relates to empathy; in this case, you are simply empathetically feeling the same feelings that the client is feeling. This type is sometimes called *concordant countertransference* (Kernberg, Selzer, Koenigsberg, Carr, & Appelbaum, 1989). The therapeutic response is to simply reflect the feelings of the client (e.g., "It sounds like you're feeling quite anxious about that.").

The second type of countertransference is about empathy as well but in a more complicated way. Here the client has mixed feelings about a situation. In the first of the previous vignettes, Laura has mixed feelings about leaving her abusive spouse. However, instead of exploring these mixed feelings, she says, "but I love him!" while the therapist focuses on the danger. In this case, both of these feelings (love and fear of danger) really belong to the client, but the client's ambivalence is being acted out between the client and the therapist. The feelings that the therapist has enacted are the ones that are most difficult for the client to tolerate (fear of her dangerous husband). Clearly Laura is worried about the situation because she is actively seeking help from a psychotherapist and has talked about her fears. This type of countertransference is traditionally called *projective identification* in the psychoanalytic literature (Gabbard, 2001a). The client's recognition of her own ambivalence will be the key to effective change, and getting the client to explore her ambivalence in therapy is the most effective intervention. This interpersonal dynamic is also commonly experienced when working with individuals with substance abuse problems. To most effectively address this type of countertransference, learn about motivational interviewing (W. R. Miller & Rollnick, 2002). In brief, address this type of countertransference by reflecting the ambivalence that you see instead of enacting it. Note that when you do find yourself enacting this type of countertransference, as you inevitably will at some point, you can always change tactics. In the previous vignette, Anita could say,

> "This seems like a terribly painful situation. I see that you love your husband and you want to stay with him, yet you are also afraid that he might hurt or even kill you, so you are uncertain about what to do."

The third type of countertransference is about reenacting the client's relationships from the past. In the second of the previous vignettes, the therapist experiences an unexpected rage reaction. He recognizes that this is not typical of him, so he hypothesizes that it is countertransference. He uses this emotion to guide the next session and discovers some important issues about trust that his client has as well as an important relationship pattern between the client and his stepfather. Had the therapist acted out the anger he had toward the client in the session, it would have been a therapeutic mistake (although a common one, according to research by Gelso, Hill, Mohr, Rochen, & Zack, 1999). This type of countertransference is called *role responsiveness* (Gabbard, 2001a), although often (confusingly) it is considered another form of projective identification.

COUNTERTRANSFERENCE BASED ON THE THERAPIST'S PERSONAL ISSUES

[In a qualitative research study] Therapist 4 possessed strong values related to independence and strength that she identified as potential sources of countertransference. The client with whom she worked for 12 sessions looked frequently to the therapist for guidance and advice, generating recurrent frustration in the therapist. Furthermore, the therapist seemed to experience difficulty identifying with the client, stating on one postsession interview, "I have never, ever, ever," been as dependent as the client. A second theme for this dyad involved death. The client's mother was in the process of dying and the therapist's mother had died within the previous year. The therapist felt some connection with the client around death but found from her own experience that it was not helpful "to get lost in the grieving." Because the therapist found information about death and dying to be helpful in her recovery process, she assumed the client would benefit from the same. Consequently, the therapist was predominately didactic and intellectual in addressing the client's concerns about her mother's impending death. (Hayes et al., 1998, p. 476)

Therapist 5 struggled for control throughout his work with a female client who looked to him for guidance and rescuing but who angrily rejected his advice because she saw it as controlling. This tapped into the therapist's countertransference issues of needing to gratify and help others and caused him to feel overly responsible for the client. The therapist struggled throughout their 17 sessions with how directive he should be, and he vacillated between empathizing with the client and distancing himself from her. (Hayes et al., 1998, p. 476)

Therapist 2 described three countertransference origins in her 17 postsession interviews: needs to nurture, perform well, and be a good parent. The therapist used her countertransference reactions [based on these three personal issues] to deepen her understanding of the client, remain patient, and nurture the client. In fact, approximately half of her countertransference manifestations [based on the therapist's personal issues] were classified as approach responses that increased closeness with her client. (Hayes et al., 1998, p. 476)

The second major type of countertransference is emotional reactions to the client due to your own personal issues. These personal issues could be related to your current life situation or your past life experiences. This type of countertransference should not be used in therapy; instead, these reactions point out areas of self-exploration for you.

The three previous quotes are from a qualitative research study in which eight psychologists were interviewed immediately following their sessions of brief therapy with eight clients (Hayes et al., 1998). The themes illustrated in the quotes emerged over time. The anonymous psychotherapists in this study showed great compassion and courage by sharing their most personal feelings with the researchers so that others could learn. These three cases (from the eight in the article) illustrate some universal issues about how countertransference (the kind that is based on a therapist's personal issues) can affect therapy.

In the first quote, therapist 4 ends up distancing herself emotionally from the dependent client with the dying mother. In the second quote, therapist 5 alternates between moving closer to the client by gratifying her desire for advice, then distancing himself when she was rejecting of him. In the third quote, therapist 2 uses her countertransference reactions to identify with and move closer to the client. Note that countertransference based on personal issues is typically manifested through moving closer to the client or distancing oneself from the client (Hayes, 2004). Distancing is generally detrimental to the therapy, while sometimes moving closer is helpful, and sometimes it is not—if one moves too close.

Note that Hayes et al. (1998) found that the therapists in the study experienced reactions toward the client that were due to their personal issues in fully 80% of sessions. This illustrates that this type of countertransference is normative and universal and cannot be avoided. Since, therefore, all of us must expect to experience this type of countertransference, we must learn to manage it appropriately. Do not try to ignore these feelings, as they will negatively affect your attitude and work with clients if you do.

RESEARCH ON COUNTERTRANSFERENCE

Unfortunately, countertransference is underresearched as a clinical phenomenon (Hayes, 2004). Perhaps this is because "countertransference emanated from psychoanalysis, a field traditionally disinclined toward empirical inquiry" (Hayes, 2004, p. 21).

Betan, Heim, Conklin, and Westen (2005) surveyed the emotional responses of a sample of psychiatrists and psychologists toward one selected client each and mathematically categorized the results into eight distinct patterns of therapist emotional reactions. These are as follows:

- Disengaged: The therapist feels distracted, withdrawn, annoyed, or bored in sessions.
- Helpless/inadequate: The therapist feels inadequate, incompetent, hopeless, and anxious.
- Overwhelmed/disorganized: The therapist desires to avoid or flee the patient and has strong negative feelings, including dread, repulsion, and resentment. Clients are likely to have borderline personality disorder or narcissistic personality disorder.
- Parental/protective: The therapist has a wish to protect and nurture the patient in a parental way above and beyond normal positive feelings toward the client.
- Criticized/mistreated: The therapist feels unappreciated, dismissed, or devalued by the client.

- Special/overinvolved: The therapist sees the client as special, relative to other clients, and has "soft signs" of problems in maintaining boundaries, including self-disclosure, ending sessions on time, and feeling guilty, responsible, or overly concerned.
- Sexualized: The therapist has sexual feelings toward the patient or experiences sexual tension.
- Positive: The therapist and client have a positive working alliance and a close connection.

Clearly, not every possible emotional reaction to clients is documented in this research. However, I include this research so that when you experience these emotions, you can be sure that you are having a common emotional reaction toward your client. Like the other research cited, this research demonstrates that it is normal to have feelings toward your clients, even negative or sexual feelings. Your challenge is to understand why you are having these feelings and use them therapeutically if appropriate. Even positive countertransference can create therapeutic challenges (see appendix 23 for more on this topic).

As part of a larger study of racial countertransference between White psychotherapists and Black clients, Constantine (2007) led focus groups to help her determine what types of racial countertransference ("racial microaggressions") the clients experienced during therapy. She found 12 types:

- Color blindness: "I don't see you as Black; I just see you as a regular person."
- Overidentification: "As a gay person, I know just what it's like to be discriminated against because of race."
- Denial of personal or individual racism: "I'm not racist because some of my best friends are Black."
- Minimization of racial/cultural issues: "I'm not sure we need to focus on race or culture to understand your depression."
- Assigning unique/special status on the basis of race or ethnicity: "You're a credit to your race" and "You're a very articulate African American."
- Stereotypic assumptions about members of a racial or ethnic group: "I know that Black people are very religious."
- Accused hypersensitivity regarding racial or cultural issues: "Don't be too sensitive about the racial stuff. I didn't mean anything bad/offensive."
- Meritocracy myth: "If Black people just worked harder, they could be successful like other people."
- Culturally insensitive treatment considerations or recommendations: "You should disengage or separate from your family of origin if they are causing you problems."

- Acceptance of less-than-optimal behaviors on the basis of racial/cultural group membership: "It might be okay for some people to cope by drinking alcohol because their cultural norms sanction this behavior."
- Idealization: "I'm sure you can cope with this problem as a strong Black woman" and "Black people are so cool."
- Dysfunctional helping/patronization: "I don't usually do this, but I can waive your fees if you can't afford to pay for counseling."

In a later phase of this research, Constantine (2007) found that these behaviors were negatively associated with clients' assessment of the therapeutic alliance and the therapists' cultural competence. This emphasizes the importance of attending to racial countertransference since numerous previous studies (Barber, Connolly, Crits-Christoph, Gladis, & Siqueland, 2000) have found that the quality of the therapeutic alliance is related to therapeutic outcome.

UNDERSTANDING COUNTERTRANSFERENCE

CT [countertransference] that is not understood or controlled by the therapist is likely to injure the therapeutic process. . . . [T]he therapist's internal experience may also be acted out in the treatment, and this is usually harmful. In such cases, the therapist is taking care of his or her own needs, enacting his or her own defenses, and not attending to the patient's issues and needs. (Gelso & Hayes, 2001, pp. 418, 419)

The previous quote illustrates some ways in which countertransference can negatively affect the therapeutic process. Judith Beck (2005) encourages you to monitor yourself during the therapy session by asking yourself questions in the following domains:

- Negative emotionality: Do I feel annoyed, angry, anxious, sad, hopeless, overwhelmed, guilty, embarrassed, or demeaned?
- Getting too close or too distant: Am I engaging in dysfunctional behaviors, such as blaming, dominating, or controlling the patient? Or am I being too passive?
- Behavior: Is my volume/tone of voice, facial expression, and body language appropriate?
- Physiological reaction: Am I feeling tense? Is my heart beating faster? Is my face becoming hot?

Before determining whether to use countertransference in therapy, you must have a good understanding of it and whether it is related to your issue, the client's, or both. Here are some questions that you can use to help understand the countertransference:

* Am I having an atypical feeling or reaction toward this client or behaving in a way that is not typical of my therapy style? If yes, clearly some kind of countertransference is operating.
* Am I having a stronger emotional reaction to this client than to other clients? This could be due either to some intense emotional issues of the client (e.g., homicidality or borderline or narcissistic traits) or to countertransference regarding your personal issues or both.
* Do I think that others in the client's life are probably having the same emotional reaction to him that I am having now? If yes, some measure of countertransference due to the client's issues is likely operating.
* Have I noticed myself feeling emotionally distant from this client or ignoring some issues? If yes, it is likely that some countertransference due to your personal issues is involved.
* Have I noticed myself becoming too involved with this client, perhaps by trying to solve problems, extending sessions too long, or doing special favors? If yes, it is again likely that some countertransference due to your personal issues is involved.
* Do I feel like the client is "pushing my buttons"? If yes, probably some countertransference regarding your personal issues is involved.

When your countertransference feelings are negative, even if you are certain that they are based on the client's issues, your interventions must be framed with care. It is okay to wait until you can discuss your reactions with your supervisor before sharing your insights with the client in a later session. The same issue will come up again if it is important. However, if you do enact the issue, all is not lost—once you realize what has happened, this can still be explored with the client after the fact.

MANAGING COUNTERTRANSFERENCE BASED ON THE THERAPIST'S ISSUES

When patients display dysfunctional behavior in session, therapists should realize that their patients' behaviors likely stem from difficult (often traumatic) life circumstances and extreme, negative core beliefs. Such a stance allows therapists to regard patients more positively, display empathy, and behave more adaptively themselves. . . . And the therapeutic relationship itself can be a vehicle for helping these patients develop a more positive view of themselves and others and learn that interpersonal problems can be solved. (J. S. Beck, 2005, pp. 43, 63)

When you identify countertransference that is based on the client's personal issues, it helps to attempt to understand the client more deeply (as Beck suggests in the previous quote). Try to understand how this pattern of difficult interpersonal interactions developed through the client's distressing negative experiences of the past. Try to understand how the client has found this (now mostly dysfunctional) way of relating to others to be helpful in some way. You can use this understanding to become more empathetic to the client and explore the issue productively in therapy rather than falling into the trap of reenacting it.

In a review of the research on countertransference management, Gelso and Hayes (2001) conclude that "the ten studies [done so far] support the idea that unmanaged CT [countertransference due to the therapist's personal issues] adversely affects treatment outcomes" (p. 419). In this review, Gelso and Hayes also concluded that research evidence supports that "awareness of CT [countertransference] feelings [due to the therapist's personal issues] was associated with fewer CT behaviors" (p. 418). Thus, an implication of this research is that when you identify countertransference that is based on your own personal issues, it is essential to work to understand your own reactions more deeply; otherwise, you will reduce your therapeutic effectiveness (Gelso & Hayes, 2001).

In a study of the effectiveness of 32 graduate student therapists, measures were made of countertransference management (Gelso, Latts, Gomez, & Fassinger, 2002). Note that in this study, the researchers were concerned with countertransference that is due to the therapist's personal issues. Countertransference management was operationalized as encompassing these five factors:

- Empathy: Being able to maintain empathy with the client despite the countertransference feelings that are also in the therapist's awareness.
- Self-insight: Understanding the origins of the therapist's personal issues that lead to the emotional reaction to the client.
- Self-integration: Maintaining healthy boundaries between the therapist and client, specifically, not acting in the therapy session on countertransference that is based on the therapist's personal issues.
- Anxiety management: Sufficient management of the therapist's anxiety.
- Conceptualizing ability: The therapist's ability to conceptualize his own reaction from a theoretical perspective.

Psychotherapy trainees who most effectively managed their countertransference based on personal issues were found to have the best psychotherapy outcomes with their clients. As you can infer from the nature of these five factors, good supervision or consultation, personal psychotherapy, and a dedication to continuing to grow one's conceptual knowledge of psychotherapy can be invaluable in developing one's ability to manage countertransference.

If you are seeing a client and you see that you are having strong emotional reactions, ask yourself these questions (derived from the five factors of countertransference management described previously):

- Can I maintain empathy with the client? Or am I acting out my feelings in a way that can interfere with therapy?
- Do I understand which of my own issues are related to the client's issues? Or do I feel distressed and confused?
- Am I able to see the client as a separate person from me? Or am I telling the client how to handle the situation based on my own personal experience— and not the client's experience?
- Am I able to stay focused during the session? Or do I feel too anxious or distressed to concentrate at times?
- Can I understand, from a theoretical perspective, why I am having the reactions that I am having? Or am I confused about why the client is "pushing my buttons"?

If you are struggling with these issues and the client's treatment is being negatively impacted, discuss this with your supervisor. The client may need to be referred to someone else, or perhaps your supervisor can help you with your conceptualizations and interventions enough that you can be effective with the client. Your struggle also indicates that you need to address these issues in your own personal therapy.

Your personal experiences—if sufficiently resolved—can help you understand your clients' difficulties more deeply and, thus, serve as a source of healing (Hayes et al., 1998). And, in fact, Hayes et al. (1998) hypothesized, based on their qualitative research, that "when therapists' countertransference is triggered by clients' family of origin issues, therapists will generally respond with compassionate understanding" (p. 478). As McWilliams (2004) states, "psychotherapy is one of the few professions in which one's greatest misfortunes can be retooled into professional assets" (p. 70).

THE FUTURE OF TRANSFERENCE AND COUNTERTRANSFERENCE RESEARCH AND THEORY

[The science of cognitive neuroscience has recognized] the existence of two ways that memory can be expressed, either explicitly (via conscious recall or recognition) or implicitly (in behavior, independent of conscious control). Explicit memory refers to conscious memory for ideas, facts and episodes. Implicit memory refers to memory that is observable in behavior but is not consciously brought to mind. . . . The existence of unconscious or implicit networks—which tend to be resistant to change because they reflect longstanding regularities in the person's experience and allow him or her to navigate the world in ways that feel predictable (even if sometimes rigid, inaccurate or otherwise maladaptive)—provides perhaps the best empirical justification for long-term therapies. . . . The connectionist notion of representations as potentials for reactivation—as sets of neurons that have been activated in the past and are hence more readily activated as a unit in the future—offers a mechanism to explain the long-held psychoanalytic position that patients are likely to express important conflicts, defenses, motives, and interpersonal patterns in their relationship with the therapist. (Westen, 2005, pp. 444–446)

The discovery of mirror neurons lends a new dimension of understanding to empathy, countertransference, and projective identification that was not previously available. Both conscious and unconscious physical processes are elicited through synchronization with clients. . . . Social psychology studies have demonstrated time and again that it is common for people to unconsciously copy one another's facial expression, synchronize breathing rates, and mimic the other's partial or complete posture. Through doing so, emotions have also been shown to be shared. This happens regularly in the therapy room as well and can go either way: therapist to client, or client to therapist. (Rothschild, 2004, n.p.)

In the first of the previous quotes, Westen (2005) relates transference to recent research findings in cognitive neuroscience. These findings have determined that there are separate brain pathways for explicit (conscious) processes and implicit (unconscious or automatic) processes. Explicit (or conscious) processes have been traditionally targeted by cognitive therapists, while implicit (or unconscious) processes (including transference) have traditionally been targeted by psychodynamic therapists (Gabbard & Westen, 2003). There is a growing consensus that addressing both types of processes is a productive therapeutic approach.

As Rothschild (2004) indicates in the second of the previous quotes, scientists are tantalizingly close to explaining how countertransference occurs. She cites a confluence of neuroscience research and social psychology research that hints toward a near-future scientific understanding of how the therapist's emotions can resonate so acutely with those of the client.

RECOMMENDED READING

Beck, J. S. (2005). *Cognitive therapy for challenging problems: What to do when the basics don't work.* New York: Guilford Press.
While Beck does not use the terms "transference" and "countertransference," she nonetheless provides a very helpful and thorough discussion of these phenomena from a cognitive therapy perspective. Note that Beck focuses on discussing the therapist's emotional reactions that are in response to the client's presentation.

Berenson, K. R., & Andersen, S. M. (2006). Childhood physical and emotional abuse by a parent: Transference effects in adult interpersonal relations. *Personality and Social Psychology Bulletin, 32,* 1509–1522.
While a bit technical, this report of contemporary transference research provides the reader with insight into how transference is detected experimentally.

Chu, J. (1988). Ten traps for therapists in the treatment of trauma survivors. *Dissociation, 1,* 24–32.
In this classic article, Chu clearly describes many countertransference challenges that confront the psychotherapist who works with trauma survivors.

Comas-Diaz, L., & Jacobsen, F. M. (1991). Ethnocultural transference and countertransference in the therapeutic dyad. *American Journal of Orthopsychiatry, 61,* 392–402.
A multitude of helpful vignettes illustrate how ethnocultural transference and countertransference can emerge in psychotherapy, even between a therapist and client of the same ethnic background. Essential reading for the therapist who wants to achieve cultural competency.

Gabbard, G. O. (2001). A contemporary psychoanalytic model of countertransference. *Journal of Clinical Psychology/In Session: Psychotherapy in Practice, 57,* 983–991.
Gabbard briefly provides an update on the current theoretical status of countertransference from a psychoanalytic perspective. Read this if you would like a more sophisticated understanding of how countertransference is a jointly created phenomenon between client and therapist.

Gabbard, G. O. (2004). *Long-term psychodynamic psychotherapy: A basic text.* Arlington, VA: American Psychiatric Publishing.
This book is written specifically for the beginning psychotherapist. Important modern principles of psychodynamic psychotherapy are outlined remarkably clearly in this text, along with ample references to research literature. Highly recommended.

Gelso, C. J., & Hayes, J. A. (2001). Countertransference management. *Psychotherapy, 38,* 418–422.
Two prominent researchers on countertransference use insights derived from their research and the research of others to describe how to effectively manage countertransference that is based on the therapist's personal issues.

Hayes, J. A., & Gelso, C. J. (2001). Clinical implications of research on countertransference: Science informing practice. *Journal of Clinical Psychology/In Session: Psychotherapy in Practice, 57,* 1041–1051.
Hayes and Gelso describe their theory and research on countertransference with an emphasis on informing the practitioner. Note that Hayes and Gelso focus exclu-

sively on countertransference that is due to the therapist's personal emotional re-
actions in this paper and in their research.

Kernberg, O. F., Selzer, M. A., Koenigsberg, H. W., Carr, A. C., & Appelbaum, A. H.
(1989). *Psychodynamic psychotherapy of borderline patients.* New York: Basic
Books.

While explicitly about treating borderline clients, this volume presents useful,
thought-provoking discussions regarding boundaries, establishing a therapeutic
contract, coping with countertransference, and addressing threats to treatment,
among other topics, that can be applied to many challenging clients.

EXERCISES AND DISCUSSION QUESTIONS

1. Can you reconcile the research on transference and countertransference discussed in this chapter with your theoretical orientation? Why or why not?

2. What characteristics of a supervisor would lead you to feel comfortable discussing your feelings toward a client? What if these feelings were embarrassing (e.g., you detest a client or feel sexually attracted to a client)?

3. How can you deal with your distressing feelings toward a client if you feel too inhibited—for whatever reason—to discuss them with your supervisor?

4. See appendix 23 if your class wishes to further discuss emotions and relationships in therapy. The appendix describes many common emotional issues between therapists and clients in therapy.

Chapter Twenty-Three

Vicarious Traumatization and Burnout

Unfortunately, you can risk some damage to your mental health by being a psychotherapist. As a beginning therapist, you should know that, and my goal is to educate you about those risks. I hope that this knowledge will help you avoid or minimize these common problems. In chapter 24, I will talk further about positive coping strategies for psychotherapists.

Many terms have been used to describe these emotional risks—vicarious traumatization, traumatic countertransference, secondary traumatic stress, compassion fatigue, and burnout—with some overlap between them (see S. Collins & Long, 2003; Jenkins & Baird, 2002). To simplify the discussion, I focus on only two of these interrelated concepts: burnout and vicarious traumatization.

BURNOUT

I could see I was burning out. I looked at the other therapists who had been with the agency longer than I had. They were apathetic, depressed and avoided work, whenever possible. The patient assignment system gave everyone new patients regularly, no matter how high their current caseload. This system rewarded those who clearly didn't care about their clients—the clients would drop out, and the clinician had less work. Those who engaged well with their clients were chronically overworked and overstressed. When staff retired or left, they were rarely replaced, resulting in higher workloads for everyone.

We never had any real input into what was going on in the agency. Occasionally, they would ask for our input, but it was clearly ignored, and the higher-ups did what they had wanted to do all along. Those with the most power were physically isolated in remote offices, and had no known contact with anyone on the "front lines." The paperwork increased significantly every year, and we joked that eventually we'd treat one patient per week and spend the other 39 hours on paperwork. We were frequently told to "do more with less."

We wondered whether anyone in charge cared if we did a good job. There were never any rewards or promotions available, and providing opportunities for professional advancement or development was never considered by the administration. A coworker posted a cartoon on her door of a door to a padded cell; the sign on the door to the padded cell said, "Do not disturb any further." We could all relate.

We wondered whether the administrators became administrators, in part, because they wouldn't have to deal with patients any more. They seemed burned out themselves. At best, the bosses were pleasant but ineffectual, at worst, they were punitive and harsh.

I got to the point that when a client talked about feeling suicidal, I felt exhausted and overburdened. I started to have difficulty caring anymore. I knew I had to leave to preserve my sanity and my professional competence. (Anonymous psychotherapist, personal communication, March 10, 2007)

This portrait of a psychotherapist who is burning out illustrates that burnout is "a prolonged response to chronic emotional and interpersonal stressors on the job, and is defined here by the three dimensions of exhaustion, cynicism, and a sense of inefficacy" (Maslach, 2003, p. 189). Most frequently found in human services workers, burnout generally includes extreme emotional fatigue, disillusionment, and apathy toward work. Gradually, productivity and concern for clients decreases. As the period of burnout progresses, the therapist may exhibit emotional problems, substance abuse, interpersonal problems, and/or increased physical illness (S. Collins & Long, 2003; Felton, 1998; Maslach, 2003).

A recent study of a random sample of psychologists found that 44% had high scores for emotional exhaustion (Rupert & Morgan, 2005), indicating that burnout is extremely common in mental health practitioners. This finding is consistent with a rate of 40% of psychologists having a high score for emotional exhaustion in the mid-1980s (Ackerly, Burnell, Holder, & Kurdek, 1988). Another recent study found that burnout can occur on the treatment team level and that this burnout results in lower patient satisfaction (Garman, Corrigan, & Morris, 2002).

Certain client issues tend to increase burnout in mental health care workers. A perception of having too many clients increases burnout, as does having more patient contact hours per week (Leiter & Harvie, 1996). Clients with potential for aggressive behavior or suicide were found to be most emotionally exhausting (Rupert & Morgan, 2005), while clients who did not improve also contributed to burnout (Shinn, Rosario, Morch, & Chestnut, 1984).

Organizational contributions to burnout have been extensively studied, and, in fact, administrative and bureaucratic factors have been found to contribute more to burnout in mental health professionals than patient care issues. Being chronically pressed for time, heavy work demands ("do more with less"), spending more time on administrative tasks and paperwork, and having less control over work activities increase burnout. Certain interpersonal issues on the job contribute to burnout as well: little appreciation for a job well done, interpersonal problems with coworkers, and abuse or harassment in the workplace. Finally, negative aspects of the organization as a whole, such as reorganization, downsizing, and a lack of resources, contribute to burned-out workers (Maslach, 2001, 2003; Rupert & Morgan, 2005). Probably because of many of these factors, mental health practitioners working in a hospital or agency have more risk of burnout than those in private practice (Raquepaw & Miller, 1989), although a recent study (Rupert & Morgan, 2005) found that male psychotherapists can be especially stressed in a group practice, while females are at greatest risk of burnout in agency settings.

VICARIOUS TRAUMATIZATION

When the main focus of my work shifted to working with rape victims . . . Suddenly, I found myself experiencing nightmares of being raped. Or I would turn a dark corner in my home and imagine a rapist coming toward me just like he had for my client. The more clients I had, the less sleep I got. I found myself becoming tense and irritable. I began to take extra safety precautions and began to view others, especially men, more circumspectly. In short, hearing other women tell me about how they were sexually assaulted was, in small ways, traumatizing and disruptive for me. . . .

I find myself thinking, "Why didn't you scream when you knew people were nearby?" or "How could you have chosen not to even tell him to stop?" I know the answers, but always have to go over them in my head to convince myself. The truth is people in danger sometimes freeze just like the rabbit in the car headlights. If she ran, she might survive, but fear has frozen her in place. And even if she had not been frozen, no one knows if it would have helped or made the situation worse. Intellectually, the answer is satisfying to me, but on a more visceral level, I find it unacceptable. If I accept this reality, I have to give up my notion of my own invulnerability and my competence to take care of myself. My schemas are challenged. I don't want to contemplate the possibility that I, too, might freeze or be unable to do anything to rectify the situation. It goes against my cherished notion that whatever bad comes my way, I will be able to handle it and overcome it. Each time I help a client accept her vulnerability and the fact that she "just froze," I have to accept that possibility for myself. I don't like it and resist it every time. . . .

When I first began working with rape victims, I found it puzzling that I experienced some symptoms of vicarious traumatization, but had never experienced this while working with other victims. As I thought about it, I came to realize that with other victims I had been able to set myself apart from them and maintain my sense of invulnerability. "Perhaps that client was abused as a child, but I am an adult and it can't happen to me." "Maybe she got caught up in an abusive relationship, but I never have, so it is unlikely that I ever will." (One might debate the latter as an illusion, but on some level, whether accurate or not, it allowed me to maintain a sense of invulnerability.) With rape, I could not maintain my distance. As I helped my clients to see that bad things happen to people randomly, I could no longer keep my invulnerability intact. I was just as vulnerable as anyone else. That realization made me more susceptible to symptoms of vicarious traumatization. It also has brought me closer to the struggles of my clients. For that I am grateful. (Astin, 1997, pp. 103, 105–106, 108)

The process of doing therapy changes us in profound ways. As you can see from the previous quote, Dr. Astin had been caught by surprise by her strong emotional reaction to the rape victims. She had treated survivors of other traumas before, she said, but had not been so personally affected until she treated the rape victims. We are all indebted to her for her honest and fearless report of her experiences. The experiences she describes perfectly illustrate the concept of vicarious traumatization (VT).

Vicarious traumatization has been characterized as "a special form of countertransference stimulated by exposure to the client's traumatic material" (Courtois, 1993). The therapist begins to take on the emotional, behavioral, and cognitive changes of her traumatized clients. This phenomenon was first described by McCann and Pearlman (1990). The previous quote illustrates these changes. While countertransference has multiple different definitions, Courtois is referring to it in the broadest of ways, as encompassing any emotional reaction the therapist has to the client. Note that VT is *not* a pathological response on the part of the therapist; rather, it is an (unfortunately) normal response that occurs in a significant proportion of therapists who treat trauma.

Vicarious traumatization can cause many changes in the therapist (McCann & Pearlman, 1990). The therapist could become more suspicious of others' motives and become cynical and distrustful. The therapist could develop a heightened sense of vulnerability and often feel unsafe. The therapist may become profoundly aware of the lack of control that we sometimes have over unexpected life events. The therapist could grow to see others as malevolent, cruel, and dangerous. The therapist may feel emotionally estranged from her loved ones by the need to keep her clients' horrors confidential. In response to a previously neutral stimulus, the therapist could be triggered to remember the client's traumatic material. Emotional numbing could occur, and the therapist could begin to engage in numbing behaviors, such as overeating, overspending, overworking, and alcohol use (Hesse, 2002).

No one is immune from the emotional impact of clients' traumas. As the quote illustrates, it is not possible to predict when any one therapist will slide from having ordinary reactions toward a client into being vicariously traumatized. We all must be prepared for this possibility.

Beginning therapists should be aware that it is impossible avoid treating posttraumatic stress disorder (PTSD) (and thus incurring some risk of VT). Why? Because of the very high prevalence of PTSD in the general population and even higher prevalence in any client population, we know that a significant number of clients in all settings will turn out to have PTSD in addition to their other difficulties. So, all clinicians must be prepared to treat PTSD clients effectively. As I've discussed earlier (chapter 9), PTSD can be a hidden problem, and the clinician can unknowingly (or unconsciously) conspire to keep it that way by not screening for it on a routine basis.

THERAPISTS AT GREATER RISK

Certain therapists are at greater risk for development of burnout and/or VT. Therapists and human services workers who have a personal history of trauma or neglect should seek personal therapy since they can be at heightened risk for VT (Nelson-Gardell & Harris, 2003; Pearlman & Mac Ian, 1995; Sabin-Farrell & Turpin, 2003). Trauma is relatively common among psychotherapists, occurring at a rate of well over 50% and even over 80% in some clinician groups (Pearlman & Mac Ian, 1995; Schauben & Frazier, 1995; VanDeusen & Way, 2006). In addition, a higher baseline level of anxiety puts one at greater risk for burnout (Maslach, 2003).

A consistent finding is that those who are younger or newer to therapy work are at increased risk of burnout or VT (Leiter & Harvie, 1996; Pearlman & Mac Ian, 1995; VanDeusen & Way, 2006). This suggests that experience and maturity are necessary to cope with the acute stresses of doing psychotherapy, especially with challenging populations like trauma survivors. Beginning therapists can be more easily overburdened by a high caseload and difficult clients until they develop more therapeutic knowledge and increased positive personal coping skills to balance their professional stresses.

A review of the literature (Sabin-Farrell & Turpin, 2003) reported that most studies found that increased exposure to traumatized clients leads to a greater risk of developing VT. It is likely that each therapist has a different tolerance for working with traumatized clients. To function effectively, it is essential that you discover what your tolerance is and keep the number of traumatized clients safely below that. Like any emotional resource, this tolerance is likely to fluctuate over time given stressors in your personal life, so don't treat too many traumatized clients at one time.

INSTITUTIONAL POLICIES TO PREVENT BURNOUT AND VICARIOUS TRAUMATIZATION

As discussed previously, burnout is more accurately seen as an organizational problem rather than an individual problem. More than 20 years ago, a study found that agencies rarely made any efforts to reduce burnout among staff (Shinn et al., 1984). Unfortunately, most agencies and hospitals have not made any progress since then. Interventions aimed at increasing individual coping to reduce burnout have had limited to no success, leading to the likelihood that reductions in burnout will be seen only if greater individual coping skills are coupled with organizational change (Maslach, Schaufeli, & Leiter, 2001).

The organization must support the psychotherapists it employs to prevent burnout and VT. Communication in healthy organizations is characterized by a democratic, informed decision-making style—instead of being exclusively hierarchical—and administrators are supportive and help provide structure as needed (Leiter & Harvie, 1996). Good health insurance that covers mental health and chemical dependency is necessary so that the therapists can seek professional help themselves to reduce the likelihood of a burned-out staff (Felton, 1998). Therapists must have some control over their workload and how their time is allocated to prevent burnout. Therapists must not be overworked since overwork often leads directly to burnout. Overwork also prevents therapists in engaging in positive coping during their personal time, which helps ameliorate the effects of hearing about clients' traumas. The organization should avoid having any therapist's caseload consist entirely of traumatized clients since this puts the therapist at increased risk of VT.

THERAPIST SELF-CARE TO PREVENT VICARIOUS TRAUMATIZATION

As a beginning therapist, you may or may not already have some personal experience with burnout in other contexts, and you are unlikely to have experienced VT yet. However, you can see that both of these conditions are risks for all of us. As a student, you should carefully monitor yourself for signs of burnout or VT and talk with your supervisors if you feel overburdened in any way by your clients or other aspects of your workload. When you have graduated, perhaps you can educate your colleagues and the administration about these issues, thereby contributing to a healthier work environment in agencies and hospitals.

The literature details a number of strategies for therapist emotional self-care, which is hypothesized to help reduce VT (McCann & Pearlman, 1990; Schauben & Frazier, 1995). These strategies include the following:

- Learn more about treating trauma. Unfortunately, the effect of further training in trauma work has not yet been examined as a protective factor regarding VT (Sabin-Farrell & Turpin, 2003). However, it is reasonable to expect that increased knowledge and mastery would help clinicians cope with the stresses of treating traumatized clients. Read up and attend workshops on how to treat traumatized clients effectively.
- Know your limits and do not treat too many traumatized clients at once.
- Balance your personal and professional lives; do not overwork.
- Use problem solving and planning to work together with your colleagues and the client to determine a plan that is likely to alleviate symptoms and distress.
- Seek emotional support and advice from colleagues, consultants, and supervisors.
- Seek out positive human experiences: art, music, supportive relationships, religion, and so on.

Finally, focus on the positive side of doing therapy. Trauma survivors often show great resilience and strength. Seeing our clients improve over time is gratifying and fulfilling. Keep in mind that this important work of healing the client will have ripple effects through the client's family, friends, and offspring for years to come.

RECOMMENDED READING

Astin, M. C. (1997). Traumatic therapy: How helping rape victims affects me as a therapist. *Women and Therapy, 20,* 101–109.
Astin powerfully describes the personal impact of working with rape victims and how she has learned to cope.

Courtois, C. (1997). Healing the incest wound: A treatment update with attention to recovered-memory issues. *American Journal of Psychotherapy, 51,* 464–496.
This classic article provides a helpful outline of the psychotherapy of incest survivors, which is applicable to any client who may be unstable and has a history of childhood trauma.

Herman, J. (1997). *Trauma and recovery: The aftermath of violence from domestic abuse to political terror.* New York: Basic Books.
In this update to her classic volume, Herman educates the reader, in an eminently readable style, about trauma and its treatment.

Hesse, A. (2002). Secondary trauma: How working with trauma survivors affects therapists. *Clinical Social Work Journal, 30,* 293–309.
Hesse provides an in-depth review of the impact of vicarious traumatization on therapists, how the therapist's reaction can affect the client, and methods of self-care.

Maslach, C., Schaufeli, W. B., & Leiter, M. P. (2001). Job burnout. *Annual Review of Psychology, 52,* 397–422.
A helpful review and explanation of the concept of job burnout by some of the most prominent researchers in the field.

EXERCISES AND DISCUSSION QUESTIONS

1. Have you met any mental health professionals who appear to be suffering from burnout and/or vicarious traumatization? Without naming any names, what signs have they given that suggest this to you?

2. Considering what you have learned from this chapter and your own personal temperament, what do you think would be most helpful to you in managing or avoiding burnout and vicarious traumatization?

Chapter Twenty-Four

Your Professional Development

As psychotherapists, our professional and personal developments are closely linked. Doing therapy is an emotionally demanding profession, and we owe it to ourselves and our clients to be up to the task. We need to learn how to be happy, healthy, and fulfilled and avoid getting burned out and exhausted.

MONITOR YOUR EMOTIONAL NEEDS

Periodic professional and personal stress is a normal part of being a practicing psychotherapist. Our work provokes many challenging emotional reactions at times and has been described as "grueling and demanding" (Norcross, 2000). It can take an emotional toll and contribute to depression, anxiety, emotional exhaustion, and disrupted relationships if appropriate self-care is not undertaken (Norcross, 2000).

Many people develop an interest in becoming a psychotherapist because of the emotional problems that they, their families, or their friends have experienced. Despite our knowledge, we are not immune to emotional distress, and, in fact, research has found that emotional problems are common in mental health practitioners and trainees. Many psychotherapists and psychotherapy trainees have experienced problems with anxiety, depression, or substance abuse (Kuyken, Peters, Power, & Lavender, 2003). Pope and Tabachnick (1993) found that over 60% of their sample of psychologists had experienced at least one episode of clinical depression, over 25% had felt suicidal at some point in the past, and almost 4% had made at least one suicide attempt. In a different study, Brooks, Holttum and Lavender (2002) found that, although a sample of British psychology trainees had better adjustment scores overall than the general population, 40% had problems in at least one of these areas: depression, anxiety, self-esteem, and work adjustment; there was also a significant proportion of the sample that had some problems with substance abuse. Other studies have cited similar results.

It is adaptive for clinicians to pay meticulous attention to detail since their clients depend on them to provide good care and assess their emergencies carefully. It is adaptive for clinicians to be active problem solvers and to often think about how to improve the care that they provide. Unfortunately, in the extreme, these adaptive traits can be maladaptive, becoming perfectionism (Wittenberg & Norcross, 2001) and self-blame (Norcross, 2000).

Ethnic minority students may also experience unique stressors during their training years, including overt and covert racism, feeling alone, worries about fitting in, lack of acknowledgment of one's identity, and feeling vulnerable (Vasquez et al., 2006). Whether compounded with ethnic differences or not, other differences between students and their teachers, peers, and clients, such as those of social class, disability status, and sexual orientation, can be challenging as well.

We need to have insight and acceptance about these stressors, and we need to be attentive to our own levels of functioning. As mental health practitioners, we have a duty to monitor our emotional functioning carefully so that we can care properly for ourselves and our clients. If our family, friends, supervisors, or peers are concerned about how we are doing, we need to listen carefully and respond mindfully and without defensiveness. As we all know, psychotherapy is a very effective treatment for all the previously mentioned issues.

UNDERSTAND YOUR TRAUMA HISTORY (IF YOU HAVE ONE)

Some clinicians may go into mental health because their own history of emotional distress has given them compassion for others who have suffered similarly. And, like any other group of adults, many mental health clinicians have a history of childhood physical or sexual abuse. The rate of childhood sexual or physical abuse for psychotherapists appears similar to or perhaps slightly greater than the rate in the general population (Feldman-Summers & Pope, 1994; Little & Hamby, 1996; Pope & Feldman-Summers, 1992). In addition, psychotherapists are not immune from other traumas, such as rape, domestic violence, and so on (Pope & Feldman-Summers, 1992).

If you are a therapist who has a history of trauma, you will have a greater intuitive understanding of what your traumatized clients have experienced. However, you also face some risks. Although it is normal to have strong emotional reactions at times when working with traumatized clients, therapists who were new to working with traumatized clients and had a history of sexual trauma displayed significantly greater emotional disruption (Pearlman & Mac Ian, 1995). Compared to other psychotherapists, therapists who have a history of childhood sexual abuse endorsed that they made more boundary mistakes in therapy and cried more with clients (Little & Hamby, 1996). They also sometimes shared their experiences of sexual abuse with clients, and they usually felt angrier with the client's perpetrator than other therapists did (Little & Hamby, 1996). If you have a history of trauma, do not share this with clients. Instead, thoroughly discuss your thoughts about taking this step with a supervisor (or a consultant) *and* your own therapist.

While sexual feelings are equally common in male and female psychotherapists, male therapists are at greatest risk for sexual boundary violations; the most recent research I found estimates that about 9% of male psychotherapists but less than 1% of female psychotherapists have had sexual relations with a client (Jackson & Nuttall, 2001). Although the number of male therapists with a history of childhood sexual abuse was relatively small, the researchers found that men with a history of childhood sexual abuse, especially those with more severe sexual abuse *and* emotional distress, are at greatest risk of sexual boundary violations (Jackson & Nuttall, 2001).

As is now clear, a significant proportion of psychotherapists have a history of trauma. If this is you, understand that you may be more vulnerable to emotional distress when working with clients, especially when you are less experienced. You must also pay very close attention to boundary issues, especially when you are tempted to self-disclose and when there is sexual transference or countertransference. Be especially mindful of when you need to seek out psychotherapy, consultation, and supervision.

GET PERSONAL PSYCHOTHERAPY

When I was a graduate student, my academic director of training recommended that I get personal psychotherapy in a rather punitive way. Later I realized that—despite its tone—this advice was some of the best I ever got. I found a nurturing and accepting therapist who helped me explore the emotional and interpersonal impact of my trauma history. The gains I made in my own psychotherapy over the years have led to fulfillment that I could never have imagined thirty years ago on that fateful day in graduate school. (Anonymous psychotherapist, personal communication, October 27, 2007)

For our own mental health and the mental health of our clients, it is essential that we monitor ourselves adequately for stress and take appropriate steps to address our emotional difficulties. For the reasons cited previously (and others), about half of psychology graduate students seek psychotherapy during their graduate studies (Dearing, Maddux, & Tangney, 2005), and at least three-fourths of psychotherapists have been in psychotherapy themselves, generally on more than one occasion (Norcross, 2005; Pope & Tabachnick, 1993). The graduate students who were studied indicated that the main barriers to seeking therapy were cost, concerns about confidentiality (with regard to their graduate program), and the time psychotherapy would take.

The potential benefits of personal psychotherapy for the psychotherapist are numerous (Norcross, 2005): improved emotional functioning, reduced countertransference potential, alleviating the stress of being a psychotherapist, demonstrating the transformative power of psychotherapy through personal experience, developing increased sensitivity to the struggles of clients, and developing clinical skills through observation of one's own therapist.

If you are interested in seeking psychotherapy, ask a trusted peer, supervisor, or colleague for some recommendations. Many private practitioners are happy to see mental health graduate students for a reduced fee, especially if you can arrange your schedule to come during the daytime hours, which are more difficult for practitioners to fill. Many graduate programs already provide all their students with a list of recommended psychotherapists in the local community. Avoid seeking psychotherapy at any agency or setting that trains students from your graduate program.

GAIN PROFESSIONAL COMPETENCE

Gaining knowledge helps to allay your anxiety about treating difficult populations, so read up on new populations and new diagnoses that you will be treating. Getting consultation or supervision can also be helpful at any stage in one's professional development. As you become more experienced and knowledgeable, your professional competence and confidence will grow. One of the advantages of being a mental health professional is that there is always something new and interesting to learn about in our field.

Professionals who work in a medical center setting are at an advantage, as there are often grand rounds and other professional presentations readily available. Professionals in medical center and university settings have ready access to professional libraries and academic search databases and search tools to help them stay current.

Important developments, both research and theoretical, occur every year, and we must figure out how to gain and use this knowledge for the benefit of our clients. Attending at least one professional conference every year or two will help keep you up on the latest developments in the field. Popular press items can be informative, including the magazines *Scientific American*, *Mind*, and *Discover* as well as the *New York Times*, especially the Tuesday science section. Reading several professional books per year is helpful. When you graduate, you might want to join or start a book or journal club so that you can keep current with the help of colleagues.

DEVELOP AREAS OF EXPERTISE

Many psychotherapy graduate students are overwhelmed by the amount of information that they do not know. It is true that the professional literature is vast, and no one of us can know any more than a fraction of it. However, competent professionals develop certain areas of practice that they are interested in and become especially knowledgeable about these topics. Perhaps you might have an intrinsic interest in a particular topic, or maybe you've had a training placement that sparked an interest in a certain client population. Go ahead and nurture this professional interest. Go to specific conferences about the topic. When you have to do a research paper, do one in your interest area whenever possible.

Your enthusiasm about your areas of interest and expertise will be helpful to you in several ways. This enthusiasm will help carry you through any difficult professional periods. You will be more motivated to keep up with the field because of your interest level. You will find it easier to get a job because you know what you are interested in and you will seek it out. Employers will appreciate your level of knowledge and your enthusiasm.

Don't worry if you don't have an area of expertise right now. If you are right for the psychotherapy field, one area of interest (or probably more than one) will make itself known sooner or later. Just be patient and be alert for it to develop.

DEVELOP SUPPORTIVE PROFESSIONAL RELATIONSHIPS

Supportive relationships with other mental health professionals are an essential portion of your professional development. It helps to have relationships with others who have various levels of experience. Many mental health professionals also end up with a life partner who is a psychotherapist as well. Greater professional support leads to better professional functioning (Kuyken et al., 2003). In addition, as a beginning therapist, open and supportive relationships with your supervisors can be invaluable in your personal and professional development.

Developing good professional relationships is also a form of networking. These relationships may help you obtain recommendations and even employment in the future.

Supportive professional relationships are particularly essential for the ethnic minority psychotherapist. Ethnic minority students and professionals often have professional challenges that White students do not (Vasquez et al., 2006). In addition, family members often tell the ethnic minority student, "You have to work twice as hard to be thought half as good" (Vasquez et al., 2006, p. 161), which can result in (understandable) workaholism and greater work stress. Ethnic minority psychotherapists can find it particularly helpful to seek out additional mentoring and supportive relationships with other professionals of similar ethnicity, even if they are at a geographic distance (Gonzalez-Figueroa & Young, 2005; Vasquez et al., 2006), and certain White mentors can be found who will have confidence in the abilities of the ethnic minority student as well (Vasquez et al., 2006). Seek these individuals out as much as possible.

Your supportive colleagues will provide helpful validation and consultation for you as you progress professionally. When you have a professional ethics question, you will have someone to call. When you need support with a difficult client, you can readily get professional consultation. When you are making a professional transition, you will have others who can advise you — and you can do the same for your colleagues.

MAKE PROFESSIONAL CONTRIBUTIONS

Making professional contributions helps you give back to the mental health community and encourages you to maintain your competence as well. You may be interested in volunteering your time and expertise at a community organization with a worthy cause. Or you may be interested in lobbying your state or federal representatives on mental health–related issues. There is a way to make a contribution for every clinician's temperament: writing, lecturing, teaching, research, supervising, and consulting. In addition, many clinicians are active in their various professional organizations.

DEVELOP RESILIENCY IN RESPONSE TO
ADVERSE PROFESSIONAL EVENTS

As psychotherapists, we are at risk of a multitude of adverse events. We might be embroiled in the legal system through malpractice suits, subpoenas, and dispositions; I have recommended a resource at the end of the chapter for giving testimony. We could experience adverse client events, such as having clients committing suicide, being stalked by a client, or being threatened by a client. Many of these adverse events are unfortunately common. For example, nearly 20% of a random sample of Australian psychologists had been stalked for at least 2 weeks by a client (Purcell, Powell, & Mullen, 2005). Having a client commit suicide is all too common, with 25% to 50% of licensed psychotherapists experiencing a client suicide (McAdams & Foster, 2000); psychiatrists have the highest risk because of the number of clients they see for medication management. Various U.S. and international studies have found that the majority of mental health practitioners will experience at least one physical assault or threat in their careers; psychiatrists and nurses are at greatest risk (Arthur, Brende, & Quiroz, 2003; Lawoko, Soares, & Nolan, 2004; Pieters, Speybrouck, De Gucht, & Joss, 2005).

Being knowledgeable about how to manage these crises from clinical, legal, and ethical perspectives can help us be prepared for whatever may happen. If the worst does happen, do not hesitate to seek support from colleagues, friends, and family. Discuss the event with sympathetic and informed colleagues to gain perspective.

KEEP BALANCED

As we all know, graduate students often tend to have a streak of perfectionism and/or workaholism. These traits are often coupled with what I call "graduate student guilt," the idea that there is work that you *should* be doing at every waking moment and that, if you aren't, you deserve to feel guilty. If you are tired, exhausted, and burned out, you will not be able to be very helpful to your clients because you don't even know how to take care of yourself.

As a graduate student, you can work on developing good habits that will help you throughout your professional life. Allow yourself designated personal time to maintain a balance between your personal and professional lives. Endeavor to set aside a significant period of time every week when you do not work on class work. If you are religious, this could perhaps be Shabbat or Sunday. If not, choose any other time period that works for you, preferably lasting at least 24 hours. You might do some housework then or spend time with your friends, children, and/or partner. Spend some time enjoying the day in whatever way works for you. Perhaps you might want to develop and pursue a hobby even if it is only for an hour every week or two. During the rest of the week, try to have a little personal or family time every day. Recharge your batteries by taking a weeklong vacation at least twice each year—and don't take any work with you.

REPLENISH YOURSELF

Keeping yourself emotionally replenished is an essential personal task for the psychotherapist. Know yourself and learn what things help you feel refreshed. Use your personal time on a daily and weekly basis for activities that replenish you. Many people find that regular exercise helps mood and energy level.

There is nothing wrong with television but use it in moderation when you choose to, not just to avoid schoolwork. If you need time away from schoolwork, try to use that time mindfully and choose activities that you will really enjoy.

There is some preliminary evidence that mindfulness practices such as yoga, qigong, and meditation can be helpful self-care practices for psychotherapists (Christopher, Christopher, Dunnagan, & Schure, 2006; Newsome, Christopher, Dahlen, & Christopher, 2006). Sitting meditation can be helpful in reducing depression and increasing positive mood states (Jain et al., 2007), and case reports suggest that meditation may help you gain perspective in difficult countertransference situations (Christensen & Rudnick, 1999; Cooper, 1999). Recent research also suggests that sitting meditation may be especially helpful in alleviating distress by reducing ruminative thoughts (Jain et al., 2007; Ramel, Goldin, Carmona, & McQuaid, 2004). Walking meditation can be a helpful alternative when you are feeling agitated, anxious, or frustrated. It can be helpful to get instruction in meditation and to meditate regularly with others to strengthen that practice.

The research in well-being and religion shows mixed and inconsistent findings (Lewis & Cruise, 2006). This research also tends to equate Christianity and/or monotheism with spirituality, which is inappropriate in our 21st-century multicultural society. For example, Hinduism, one of the world's five major religions, is polytheistic, as are many indigenous religions, and some Buddhists consider themselves agnostic or atheist. Of course, you are the best judge of whether religious practice would be an uplifting and replenishing experience for you; if so, make time to participate actively with your preferred religious group.

NURTURE YOUR OWN HAPPINESS

Until recent times, our professions have focused entirely on alleviating suffering. However, recent research sheds some light on what actually makes people happy (Haidt, 2005). As therapists, we can apply the scientific study of happiness to ourselves and our clients.

Our clients implicitly ask two things of us: to alleviate their suffering and to help them live a happy life. Many clients lament that others seem to be living a happy life but that they do not seem to be able to. Our insights and knowledge can help us guide our clients to the happiness they have longed for.

People have many ideas about what will make them happy, but they are often wrong (Gilbert, 2006). Having more money, above a level sufficient for a modest middle-class (non-poverty) lifestyle, does not result in significantly greater happiness (Diener & Seligman, 2005; Kahneman, Krueger, Schkade, Schwarz, & Stone, 2006), although having an education above the high school level does (Easterlin, 2003). More possessions do not make people happy either (Easterlin, 2003), as people get used to what they have and then desire even more. Youth doesn't make people happier either; in fact, older people generally are happier than the young, although happiness can decline after the mid-70s (Mroczek, 2001).

However, there are some simple things that do actually increase happiness, or subjective well-being, as some authors prefer to call it. People who are more socially connected (Kawachi & Berkman, 2001) tend to be happier. People who consciously practice gratitude are happier (Seligman, Steen, Park, & Peterson, 2005). Flow experiences increase happiness. Flow is "a particular kind of experience that is so engrossing and enjoyable that it becomes . . . worth doing for its own sake even though it may have no consequence outside itself. Creative activities, music, sports, games and religious rituals are typical sources for this kind of experience" (Csikszentmihalyi, 1999, p. 824). People who experience flow are invigorated and have a greater sense of well-being (Csikszentmihalyi, 1999). Meditation may cause changes in brain functioning that increase positive affect (Davidson et al., 2003).

APPRECIATE THE REWARDS OF BEING A PSYCHOTHERAPIST

Despite the many challenges, there are profound rewards that come from a career as a psychotherapist. I will leave you with the words of a colleague and the words of two prominent therapists, teachers, and writers on the subject.

> On a regular basis I'm given the chance to bear witness to the most personal, moving and ultimately the most profound struggles that are part and parcel of the human condition for all of us. I'm allowed to participate in and to influence in some small—and at times not so small—way the unfolding of another person's life, all the while being profoundly influenced myself by the whole process. This work has brought a depth and breadth to my own life and personhood that I can't imagine being afforded to me in any other line of work. How lucky is that? (M. E. Bratu, personal communication, June 8, 2007)

> To my mind, the ultimate satisfaction in being a therapist is the opportunity to earn a living by being honest, curious, and committed to trying to do right by others. . . . While many professions involve service to others, the vocation of

psychotherapy allows for a particularly intimate, organic, integrated kind of helping that makes one's work meaningful and fulfilling, no matter how tiring. I am grateful that such a role exists in my era and culture, a role that allows me to earn a living by doing what I enjoy doing and find consonant with my temperament.... Watching a client grow psychologically is the closest analogue we have in professional life to the experience of watching a beloved child change into a self-assured adult. There is nothing like it. (McWilliams, 2004, pp. 282–283)

Those who are cradlers of secrets are granted a clarifying lens through which to view the world—a view with less distortion, denial and illusion, a view of the way things really are.... When I turn to others with the knowledge that we are all (therapist and patient alike) burdened with painful secrets—guilt for acts committed, shame for actions not taken, yearnings to be loved and cherished, deep vulnerabilities, insecurities and fears—I draw closer to them. Being a cradler of secrets has, as the years have passed, made me gentler and more accepting. When I encounter individuals inflated with vanity of self-importance, or distracted by any of a myriad of consuming passions, I intuit the pain of their underlying secrets and feel not judgment but compassion, and above all, connectedness.... [W]e are the midwife to the birth of something new, liberating and elevating. We watch our patients let go of old self-defeating patterns, detach from ancient grievances, develop zest for living, learn to love us, and through that act, turn lovingly to others.... What a treat it is to watch them open doors to rooms never before entered, discover new wings of their house containing parts in exile—wise, beautiful, and creative pieces of identity. (Yalom, 2002, pp. 257–258)

CONCLUSION

I began the introduction of this book by telling you about my feelings of anxiety as well as my hunch that I was somehow ill prepared when I saw my first psychotherapy client as a graduate student. Since then, as a teacher and supervisor, I have thought long and hard about what beginning students need to know when they walk into that first psychotherapy session. This book has been the culmination of those thoughts. My sincerest hope is that this book helps you, in some way, on your journey to become a well-prepared, competent, and confident psychotherapist.

RECOMMENDED READING

Brodsky, S. L. (1991). *Testifying in court: Guidelines and maxims for the expert witness*. Washington, DC: American Psychological Association.

Brodsky's books, including this one, provide helpful and practical advice for any mental health professional (whether you are an expert witness or not) who has become embroiled in the legal system. If you are ever subpoenaed and you have to give testimony in court or give a deposition, read this first. In addition, talk to a lawyer about the difference between an expert witness and a witness of fact.

Csikszentmihalyi, M. (1999). If we are so rich, why aren't we happy? *American Psychologist, 10,* 821–827.

In this well-written article, Csikszentmihalyi summarizes much of the research on happiness, income, and flow and draws some profound conclusions about human existence and well-being.

Glinkauf-Hughes, C., & Mehlman, E. (1995). Narcissistic issues in therapists: Diagnostic and treatment considerations. *Psychotherapy, 32,* 213–221.

Despite its off-putting title, this article is simply about gaining insight into common emotional issues among psychotherapists, such as parentification, perfectionism, and the imposter phenomenon.

Gelso, C. J., & Hayes, J. A. (2007). *Countertransference and the therapist's inner experience: Perils and possibilities.* Mahwah, NJ: Lawrence Erbaum Associates.

This book provides a helpful perspective on current thinking and research regarding the emotions and reactions of the therapist towards the client. In this relatively brief volume, the authors explore the subject from all angles: historical, theoretical, conceptual, and empirical.

Nhat Hanh, T. (1975). *The miracle of mindfulness: A manual on meditation.* Boston: Beacon Press.

A short classic volume to introduce the reader to basic meditation practices.

Norcross, J. C., & Guy, J. D. (2007). *Leaving it at the office: A guide to psychotherapist self-care.* New York: Guilford Press.

The authors discuss helpful issues for therapists, such as nurturing relationships, setting boundaries, fostering creativity and growth, and others.

WEB RESOURCE

http://www.authentichappiness.sas.upenn.edu

This is the website for the University of Pennsylvania Positive Psychology Center, which has numerous interesting resources regarding the psychological study of happiness.

EXERCISES AND DISCUSSION QUESTIONS

1. What are the rewards and the costs to you of being a psychotherapist?

2. How has the process of becoming a psychotherapist changed you personally? Has it changed your personal relationships? How?

Afterword

One of my struggles in writing this volume was a striking lack of literature about certain practical issues. Some authors helpfully shared their personal experiences and insights, and I referenced these when possible.

However, there is little to no research about certain clinically important topics. I have listed some of my questions about those topics here. I hope that this might inspire research and further writing by mental health professionals.

- What do clients think about what their therapists wear? Do they care about earrings and tattoos? Do these opinions change with the client's age?
- What coping strategies—adaptive and maladaptive—do therapists use to cope with their clients' emotional pain? Can trainees be taught these coping strategies?
- How do clients react to the therapist's office decor? What about plants? Family pictures? Religious symbols? Color schemes? Presence or absence of "ethnic" art? Does it matter whether this "ethnic" art matches the client's ethnicity?
- What are typical attendance, cancellation, no-show, and fee policies in different therapy settings? What is the impact of different policies on client retention?
- What factors predict no-shows and cancellations? What methods of addressing these in therapy are most effective?
- How do clients react to therapists' pregnancies? Do these reactions differ by client? How? Do men have any similar issues with taking paternity leave?
- What are common boundary crossings in therapy (e.g., gifts, hugs, and attending client events)? How often do they occur? How are these typically

handled? Why did the therapist allow the boundary crossing, and what was the effect on therapy?

- Which personal questions are clinicians willing to answer, and which ones do they refuse? How much does this vary by theoretical orientation?
- How many therapists have a history of treatment for more serious mental illnesses (e.g., major depression, bipolar disorder, schizophrenia, or post-traumatic stress disorder)? Do these therapists ever reveal this to their clients? Under what circumstances?
- How often do mental health professionals have to cope with prejudicial behavior on the part of clients? What are the best ways of coping with this?
- How much do psychotherapists typically tell their partners, friends, and relatives about their work? Does this differ depending on whether the partner is a psychotherapist as well? How much is unavoidable? When is it too much?
- What kind of personal Web presence do psychotherapists have? What do they think is appropriate? Does this vary by age?
- What do psychotherapists say to start a psychotherapy session? Do they say the same thing every time? What are the differences in how therapy sessions start by theoretical orientation?
- How much do beginning therapists suffer from vicarious traumatization and burnout? How much do they simply feel overwhelmed?

And, finally, while there is some interesting and informative research on transference and countertransference, far too few researchers are working on it, and there is clearly promise for interdisciplinary work with cognitive neuroscientists and social psychologists that remains to be done.

APPENDICES

Appendix One

Questions for Your New Supervisor

Whenever you get a new supervisor or go to a new training site, there are some questions that are helpful to ask. I have suggested questions throughout the text but have summarized many of them here for your convenience when meeting with a new supervisor.

ADMINISTRATIVE AND PROCEDURAL ISSUES

- What is the administrative structure at this site? How do I fit into that?
- Who do I need to know? Can you introduce me?
- How are fees dealt with in this setting?
- How are new clients assigned?
- How is informed consent obtained at this facility?
- How are clients educated about limits to confidentiality?
- Where are the HIPAA (Health Insurance Portability and Accountability Act) forms?
- Do I discuss audiotaping verbally with clients, or is there a form they need to sign as well?
- What are the guidelines for release of information at this facility?
- What should I do if I get sick or have a personal emergency and need to cancel my clients?
- What are arrangements for vacation coverage for my clients?
- What are the clinic policies if a client brings me a gift?

DOCUMENTATION AND COMMUNICATION ISSUES

- How are progress notes done at this facility? Do you require that I keep process notes? Are they discoverable in this state?
- How are initial intake interviews done at this facility? Are there any forms or templates that I need to fill out?
- How are treatment plans written and documented here? Can you show me a sample that has been done well?
- How do I find and access medical records at this facility?
- Can I send e-mails to other clinicians about clients securely at this site?
- What do you recommend about client contact by e-mail?

SUPERVISORY ISSUES

- What is your theoretical orientation? How do you work with students who are trained in another orientation?
- How are evaluations done in this setting?
- If I am having problems, what is the process for remediation?

CLIENT CARE ISSUES

- Do you need me to do a Mental Status Exam? Can you teach me how?
- What diagnoses are particularly common in this client population? Do you have any recommended reading for me to learn more?
- What referrals are commonly made from this facility? Do you have brochures, business cards, or contact information for those facilities?
- How do you recommend that I deal with no-shows and cancellations?
- How do you suggest that I deal with attendance problems?
- What thoughts do you have about self-disclosure with this client population?
- What are your thoughts about clients' requests for hugs?
- What do you think about attending client events?
- [If you feel this is pertinent to you] What should I do if a client appears prejudiced toward me?

CRISIS ISSUES

- What are the procedures for outpatient commitment [if your state has it]?
- How can I find you if I'm having a client emergency? Who should I talk to if I can't find you?
- How are clients hospitalized voluntarily and involuntarily at this site? How are involuntary clients managed here?
- What if a client gets violent? Should I try to help intervene after I call the police or security?

Appendix Two

Verbal Informed Consent

Remember the main points in the informed consent process:

- A mentally competent client
- Education about the treatment process and treatment options
- Voluntary consent to treatment
- Documentation of all this

STEP 1: DISCUSS/EDUCATE

A. Knowledge About Psychotherapy

- Nature of treatment (e.g., weekly psychotherapy sessions, lasting about 50 minutes, discussing which likely topics)
- Estimated duration of treatment
- Risks and benefits to psychotherapy and that results cannot be predicted with certainty but depend in large part on the engagement and effort of the client
- Confidentiality—see appendix 3
- Financial issues: fees and insurance
- Supervision and need for audiotaping or videotaping
- Therapy can be discontinued at any time
- Questions can be answered at any time
- Opportunity for questions

B. Knowledge About Alternatives to Psychotherapy

- What the alternatives are, including doing nothing
- The benefits and risks of these alternatives
- If uncertain, the client can seek more information on own or through a second opinion

STEP 2: THINK

- Is the client mentally competent to engage in the informed consent process?
- Can the client comprehend relevant information, appreciate the relevance of the information, and weigh the risks and benefits against alternatives?
- Has the client made a voluntary choice to participate?
- If you are unsure, talk to your supervisor about how to proceed.

STEP 3: DOCUMENT

- Indicate in the client's chart that your professional opinion is that the client is mentally competent to engage in the informed consent process
- Then list the informed consent issues that you discussed with the client and any notable interactions with the client about these issues and that the client consents to treatment

SCRIPT

"I'd like to give you some information about our work together and see if you have any questions. My recommendation is that you attend weekly individual psychotherapy sessions that last for 45 to 50 minutes. The clinic requires that you pay your fee at the desk when you come in each time. If you need to cancel, please call me as soon as possible, at least 24 hours in advance. Do you have any questions?

"In therapy, we will address your current life difficulties and attempt to help you with them. I don't know how long treatment is likely to take, but I can give you some feedback on that when I get to know you better. I can't say for sure how much you are likely to improve, but I can tell you that most clients with similar problems improve significantly if they attend their appointments regularly and make their best effort. There is some risk that your condition may worsen, but that might also happen if you don't come to therapy. In addition, there is some risk that you may decide to make changes that important people in your life may not like, and they might have some reactions to that. Do you have any questions about the risks and benefits of therapy?

"Some people with similar problems to yourself prefer to take medications than to come to therapy, and some people prefer to do both. What are your thoughts about that?

"Of course, if you want to stop therapy, you can do so at any time; however, if you've decided to stop, I'd appreciate it if we could discuss it first. If at any time you want a second opinion, please let me know. Do you have any other questions? Let me know any time you want to discuss any of these issues again, okay?"

References: Beahrs and Gutheil (2001); Braaten, Otto, and Handelsman (1993); Eyler and Jeste (2006); Zuckerman (2003).

Verbal Education on Limits to Confidentiality

You may need to adapt the following script to your specific state laws and the situation at your training site. In summary, you will want to discuss these topics:

- What the legal limits to confidentiality are:
  - Child abuse
  - Elder abuse
  - Any other limitations specific to the state where you are practicing, such as *Tarasoff*
  - That you cannot predict exactly what would happen if the client gets embroiled in legal or criminal problems
- Limits to confidentiality specific to the site that the client may not be aware of with respect to charting and discussions between clinicians
- That you are a student and you will be discussing the client's treatment with your supervisor

SCRIPT

"Some people think that everything we discuss in therapy is strictly confidential. Generally this is true, but I wanted to let you know that there are a few legal limitations to your confidentiality. I bring this up because I want you to be fully informed. For example, if I hear anything from you that leads me to believe that a child, dependent person, or elderly person is being harmed, I would need to report that to the state for investigation. In addition, if you are involved in any legal or criminal proceedings or if you plan to hurt someone, there is some risk that I might need to disclose information to the police or to a court. Do you have any questions? [Depending on the complexity of the question, you might need to advise the client to seek legal counsel.]

"In addition I wanted to let you know that at this site, you have one electronic record that all the staff have access to. Anyone who is treating you will be able to see the progress notes that I write about our work. However, I want to assure you that I keep these notes brief and to the point. If at any point you would like to see them, please let me know. Do you have any questions? [Modify this paragraph to suit the specific situation at your site.]

"I also will discuss your difficulties with your psychiatrist and the rest of the treatment team as needed. This is so we can work together as a team to help you. Since I am a trainee, I will need to discuss our work together with my supervisor, and we will sometimes review the audiotapes that I make of our sessions. Do you have any questions?"

Appendix Four

Outline of Intake Interview

Keep in mind the four primary goals for the intake interview:

- Establish rapport
- Obtain informed consent, including providing information on confi-dentiality (depending on the population and the specific client, this can be done in writing prior to the session, with an opportunity for questions within the session)
- Determine the presenting problem
- Evaluate the client for suicidality and other crises

The most important issues for the first session are in *italics*. The other topics are essential information that you should gather to appropriately assess and diagnose the client but can generally be postponed until the second session if you run out of time.

PRESENTING COMPLAINT

- Current problems, including intensity, frequency, and duration of symptoms
- Why coming for help now
- Ask questions as needed if client is vague

INTERPERSONAL AND COPING PROBLEMS, INCLUDING ASSESSING LEVEL OF DISTRESS

- Legal problems
- Relationship problems
- Parenting problems
- Interpersonal problems
- Job/school problems
- How is the client coping effectively and ineffectively?
- How are symptoms affecting functioning?

CRISIS EVALUATION

- Suicidal ideation or behavior, self-harm
  - Are you having any thoughts about hurting yourself?
  - Has that ever been a problem for you?
  - Have you been feeling hopeless?
  - Have you had any family members who have committed suicide?
- Homicidal and/or violent ideation or behavior
  - Are you having any thoughts of hurting anyone? Ask follow-up questions as needed to ascertain exactly what violent or threatening behavior, if any, has already transpired recently.
  - Have you ever been violent in the past? When? Can you tell me more about what happened?
  - Have you ever had any legal problems? If so, ask the following questions: Have you ever been arrested? Have you ever been in jail or prison? What were the charges?

DIAGNOSE MENTAL ILLNESSES AND ASSESS ALL PSYCHOLOGICAL SYMPTOMS, ESPECIALLY THE FOLLOWING

- Anxiety symptoms
  - Agoraphobia without panic (panic disorder has a 2% to 3% lifetime prevalence)
  - Generalized anxiety disorder
  - Obsessive-compulsive disorder
  - Panic disorder
  - Post-traumatic stress disorder

- ◦ Simple/specific phobia
- ◦ Social phobia
- Substance use or abuse
  - ◦ Alcohol abuse/dependence
  - ◦ Drug abuse/dependence
- Mood symptoms
  - ◦ Bipolar I or II
  - ◦ Dysthymia
  - ◦ Major depression
- Psychotic symptoms
- Other diagnoses and symptoms
  - ◦ Adjustment disorder
  - ◦ Attention-deficit/hyperactivity disorder
  - ◦ Eating disorders, if common in the client population
  - ◦ Self-harm behavior
  - ◦ Diagnoses common to the specific population at your site
  - ◦ Other diagnoses suggested by the client's presentation

Note that this list includes the most common diagnoses in the U.S. population (see chapter 9) as well as those that are most associated with suicidality (see chapter 19).

MEDICAL PROBLEMS

- Do you have any medical problems?
- Are you taking any medications? What is that for?
- Do you have any pain? Where is it? What is causing that? How much does it bother you? How much does the pain interfere with your activities?
- Medical history

MENTAL HEALTH HISTORY

- Previous psychotherapy, when last seen, for how long, and how many previous therapists
- Psychiatric hospitalizations, number of hospitalizations, date of first, date of most recent, why hospitalized
- Is client under the care of a psychiatrist? If so, get client to sign a release of information so that you can coordinate care.

- Other past treatment, such as substance abuse or intensive outpatient
- Family history of mental illness and substance abuse

SOCIAL HISTORY

- Family of origin, including ethnic background, religion, number of siblings, and family relationships
- Any history of childhood abuse, mistreatment, or neglect
- Other adult or childhood traumas
- Education, including problems suggestive of a learning disability
- Military service, including whether client observed or participated in combat
- Criminal history and legal problems
- Religious beliefs and involvement
- Leisure activities, hobbies, and active participation in organizations
- Current living situation, including everyone in the home
- Children, including where they are living
- Social network and support system
- Relationship status, including sexual orientation and marital history
- Work history, including current occupation

OBSERVE

- Behavior
- Verbalizations and thought processes, including coherence, memory, attention, and concentration
- Apparent verbal intelligence
- Physical characteristics
- Alertness
- Orientation
- Clothing and hygiene
- Motor activity
- Voice
- Attitude toward you
- Affect
- Mood
- Judgment
- Insight

GIVE FEEDBACK ABOUT THE FOLLOWING

- Diagnoses
- Treatment

MAKE REFERRALS

- Health related
- Mental health treatment

References: Choca and Van Denburg (1996); Moline, Williams, and Austin (1998); Morrison (1995, 2007); Simon (2004).

Appendix Five

Screening Questions and Diagnostic Hypotheses About Sleep

QUESTIONS ABOUT SLEEP

When asking about sleep, you can simply say, "How has your sleep been lately?" Let the client tell you about any current sleep problems. Most of this information will be useful to you. If the client is having sleep problems but is having difficulty articulating what they are, you might ask some of the following questions:

- What happens when you get into bed? If I had a video of you at bedtime, what would I see?
- How do you feel when you wake up in the morning? Is your sleep restful?
- Are you able to get to sleep at night when you want to? [If not:] Is this because you are lying awake worrying about your problems?
- Can you sleep through the night? How often do you wake up? How long does it take you to get back to sleep once you're awake?
- Do you wake up earlier than you had planned?
- How many hours of sleep are you getting? [If less than 8:] Is that enough for you? (If sleep is limited but client looks energetic, ask about manic symptoms right away.)
- Do you have any nightmares or bad dreams? How often? About how many times do you have nightmares in a week (or month)? Do they ever wake you up? What are they about?
- Does your partner say that you snore?
- Does your partner say that you kick or move around a lot at night?

As you can tell in Table A5, each of these sleep problems is commonly associated with a different diagnosis. The clues you get from the client's sleep pattern will help you zero in the client's problems and diagnosis more quickly.

References: American Psychiatric Association (2000); Morrison (2007).

Table A.5. Sleep Problems and Diagnostic Hypotheses

Sleep Problem	Diagnostic Hypothesis to Consider
Nightmares or disturbing dreams	PTSD
Fearful of going to sleep	PTSD
Difficulty getting to sleep because of rumination	Depressive or anxiety disorders
Insomnia	Depressive or anxiety disorders
Poor quality of sleep and/or doesn't sleep soundly	Depressive or anxiety disorders, sleep disorders
Wakes up in night, can't get back to sleep promptly	Depressive or anxiety disorders
Early morning awakening	Melancholic depression
Not feeling a need for more than 2 to 3 hours of sleep, still full of energy	Mania or hypomania. In *very* rare cases, this little sleep can be normal for an individual who has no mania.
Inability to sleep or excessive drowsiness	Drug or alcohol intoxication or withdrawal can cause these problems.
Doesn't sleep soundly, partner states that client snores loudly	Sleep disorder (sleep apnea) quite likely; however, emotional problems may be adding to sleep disturbance.
Doesn't sleep soundly, partner states that client is a very active sleeper, kicks or moves frequently while asleep	Sleep disorder (periodic limb movement disorder) quite likely; however, emotional problems may be adding to sleep disturbance.
Falls asleep suddenly in the middle of daily activities	Sleep disorder (narcolepsy) quite likely; in addition, there is some possibility of other medical issues, such as previously undetected seizures.
Sleep schedule changes from day to day, frequent napping, complains of tiredness	No clear diagnostic implications; however, behavioral interventions to improve sleep habits are very likely to be helpful (see appendix 18). Will need to reevaluate sleep after implementing these.
Emotional problems are mild (for example, no other disorder than adjustment disorder), no reported sleep problems, good sleep habits, yet client complains of daytime tiredness	Consider referral for evaluation of sleep disorders and be sure that the client is evaluated by physician for possible medical problems.

Appendix Six

Screening for Post-traumatic Stress Disorder

OVERVIEW

Screen routinely for post-traumatic stress disorder (PTSD) when first see-ing a client, even if the client has a well-documented mental health his-tory. Post-traumatic stress disorder is often comorbid with other mental illnesses, most commonly depression, anxiety, and substance abuse but also including seemingly unlikely ones such as schizophrenia (Resnick, Bond, & Mueser, 2003). Clients who present for other difficulties often have their PTSD missed by clinicians (Sheeran & Zimmerman, 2002). Post-traumatic stress disorder has a high lifetime prevalence of 6.8% of the U.S. population—meaning that 1 out of 15 people has a past or cur-rent diagnosis of PTSD (National Comorbidity Survey; R. C. Kessler, Berglund, Demler, Jin, & Walters, 2005).

Franklin, Sheeran, and Zimmerman (2002) determined that simply asking "Have you ever experienced a traumatic, life threatening, or ex-tremely upsetting event?" is a very effective screening question (see the section "Screening Alternative 1"). Prins et al. (2004) have developed a useful four-item screening questionnaire that clients can fill out them-selves (see Table A.6). You can also ask these four questions verbally as screening questions for PTSD during an initial interview.

After administering the screening questions, if the client appears likely to have PTSD follow up with further questions about PTSD using the symptoms described by the *Diagnostic and Statistical Manual of Mental Disorders* (4th ed., text revision; *DSM-IV-TR*; American Psychiatric As-sociation, 2000). Clients usually tolerate questions about PTSD symp-toms well, even if they may not tolerate discussion of the trauma. Be sure to document the frequency of nightmares, flashbacks, and intrusive memories as well as you can.

A CAUTIONARY NOTE ABOUT PTSD AND TRAUMA ASSESSMENT

Use care when assessing the trauma history. Get just enough basic facts to document the presence of a trauma history. It is best to use behaviorally based, closed-ended (yes or no) questions to assess trauma history in the first session.

Premature and overly detailed discussion of the trauma can destabilize some clients (Courtois, 1997). Clients with PTSD can have their symptoms worsened by too aggressive questioning of the details of their trauma histories. Stop the client if the client is volunteering details about the trauma history: "I'd like to stop you for a minute before we go on. This information that you are giving me is very important. However, I'm realizing that you don't know me very well yet, and I'm thinking you might feel safer waiting to discuss this in detail until we know each other better. What do you think?" In addition, don't let a client that you hardly know tell you a lot of details about a trauma since he or she may feel too exposed and vulnerable after the session and not return.

SCREENING ALTERNATIVE 1: PTSD SCREENING QUESTION FROM THE STRUCTURED CLINICAL INTERVIEW FOR THE DSM-IV-TR

Have you ever experienced a traumatic, life-threatening, or extremely upsetting event?

Note: For a written version to administer to clients, copy table A.6, cut off everything but the questions, then copy again and give to client. Or you can ask these questions of the client verbally during the intake interview.

References: First, Spitzer, Gibbon, and Williams (2002); Franklin, Sheeran, and Zimmerman (2002); Kimerling, Trafton, and Nguyen (2006); Prins et al. (2004).

Table A.6. Screening Alternative 2: The Primary Care PTSD Screen (PC-PTSD)

In your life, have you ever had any experience that was so frightening, horrible, or upsetting that, *in the past month, you* . . .

1. Had nightmares about it or thought about it when you did not want to?	YES	NO
2. Tried hard not to think about it or went out of your way to avoid situations that reminded you of it?	YES	NO
3. Were constantly on guard, watchful, or easily startled?	YES	NO
4. Felt numb or detached from others, activities, or your surroundings?	YES	NO

Scoring:
3–4	PTSD diagnosis likely; ask further questions about symptoms
2	PTSD diagnosis unlikely but follow up as indicated clinically
0–1	Probably no PTSD

Reference: Prins et al. (2004)

Appendix Seven

Screening for Bipolar Disorder

OVERVIEW

The lifetime prevalence in the U.S. population of bipolar I or II disorders is 3.9% (National Comorbidity Survey; R. C. Kessler, Berglund, Demler, Jin, & Walters, 2005). This means that 1 out of 20 people has bipolar disorder. We expect that anyone with a history of bipolar mood episodes will have a recurrence without treatment.

Rarely do persons who are manic understand that they are mentally ill, even in retrospect when they are no longer manic. Thus, they will not volunteer a history of manic symptoms. Strangely, many people with bipolar disorder characterize mania as "feeling like myself." They feel great—motivated, brilliant, and full of life and ideas. A client of mine once described mania as life being "all sparkly." When they are feeling euthymic (e.g., normal), they think life is "blah." They do, however, understand accurately when they have major depression.

At least one-third of clients who present with major depression will have underlying bipolar disorder (Bowden, 2005), Therefore, every client who comes in with present or past major depression must be screened for a history of manic symptoms. Some screening questions for mania are presented for your use in this appendix.

Hypomania (a briefer and milder form of mania, as seen in bipolar II) is especially easy to miss. Recent research has pinpointed that the modal hypomanic episode lasts for 2 days (which is less than specified by the *Diagnostic and Statistical Manual of Mental Disorders* [4th ed., text revision; American Psychiatric Association, 2000] for diagnosis of the condition). These episodes can have mild symptoms, and thus the client can confuse hypomania with simply "feeling good"; therefore, the brevity of the hypomanic episodes and the client's lack of concern about them makes them difficult to detect by clinicians. In bipolar II, hypomanic symptoms often occur either before or after depressive episodes. Research suggests that clients may be more accurate recalling their hyperactive behavior during manic episodes rather than their irritable or expansive mood. Thus, behaviorally based questions ("Did you stay up all night and hardly need any sleep?") will more likely elicit manic symptoms than mood-based questions ("Did you feel 'on top of the world'?"). The Mood Disorder Questionnaire in appendix 8 may be helpful in that regard.

To add to the diagnostic confusion for the clinician, there is support for the existence of a disorder in which only manic episodes are present, without any identifiable history of depressive episodes (Cuellar, Johnson, & Winters, 2005). A final diagnostic issue with bipolar disorder is that there is evidence that attention-deficit/hyperactivity disorder and the manic phase of bipolar disorder are often mistaken for each other in children (Kim & Miklowitz, 2002).

A few bipolar clients are easy to diagnose. These are the ones with extreme mania that necessitates hospitalization or acute treatment. Any past or present diagnosis of mania or hypomania necessitates a diagnosis of bipolar disorder.

HISTORY SUGGESTIVE OF UNDERLYING BIPOLAR DISORDER (BOWDEN, 2001, 2005)

- Earlier age of onset (mean of 18 for bipolar disorder versus mean of 25.5 for unipolar depression)
- High frequency of depressive episodes
- Greater proportion of time ill
- First-degree relative with bipolar disorder (e.g., parent, sibling, or child)
- Many family members with mood disorders
- Comorbid substance abuse (60% of bipolar clients have substance abuse)

SYMPTOMS SUGGESTIVE OF UNDERLYING BIPOLAR DISORDER (BOWDEN, 2005)

- Relatively acute onset and/or abatement of symptoms
- Less anger and anxiety, fewer physical complaints, less psychomotor

agitation, and less likely to lose weight in bipolar disorder compared to unipolar depression
- More social withdrawal, psychomotor retardation, and hypersomnia in bipolar disorder
- Self-description indicative of mood lability ("Everyone says I'm moody.")
- Development of mania or hypomania in response to antidepressants

SCREENING QUESTIONS FROM THE MOOD DISORDER QUESTIONNAIRE

You can use the first two questions from the Mood Disorder Questionnaire in appendix 8 as screening questions, then administer the questionnaire or ask further questions as needed:

"Has there ever been a period of time when you were not your usual self and you felt so good or so hyper that other people thought you were not your normal self or you were so hyper that you got into trouble?"

"Has there ever been a period of time when you were not your usual self and you were so irritable that you shouted at people or started fights or arguments?"

I also like this screening question for mania:

"Have you ever had a period of a couple days to a week where you only needed a few hours of sleep every night yet you were full of energy?"

If any of these questions are answered yes, follow up with further symptoms of mania/hypomania. Or you can follow up with manic/hypomanic symptoms anyway if you suspect there may be a history of mania and the client may be in some denial about that.

Mood Disorder Questionnaire

SCORING ALGORITHM FOR THE
MOOD DISORDER QUESTIONNAIRE

Client gets a positive screening result IF:
  At least 7 of the 13 symptom questions must be answered yes
  AND
  Question 2 is answered yes
  AND
  Question 3 is answered Moderate problem or Serious problem

Reference: Hirschfeld et al. (2000). Reproduced with permission.

Table A.8. The Mood Disorder Questionnaire

1. Has there ever been a period of time when you were
   not your usual self and

. . . you felt so good or so hyper that other people thought you were not your normal self or you were so hyper that you got into trouble?	YES	NO
. . . you were so irritable that you shouted at people or started fights or arguments?	YES	NO
. . . you felt much more self-confident than usual?	YES	NO
. . . you were much more talkative or spoke faster than usual?	YES	NO
. . . you got much less sleep than usual and found you didn't really miss it?	YES	NO
. . . thoughts raced through your head or you couldn't slow your mind down?	YES	NO
. . . you were so easily distracted by things around you that you had trouble concentrating or staying on track?	YES	NO
. . . you had much more energy than usual?	YES	NO
. . . you were much more active or did many more things than usual?	YES	NO
. . . you were much more social or outgoing than usual; for example, you telephoned friends in the middle of the night?	YES	NO
. . . you were much more interested in sex than usual?	YES	NO
. . . you did things that were unusual for you or that other people might have thought were excessive, foolish, or risky?	YES	NO
. . . spending money got you or your family into trouble?	YES	NO

2. If you checked YES to more than one of the above,   YES   NO
   have several of these ever happened during the same
   period of time? Please circle one response only.

3. How much of a problem did any of these cause you—
   like being unable to work; having family, money, or legal
   troubles; or getting into arguments or fights? Please circle
   one response only.

No problem	Minor problem	Moderate problem	Serious problem

Appendix Nine

Screening for Major Depression

OVERVIEW

Major depression has a very high lifetime prevalence of 16.6% in the U.S. population—meaning that one out of six individuals has current or past major depression (R. C. Kessler, Berglund, Demler, Jin, & Walters, 2005). Questions about vegetative symptoms of depression early in an interview are nonthreatening to clients, and it is wise to screen for depression in all settings. Thus, a good place to start an interview would be asking about vegetative symptoms of depression, specifically, appetite, weight gain or loss, energy level, and sleep. These questions are similar to what the client might be asked by the primary care physician. A list of these questions follows. Alternatively, you can start with screening questions for mood and *anhedonia* (lack of interest in pleasurable activities).

VEGETATIVE SYMPTOMS OF DEPRESSION

- "How has your sleep been lately? Have you been having any difficulties with your sleep? What are they?"
- "How is your appetite?"
- "How is your energy level? Do you have enough energy to do everything you need to do?"

MOOD AND ANHEDONIA

- "Have you ever had a period of a couple weeks when you felt down most of the time? When was that?"
- "Have you ever had a period of a couple weeks when you just weren't interested in your usual activities? When was that?"

If the client answers yes to either of these questions, ask further questions about depressive symptoms.

Reference: American Psychiatric Association (2000).

Appendix Ten

Screening Questions About Seasonal Affective Disorder

OVERVIEW

Seasonal affective disorder (SAD) is considered to be a subtype of major depression. Rosenthal (1998), himself a sufferer of SAD, suggested that a diagnosis should be made when the client has major depression for at least two consecutive winters.

SAD has a characteristic symptom profile that differs from nonseasonal major depression:

- Extreme fatigue and exhaustion.
- Strong carbohydrate cravings and, consequently, increased carbohydrate consumption, often causing the afflicted client to gain weight in the winter.
- Paradoxically, carbohydrates increase energy in SAD clients, while other people just get sleepy.
- Client wants to sleep in too late and go to sleep too early.
- Hypersomnia accompanied with poor quality of sleep and frequent awakenings.
- Low sex drive.
- Poor concentration, difficulties thinking clearly, and feeling "in a fog" mentally.
- Relationships suffer because "people with SAD often just want to curl up in a secluded place and be left alone" in the winter (Rosenthal, 1998, p. 59).
- Some clients with SAD feel extremely sad, whereas in others the previously mentioned symptoms are much more prominent.

SAD can be effectively treated with light therapy and/or psychotropic medications. Light therapy entails daily exposure to bright light through a special light fixture or light box. According to Lam and Levitan (2000), "Clinical consensus guidelines have recommended light therapy as a first-line treatment for SAD, based on the evidence of numerous studies showing efficacy, including large randomized controlled trials and meta-analyses" (pp. 469–470). So bright-light therapy is a well-validated treatment. However, one study found that the subjects' mood improvements in SAD due to light therapy were not as great as the subjects' mood improvements during the following summer (Postolache et al., 1998).

SCREENING QUESTIONS FOR SAD

When your client presents with depression in the winter, try to ascertain the onset of the depression and the time frames of past depressive episodes:

- "When did you start getting depressed?"
- "When was the last time you were depressed? Have you been depressed in the winter before? When was that?"
- "At what time of year did you start feeling better?"

In addition, ask questions that might elicit typical symptoms and emotions of SAD:

- "When are you going to bed? How much are you sleeping? How is the quality of your sleep?" (SAD sufferers will go to bed early, then sleep fitfully all night, perhaps awakening for a while in the middle of the night.)
- "Have you been having any food cravings? For what?"
- "How has your concentration and thinking been?"
- "Do you feel any different on a sunny winter day or an overcast day?"

You might find that clients have taken steps that are partially effective at dealing with the situation, without really knowing what it is: going for tanning in the winter (intense tanning light lifts mood temporarily), vacationing as long as possible in sunny climates, or volunteering for business trips to sunny locales.

LIGHT THERAPY TREATMENT

Here are two reputable sources for high-intensity lights to treat SAD:

* http://www.northernlighttechnologies.com
* http://www.sunbox.com

The client's insurance may not pay for a high-intensity light to treat SAD; however, you can call the company and ask for a discount for your clients. Then when the client calls, the client can give your name and get the discount. It is best for the client to get either an actual light box or one of the lamps that looks like a terribly ugly desk lamp. The other items offered (visors and dawn-simulating clocks) may not be as well validated by research.

In order to treat clients with high intensity light, you should read more on the subject. However, here are a few guidelines for your information:

* The client should use the light box as soon as possible after awakening.
* The amount of time needed by each client varies from 20 to 90 minutes.
* If the client feels sleepy too early at night, evening light can be added.

Again, note that not every client with SAD responds sufficiently to bright-light treatment, and psychotropics may be needed instead or as a supplement.

References: American Psychiatric Association (2000); Burgess, Fogg, Young, and Eastman (2004); Rosenthal (1998).

Identifying Adult Attention-Deficit/ Hyperactivity Disorder

OVERVIEW

Unfortunately, while the *Diagnostic and Statistical Manual of Mental Disorders* (4th ed., text revision; *DSM-IV-TR*; American Psychiatric Association, 2000) allows for the possibility of adult attention-deficit/hyperactivity disorder (ADHD), it provides little effective guidance toward making the diagnosis (Resnick, 2007). The criteria are worded in such a way that they are developmentally inappropriate for adults for example, "runs and climbs excessively" and "has difficulty playing . . . quietly" (McGough & Barkley, 2004). The Structured Clinical Interview for the *DSM-IV-TR*, an important structured diagnostic interview, has no module for adult ADHD (M. First, personal communication, May 3, 2007).

Nonetheless, research suggests that 50% to 80% of ADHD persists to adulthood (McGough & Barkley, 2004). These adults have continued interpersonal, vocational, and educational impairment. The rate of adult ADHD has been assessed as 4% of the U.S. population (R. C. Kessler, Chiu, Demler, & Walters, 2005). Effective behavioral and pharmacotherapy treatments are available that will help the client cope with symptoms (Ramsay & Rostain, 2005). Therefore, here are some tips gleaned from the literature on identifying adult ADHD.

ADULT BEHAVIORAL CORRELATES WITH ADHD

Adults with ADHD often present for treatment with anxiety and/or depression (Ramsay & Rostain, 2005). Research has found that the problems listed in the following are more common in adults with ADHD (McGough & Barkley, 2004; Ramsay & Rostain, 2005; Weiss & Murray, 2003). When you see these problems in clients, consider evaluating for adult ADHD:

- Relationship problems
- Unsafe driving history, perhaps including a motor vehicle crash
- Substance abuse
- Chronic academic and/or vocational problems and possibly having been fired
- Affective instability and poor emotional regulation
- Feels like a failure and has low self-esteem
- Loses track of details, has difficulty keeping up with the daily demands of life, and has poor time management
- Poor medical health, probably due to poor follow-through with appointments and treatment
- Family history of ADHD

Note that clients with ADHD are distractible only when they are bored and not fully engaged in a task, and they are unlikely to be bored during individual psychotherapy sessions. Thus, in many cases, you will not observe significant distractibility during the session and will need to rely on the client's report of behavior out of the session.

CORE SYMPTOMS

As noted in the *DSM-IV-TR* criteria, some individuals may have all three types of symptoms, while others may be of the mainly inattentive type and others of the impulsive-hyperactive type. I have included some adult behavioral examples for each core symptom (informed by R. J. Resnick, 2007):

- Inattention: Forgets appointments or family activities, is often late for meetings, doesn't get refills of medications in a timely manner, has poor attention to personal health care issues, partner complains that client does not listen, has poor attention to social cues, personal finances are a mess, and has inability to sustain attention on boring tasks
- Impulsivity: Takes first action that comes to mind instead of carefully considering all alternatives, blurts out inappropriate comments during social situations, makes "careless errors" frequently, has temper out-

bursts, shows inappropriate irritability toward others at work, and has low frustration tolerance

• Hyperactivity: Leaves tasks in the middle and may never finish, talks excessively without listening to others, gets frustrated when has to wait, and feels "squirmy" or restless during long meetings, especially when bored

DIAGNOSTIC TIPS

Adults with ADHD must have had ADHD as a child, whether diagnosed or not. A third party, such as a parent, can provide valuable information about the client's behavior as a child (McGough & Barkley, 2004). When evaluating for adult ADHD, consider all settings for behavior, not just work and school settings as specified by the *DSM-IV-TR* criteria but also dysfunction in any setting that the adult may be in, including financial management, child rearing, relationship with significant other, following through on health maintenance behaviors, and so on (McGough & Barkley, 2004). In addition, adults with fewer than six symptoms (the threshold for the diagnosis of ADHD) may still have significant impairment and need treatment (McGough & Barkley, 2004).

WEB RESOURCE

http://www.hcp.med.harvard.edu/ncs/asrs.php
   The National Comorbidity Survey at Harvard University has posted self-report screening questionnaires for adult ADHD that were developed in conjunction with a World Health Organization work group. This symptom checklist (the Adult ADHD Self-Report Scale) is in the public domain. There is a 6-item and an 18-item version, and it is in many different languages. This checklist operationalizes ADHD symptoms in terms of adult behaviors, assisting the clinician in making a diagnosis. I strongly recommend that you use it when you suspect adult ADHD.

Screening for Psychosis

The prevalence of some lifetime history of hallucinations and delusions in the general population is 9.1%, although most of those reports were fleeting visions or briefly hearing the voice of a departed loved one (National Comorbidity Survey; R. C. Kessler, Berglund, Demler, Jin, & Walters, 2005). The prevalence of psychotic disorders (schizophrenia, schizophreniform disorder, schizoaffective disorder, delusional disorder, and psychosis not otherwise specified) was found in a recent U.S. national survey to be 0.5% (National Comorbidity Survey; R. C. Kessler et al., 2005), but that is almost certainly an underestimate since many individuals with psychosis are not in a household setting (e.g., hospitalized, in a long-term institution, or in prison). Research that examined institutions as well as households finds twice the rate of psychotic disorders in the population (Goldner, Hsu, Waraich, & Somers, 2002). *Thus, a reasonable rule of thumb would be to expect about or at least a 1% prevalence of psychotic disorders in the U.S. population.*

Screening for psychosis is not easy because psychotic disorders are extremely heterogeneous. To make a diagnosis of schizophrenia according to the *Diagnostic and Statistical Manual of Mental Disorders* (4th ed., text revision; American Psychiatric Association, 2000), the client must have two of these: hallucinations, delusions, disorganized speech, disorganized or catatonic behavior, and negative symptoms. Hallucinations can occur in any sensory modality, and if you are being thorough, you will ask about each possible sense. Delusions are very heterogeneous as well, although there are six or so common categories of them. Disorganized speech is generally diagnosed by observation, although if you haven't seen it before, it can be difficult to diagnose. In addition, clinically, I have found that some clients with psychotic symptoms have very mild thought disorder symptoms that may interfere with their cognition and/or functioning but that might not be obvious to the clinician. I discuss screening questions only for hallucinations and delusions in this appendix, as the other symptoms require observation and consultation with experienced clinicians to diagnose.

Screening for psychosis is recommended for every client but can be overly intrusive and time intensive when the client is high functioning and has a very low probability of psychosis. Thus, in practice, how does one balance these considerations? As a practical matter, research has shown that auditory hallucinations are by far the most common type of hallucination experienced by inpatients with schizophrenia or bipolar disorder (Baethge et al., 2005), with visual hallucinations coming in a distant second, and that persecutory delusions are the most common delusions. This might suggest that observing the client for thought disorder, coupled with screening for auditory and visual hallucinations and paranoia, might be sufficient in a high-functioning population. In a lower-functioning population, a more thorough screening should be considered. However, note that there is no research to guide us.

Here I list the screening questions for hallucinations in each sensory modality, along with a description of how the client will commonly experience or describe the hallucinatory experience:

- Auditory: "Have you been hearing any voices?" If no, you can also try, "Does it seem that other people are commenting on your behavior? Tell me about that." Clients with psychotic disorders may hear voices commenting on their behavior or thoughts. Often voices comment on clients' behavior in some way. The voices might tell them what to do, although they may not act on it. The voices may talk almost all the time, or they may talk just occasionally. In milder cases, the client might hear what sounds like mumbling but cannot make out the words. Or the client might hear a voice calling her name when no one is present.
- Visual: "Have you been seeing any visions?" Visual hallucinations are almost always visions of humans or humanlike beings. Usually visual hallucinations happen less frequently than auditory ones.
- Tactile: "Have you been having any unusual feelings on your body or skin?" Tactile hallucinations are often described as feelings of electricity or crawling on the skin. Occasionally, a client may have a sensation within the body or under the skin that often accompanies a delusion of parasitic infestation.

- Olfactory: "Have you been experiencing any unpleasant smells that others don't notice?" Olfactory hallucinations are extremely common. Usually, the client cannot articulate what the smell is but does state that it is unpleasant and realizes that others do not smell it.
- Gustatory: "Have you been experiencing any unusual bad tastes lately that others don't notice?" Gustatory or taste hallucinations are generally experienced as a bad taste. Sometimes these are accompanied by a delusion that the client is being poisoned.

In addition, you may notice that the client is looking around the room for something that is not there or seems distracted. In these cases, the client may be experiencing hallucinations during the interview and is responding or attending to them.

Here are some screening questions for paranoid delusions and delusions of reference:

- "Does it seem like people are talking about you?"
- "Are people paying special attention to you?"
- "Do you feel that people are out to get you?"
- "Does it ever seem that the television or radio is talking specifically to you? Tell me about that."

Here are some questions for some other, less common delusions:

- "Do you feel that you have any special abilities? What are those?"
- "Do you feel that you have some special importance? What is that?"
- "Have you ever felt that you could read people's minds or that they could read your mind?"

Clients might also have erotic delusions and somatic delusions, but these seem to be much less frequent. Somatic delusions (delusions of illness) often seem to be accompanied by tactile hallucinations. Delusions of being poisoned often seem to be accompanied by gustatory hallucinations.

Reference: American Psychiatric Association (2000).

Appendix Thirteen

Screening for Anxiety Disorders

PANIC DISORDER

Panic disorder is very common (4.7% lifetime prevalence; National Co-morbidity Survey; R. C. Kessler, Berglund, Demler, Jin, & Walters, 2005), and many clients will often be well aware that they are having panic attacks. In a higher-functioning population, you can often simply ask these questions:

"Have you ever had a panic attack? [If yes:] What sensations were you having physically and emotionally during the attack?"

Or you can ask a more descriptive question:

"Have you ever had a brief period when you felt intensely fearful or distressed? What was that like?"

Keep a copy of the criteria of the *Diagnostic and Statistical Manual of Mental Disorders* (4th ed., text revision; *DSM-IV-TR*; American Psychiatric Association, 2000) handy and follow up with asking about specific symptoms until you have a complete description of the client's experience during the panic attack and you can make a diagnosis if warranted. Check to see if the client has developed agoraphobia as well:

"Have you been feeling fearful of being in certain locations outside your home? What locations make you fearful?"

Typical fears include going outside at all, being in a crowd, being on public transportation, or being in any confined space.

405

0000000

so0n

SOCIAL PHOBIA

Social phobia is very common (12.1% lifetime prevalence; National Co-morbidity Survey; R. C. Kessler et al., 2005). Again, clients are often aware that they have problems in this area, although they may not be aware that it is classified as a mental illness. Here is a screening question for social phobia:

"Are you worried about certain social situations? Tell me more about that."

If the client answers yes, ask for a description of the experience and ask sufficient follow-up questions to make a diagnosis. This question is general enough that other worries will be elicited, so you will need to be careful about making a diagnosis.

SPECIFIC PHOBIA

Specific phobias are among the most common mental illnesses (12.5% lifetime prevalence; National Comorbidity Survey; R. C. Kessler et al., 2005), and most people are aware of any phobias that they may have. In many cases, they do not have a significant negative impact on a person's life, but it can be helpful at times to know if your client does have a phobia. Here is a screening question you can use:

"Are there any particular situations or events that make you very fearful, like heights, spiders, being in an airplane, and so on?"

OBSESSIVE-COMPULSIVE DISORDER

Obsessive-compulsive disorder (OCD) is a less common anxiety disorder (1.6% lifetime prevalence; National Comorbidity Survey; R. C. Kessler et al., 2005). Some clients are aware that they have OCD, while others are not. Thus, it is helpful to ask behaviorally based screening questions. To have a diagnosis of OCD, the client can have either obsessions, compulsions, or both. Here is a screening question for obsessions:

"Have you been bothered by distressing thoughts that you can't get out of your head? What were those thoughts?"

It can sometimes be difficult to tell the difference between rumination and obsessive thoughts—however, the client with obsessive thoughts will experience them as intrusive—whereas clients who ruminate often hold the (irrational) belief that continuing to ruminate is somehow helpful.

Here is a screening question for compulsive behaviors (and mental acts):

"Do you ever feel driven to repeat certain things over and over such as checking the stove, hand washing, counting, or other activities?"

Be aware that some clients with post-traumatic stress disorder will repeatedly check doors and windows to be sure that they are locked. If this is the only compulsive behavior that the client has and if there are no obsessions, the checking could be due to hypervigilance instead of OCD.

GENERALIZED ANXIETY DISORDER

Generalized anxiety disorder (GAD) is very common (5.7% lifetime prevalence; National Comorbidity Survey; R. C. Kessler et al., 2005). Here are some screening questions:

"Have you been feeling anxious or nervous? Do you have a lot of worries? How much is that bothering you? How long has that been going on?"

Duration should be at least 6 months for GAD diagnosis. If the client indicates that anxiety and worry is a significant problem, follow up with asking about more specific GAD symptoms from the *DSM-IV-TR*.

Appendix Fourteen

Screening for Alcohol Use Problems

Alcohol use is by no means universal in the U.S. population. Nearly one-half of the population either does not drink any alcohol at all or drinks fewer than 12 alcoholic drinks per year (Dawson, 2003). Yet nearly 20% of the population has a lifetime prevalence of alcohol abuse or dependence (National Comorbidity Survey; R. C. Kessler, Berglund, Demler, Jin, & Walters, 2005). The Department of Health and Human Services (2005a) recommends a maximum of one drink per day for women and two drinks per day for men.

CAGE

The CAGE was developed by Ewing (1984) to assess alcohol misuse. Since then, it has been widely used as a screening measure for alcohol abuse in a wide variety of settings. The CAGE consists of four questions about alcohol use. CAGE is an acronym that stands for a key word representing each question. The four questions are the following:

- "Have you ever felt that you ought to Cut down on your drinking?"
- "Have people Annoyed you by criticizing your drinking?"
- "Have you ever felt bad or Guilty about your drinking?"
- "Have you ever had a drink first thing in the morning to steady your nerves or to get rid of a hangover (Eye-opener)?"

Some studies have used cutoffs of one yes answer to indicate alcohol problems, while others have used a cutoff of two (Dhalla & Kopec, 2007).

In a clinical setting, you may wish to follow up each yes answer with further questioning ("tell me about that") so you can further evaluate the client's drinking behavior on an individualized basis.

In a review of the reliability and validity of the CAGE, Dhalla and Kopec (2007) indicate that the CAGE generally has adequate psychometric properties. However, they caution that it is not a very sensitive instrument and may miss binge drinking or more subtle signs of alcoholism.

FURTHER QUESTIONS ABOUT ALCOHOL USE

The effectiveness of the CAGE as a screening tool depends on the population (Dhalla & Kopec, 2007). The CAGE is well validated with these populations: medical outpatients, psychiatric inpatients, and medical or surgical inpatients. The CAGE is not sensitive enough to detect problem drinking in these populations: college students, White women, and pregnant women. For this reason, various studies have attempted to augment the CAGE. Here I list some additional follow-up questions you might want to use (derived from studies cited by Dhalla & Kopec, 2007):

- "Have you ever driven under the influence?"
- "Have you ever had a drinking problem?"
- "How many drinks does it take to make you feel high?" (more than two indicates tolerance)
- "How often do you have a drink containing alcohol?"
- "How many drinks containing alcohol do you have on a typical day when you are drinking?"
- "Have you ever gotten into trouble at work because of your drinking?"
- "Have you ever been told you have liver trouble such as cirrhosis?"
- "Have you ever been hospitalized because of your drinking?"

The following question is also recommended as a screening question for heavy drinking:

- "How many times in the past year have you had [five for men, four for women] or more drinks in a day?"

If the client has had at least one heavy drinking day in the past year, the client is considered an at-risk drinker (National Institute on Alcohol Abuse and Alcoholism, 2007).

ALCOHOL USE DISORDERS IDENTIFICATION TEST

Since signs of alcoholism or problem drinking may be too subtle to be detected on the CAGE, an excellent alternative is a longer well-validated measure, the Alcohol Use Disorders Identification Test (AUDIT). The AUDIT is in the public domain and can be found at http://whqlib-doc.who.int/hq/2001/WHO_MSD_MSB_01.6a.pdf, or by conducting an Internet search. There are interview and self-report versions of the AU-DIT readily available on that website along with ample documentation that is helpful in interpreting the results.

BREATHALYZERS

Your training site may have breathalyzers. They are easy to use, and an experienced clinician can show you how to use one and interpret the results in a few minutes. If breathalyzers are used in your setting, discuss with your supervisor how and when to implement this intervention with your clients. Note that you will detect alcohol with a breathalyzer only if the client has been drinking the same day or, in some instances, if the client drank heavily the day before.

Appendix Fifteen

Screening for Drug Use Problems

A federal government study found that in 2005, 8% of the American population 12 years of age and older used an illegal drug in the past month or used a prescription drug to get high (Department of Health and Human Services, 2005b). Slightly more than half of those drug users used only marijuana. The lifetime prevalence of drug abuse or dependence has been found to be slightly over 10% (National Comorbidity Survey; R. C. Kessler, Berglund, Demler, Jin, & Walters, 2005).

Three methods are used to screen for drug use problems. First, the client can be interviewed about the drug use. Second, a questionnaire can be used. Third, the client can be sent for a urine toxicology test to detect the presence of illegal drugs.

INTERVIEW QUESTIONS

You will want to know about any illegal drugs that the client may be using. This tells you important information about the client's lifestyle and the client's ability to cope effectively with problems.

- "Have you ever used any illegal drugs? When was the last time? What did you use?"
- "Have you ever used any prescription drugs that weren't prescribed to you or used prescription drugs to get high?"
- "How do you find it helpful to use [drug]?"
- "How often do you use [drug]? How much do you use?"
- "When was the last time you did without [drug]? How did that go?"

Observe the client's responses for signs of abuse and addiction (American Psychiatric Association, 2000) and ask further questions as needed:

- Do you need to take more [drug] over time to get the same high?
- Do you feel sick or have withdrawal symptoms if you don't have [the drug]?
- Do you sometimes end up taking more of [the drug] than you intended to?
- Have you tried to limit your use of [drug]? How did that go?
- Have you tried to quit using [drug]? How did that go?
- Do you end up using when you could be spending time with [partner, children, family, friends]? Do you use instead of [hobbies, leisure interests]?
- Do you have any medical or emotional problems? How does your drug use affect these problems?

DRUG ABUSE SCREENING TEST

One questionnaire that is commonly used is the Drug Abuse Screening Test (DAST), which comes in versions of various lengths. This test is in the public domain and is widely available on the Internet (conduct a search of its name to find it). Cocco and Carey (1998) found in a study of severely mentally ill psychiatric outpatients the 10-item DAST to have adequate psychometric properties.

URINE TOXICOLOGY SCREENING

The urine toxicology screen is the gold standard for detection of drug use. The client gives a urine sample and may be observed doing so by a nurse or physician if needed. Commonly, cannabinoids (marijuana and hashish), amphetamines, PCP, cocaine, and opiates are screened for, although the panel could be smaller or larger, depending on the facility. Most illegal drug use is detected only for the past 1 to 3 days, depending on the drug (Laboratory Corporation of America, 2007), but prolonged use of marijuana, benzodiazepines, or PCP can result in positive results (results indicating that the client used drugs) after a month or more.

Appendix Sixteen

Screening for Eating Disorders

Estimates of the lifetime prevalence of anorexia (0.3% to 3.7%) and bulimia (1.0% to 4.2%) among women vary significantly between studies (Work Group on Eating Disorders, American Psychiatric Association, 2006). Rates of these eating disorders among men are significantly lower. The SCOFF (Morgan, Reid, & Lacey, 1999) provides five helpful screening questions for eating disorders:

- "Do you make yourself Sick because you feel uncomfortably full?"
- "Do you worry you have lost Control over how much you eat?"
- "Do you believe yourself to be fat when Others say you are too thin?"
- "Have you recently lost more than Fourteen pounds in a 3-month period?"
- "Would you say that Food dominates your life?"

Two or more answers of yes indicate a likely diagnosis of anorexia nervosa or bulimia. Note that, as with all screening questions, further information will be needed to make a diagnosis according to the *Diagnostic and Statistical Manual of Mental Disorders.*

Common Abbreviations in Mental Health Progress Notes

This list concentrates on abbreviations commonly used by mental health practitioners. It is possible that your training site will have a list of approved abbreviations; if so, be sure to get a copy and don't use any abbreviations that are not on the list. In addition, some sites do not allow any abbreviations in charts. Ask your supervisor about the policy at your training site.

For medical abbreviations, conduct an Internet search for "medical abbreviations" to find various lists for interpreting the medical information in the client's chart. Be cautious when interpreting medical abbreviations and ask your supervisor for help as needed. Many medical abbreviations are common, but there is no standardized list, and, as you can see, some abbreviations may mean one thing in one context and another in another context.

MEDICATION DOSING ABBREVIATIONS

b.i.d.: twice daily
h.s.: at nighttime
prn: as needed
q.d.: every day
q.h.s.: at nighttime
q.i.d.: four times daily
t.i.d.: three times daily

417

OTHER COMMON MENTAL HEALTH ABBREVIATIONS

A: assessment—generally a section title for a progress note

AA or A/A: African American

A&O: alert and oriented

ADHD: attention-deficit/hyperactivity disorder

ADL: activities of daily living, such as dressing self, feeding self, grooming self, and so on

AMA: against medical advice, such as "patient was discharged AMA"

bf: boyfriend

BP: bipolar, or, more commonly, blood pressure

BPD: borderline personality disorder

CO or c/o: complains of, meaning verbalizes symptoms, such as "patient c/o frequent auditory hallucinations"

D: data, a substitute for S/O—generally a section title for a progress note

d/c: discharge or discontinue, depending on context

DD: developmental disorder

DOB: date of birth

dx: diagnosis

ETOH: short for ethanol or alcohol

F: commonly female, but also father, depending on context

GAD: generalized anxiety disorder

gf: girlfriend

H: husband

HA: headache

H&P: history and physical, a type of standardized medical screening exam

HI or H/I: homicidal ideation

HO or H/O: history of

hx: history

L: left

M: commonly male, but also mother, depending on context

MD: could be major depression or manic depression, depending on context (because of this, it is best not to use this one yourself)

MDD: major depressive disorder

mj: marijuana

NKA: no known allergies

NKDA: no known drug allergies

O: objective—generally a section title for a progress note

OCD: obsessive compulsive disorder

OD or O/D: overdose

OX3: oriented times three; in other words, client knows own name, where client is, and what the date is.

P: plan—generally a section title for a progress note

PA: generally panic attack, also could be physical abuse, depending on context

PMH: previous medical history

pt: patient

PTSD: post-traumatic stress disorder

R: right

R/O: rule out, such as "R/O PTSD," meaning that the clinician should continue to consider whether the diagnosis of post-traumatic stress disorder applies to this patient

ROI: release of information

RTC: return to clinic (generally followed by a date), specifies the time of the next appointment.

Rx: medication

S: subjective—generally a section title for a progress note

SA: substance abuse or sexual abuse, depending on context (another one you should not use because of ambiguity)

SAD: seasonal affective disorder, otherwise known as major depression, with seasonal pattern

SI or S/I: suicidal ideation

S/O: subjective/objective—generally a section title for a progress note

Sx: symptoms

tx: treatment

UTS: urine toxicology screen, administered to detect illegal drugs (but not alcohol)

VI or V/I: violent ideation

W: wife or White, depending on context

x: times

yo: years old

Appendix Eighteen

Sleep Hygiene and Stimulus Control Interventions for Insomnia

SLEEP HYGIENE INSTRUCTIONS

1. Refrain from caffeine after noon.
2. Avoid exercise within 2 hours of bedtime.
3. Avoid nicotine within 2 hours of bedtime.
4. Avoid alcohol within 2 hours of bedtime.
5. Avoid heavy meals within 2 hours of bedtime.

STIMULUS CONTROL INSTRUCTIONS

1. Go to bed only when sleepy.
2. Do not use your bed or bedroom for anything but sleep or sex; do not read or watch television in bed.
3. If you do not fall asleep within about 20 minutes, leave the bed and do something in another room and return to bed only when you feel a strong urge for sleep.
4. If you do not fall asleep quickly on returning to bed, repeat instruction 3 as many times as necessary.
5. Use your alarm to awaken at the same time every morning regardless of the amount of sleep obtained.
6. Do not nap during the day.

The rationale for the stimulus control instructions is to train the body to associate the bed with sleep rather than insomnia. Thus, when the client feels awake, the client gets out of bed. Naps often interfere with the next night's sleep. Awakening at the same time every morning helps reset the client's sleep to a normal healthy schedule.

Warn the client of the necessity to be rigorous about sticking to these instructions until sleep has normalized and that it may take several weeks for sleep to normalize.

References: Harvey and Tang (2002); Taylor, Lichstein, Weinstock, Sanford, and Temple (2007).

Appendix Nineteen

Discredited Treatments for Mental/Behavioral Disorders

All of the "treatments" listed here have no evidence of effectiveness. In addition, there is evidence that some of these can cause emotional harm. Do not engage in or recommend any of these treatments to clients. These treatments are from the "Certainly Discredited" and "Probably Discredited" categories from the reference given at the end of this appendix.

Age-regression methods for treating adults who may have been sexually abused as children
Angel therapy
Aromatherapy
Bettelheim model for treatment of childhood autism
Chiropractic manipulation for mental/behavioral disorders
Color therapy
Craniosacral therapy (manipulation of the skull bones) for treatment of anxiety and depression
Crystal healing
Dolphin-assisted therapy for treatment of developmental disabilities
Healing touch (not massage therapy)
Holding therapy for reactive attachment disorder
Orgone therapy (use of orgone box or orgone energy accumulator)
Past lives therapy/future lives therapy
Preventive intervention for "born criminals"
Primal scream therapy
Psychological treatments of schizophrenia based on the schizophrenogenic theory of schizophrenia
Rebirthing therapies

Reparenting therapies for treatment of mental/behavioral disorders
Sexual reorientation/reparative therapy for homosexuality
Standard prefrontal lobotomy
Thought Field Therapy
Treatments for mental disorders resulting from Satanic ritual abuse
Treatments for post-traumatic stress disorder caused by alien abduction
Use of pyramids for restoration of energy

Reference: Norcross, Koocher, and Garofalo (2006).

Assessing Suicide Risk Levels: Case Vignettes and Discussion

The following case vignettes and discussions are to assist you in developing your own ability to assess suicidality risk levels in clients.

NOT AT RISK

Karen Price, a 30-year-old White female, presents at the clinic with depression. She has no history of previous depression but is undergoing a stressful divorce and is now a single mother of a 3-year-old boy. She denies any current suicidal ideation. She had passive thoughts of suicide when 15 years old but never engaged in any suicidal behavior or self-harm. She is doing well at work and has a network of friends who have been a great comfort to her.

This is a typical client who is not at risk. She denies any suicidal ideation and has no history of suicidal behavior. No further action is needed other than psychotherapy as usual.

NO RISK AT THIS TIME

Emily Chu, an 18-year-old Asian female, presents to the student counseling center with depression of recent origin. She is separated from her family for the first time and is having some difficulty meeting others. She states that she has never been depressed before, nor has she ever had suicidal ideation, but she is now occasionally wishing that she were dead. She denied any intent to hurt herself and does not have a plan.

She said that suicide would devastate her family and that she is close to them and would never do that to them. She readily agreed to attend psychotherapy and a support group at the counseling center. She looked much brighter at the end of the session, smiling and saying that she felt encouraged because she knows that there is help available to her.

This is an example of a client who has no risk at this time. Like Emily, these clients have only passive suicidal ideation of recent origin and no history of previous suicidal attempts. Low-risk clients adamantly and believably deny any suicidal intent. They have no significant risk factors. These clients have an excellent level of engagement in treatment. They readily verbalize reasons to live, engage well in therapy, and adhere to treatment recommendations.

No special action is needed. Psychotherapy as usual is sufficient, with an emphasis on building social support, good coping skills, and hope. But continue to assess suicidality periodically, and anytime the client looks worse, until the passive suicidal ideation stops and as needed thereafter. Depending on the level of symptoms, you might consider referral for psychotropic medications.

LOW RISK

Fred Watson is a 50-year-old White male with a long-standing diagnosis of schizophrenia. Voices have been telling him to kill himself, but he tells the clinician that he understands that he shouldn't do that and that he has no intention of acting on this. He has a history of taking his medications reliably, but he and his family moved recently, and he missed a few doses. He states that he understands that this is why the voices have returned but that he just wanted to let the therapist know. He has no history of suicide attempts and has only once before had these problems with voices telling him to kill himself; at that time, also, he sought out help appropriately and promptly and did nothing to hurt himself.

Toni Howard is a 35-year-old African American female with a long-standing diagnosis of borderline personality disorder. She has been in treatment for 6 months and is well engaged with her therapist. She has denied any suicidal ideation and self-harm consistently for 2 months. She talks frequently about her desire to be a good mother to 10-year-old daughter. However, she has a history of five psychiatric hospitalizations, two suicide attempts, cutting, and chronic suicidal ideation.

Fred is an example of a low-risk client who has passive suicidal ideation with no previous attempts. Toni is another type of low-risk client. She has a history of multiple suicide attempts with no current ideation. Note that both clients adamantly deny intent. Low-risk clients may have risk factors of concern, perhaps a self-harm history with previous attempts (e.g., Toni) or a White male with a high-risk diagnosis (e.g., Fred). Low-risk clients are well engaged in therapy. They readily verbalize reasons to live and adhere to treatment recommendations.

For the client's safety, discuss a suicide prevention plan and ascertain verbal agreement to comply. However, the only needed action for low-risk clients is continued outpatient psychotherapy that addresses triggers for suicidal ideation until it improves. Reframe the suicidal ideation as a sign that the client is in distress and needs help; this reframe will generally be readily accepted. Again, focus on building social support, good coping skills, and hope. Assess suicidality regularly until suicidal ideation stops and as needed thereafter. Psychotropics may well be needed.

MODERATE RISK

Eugenie Gardner is a 25-year-old White female graduate student with a history of chronic depression and post-traumatic stress disorder (PTSD) from childhood sexual abuse. As a teenager, she often cut herself and occasionally still resorts to this at times of stress. She was hospitalized for as suicide attempt at 23 years old. She has been in treatment at the college counseling center for 4 months. Over that time, her mood has improved, and she has demonstrated improved coping skills and decreased cutting. However, she attended a keg party last weekend with her younger roommates. One of the men at the party offered to walk her home and raped her. She came to the clinic today with suicidal ideation and fresh self-inflicted cut marks on her arms. After discussion with her therapist, she agreed to an appropriate suicide prevention plan and more frequent outpatient psychotherapy sessions. She assured the therapist that she would not hurt herself.

Robert Coleman is a 57-year-old White male whose wife of 20 years died 2 weeks ago from cancer. The cancer came on suddenly a few months ago. He apparently coped adequately throughout the illness. His three children live at least 400 miles away. His wife always arranged their social outings, and he hasn't telephoned any friends on his own in years. He hasn't been going to church since her illness and feels that God has abandoned him. He states that there isn't any hope for him without his wife. He denies any history of depression or suicidality but has been having suicidal ideation since her death 2 weeks ago. He denies any suicidal intent but states that his children would be fine without him. He agrees to attend a partial hospitalization program starting tomorrow, agrees to a suicide prevention plan, and states that he knows his wife would not have wanted him to hurt himself.

Eugenie and Robert are examples of clients with multiple risk factors and passive suicidal ideation. Eugenie's risk factors include her history of cutting, her hospitalization, and her high-risk diagnoses. Robert's risk factors are that he is a widowed, older White male.

Moderate-risk clients believably agree to a suicide prevention plan. These clients can articulate at least one significant reason to live and/or positive plans for the future. They agree to follow the treatment plan recommended by the therapist. The therapist's assessment is that the moderate-risk client has sufficient emotional resources and motivation to comply with the treatment plan.

The moderate-risk client needs frequent and intensive treatment. Consider two individual sessions per week plus group therapy, partial hospitalization, and/or hospitalization. If the client is treated as an outpatient, start psychotropics immediately, mobilize the client's social support system as much as possible, reassess risk every time seen, and aggressively address stressors and symptoms in sessions.

HIGH RISK

Danny Griffin is a 35-year-old White male with bipolar disorder and a long-standing history of alcohol and cocaine abuse. He is uncertain how many psychiatric hospitalizations he has had but thinks it is more than 15 and less than 20. He says that he hasn't liked any of the outpatient therapists he has been assigned in the past, so he just stops going to see them. He comes in to the emergency room stating that he thinks he should kill himself. He feels that nobody would care if he did so. The intake worker thinks he is having a mixed-mood episode: He is agitated, can't sleep, and has been feeling very sad and distressed.

Al Young is a 22-year-old African American male with a history of multiple suicide attempts and recurrent major depression. He has PTSD from childhood physical abuse at the hands of his biological mother, a heroin addict. He was taken from her home at 6 years old and spent the next 8 years in various foster homes before he was placed in a facility for emotionally troubled youth at 14 years old. He has been staying with his 39-year-old biological mother, who maintained sporadic contact with him throughout the years, but says that they argue all the time. He says he doesn't have any friends and doesn't want to. He drinks about six beers every night in order to sleep. He can't find a job. He took half a bottle of pills last night to kill himself and went to sleep but woke up this morning and came to the emergency room. He says he can't commit to a suicide prevention plan since he just wants to die.

Both Danny and Al are high-risk clients. They have active suicidal ideation and multiple serious risk factors. Both are male with no significant social support. Additionally, both clients show signs of being overly impulsive: Danny because he is abusing substances and in a bipolar mixed episode and Al because of substance use and his recent suicide attempt.

Engagement is a problem, as neither client appears to be able to engage interpersonally with the therapist or anyone else at this point. For this reason, it is uncertain whether they could be relied on to attend intensive outpatient treatment, even if agreed to. Al cannot commit to a suicide prevention plan. Danny is unlikely to follow through, given his past history and unstable mood state. Both of these clients should be hospitalized.

As an aside, I suggest that you not label a client as high risk if you are planning on treating the client as an outpatient. If you think the client can be treated as an outpatient, will comply with treatment, and will not kill him- or herself, then classify the client as moderate risk. If you really think the client is high risk, then hospitalize. Think about the worst-case scenario: Would you like to sit in the witness box and be asked by a prosecutor why you did not hospitalize a client whom you documented was high risk?

Appendix Twenty-One

Examples and Signs
of Child Maltreatment

PHYSICAL ABUSE

- Eyewitness observations of a parent's abusive or neglectful behavior (e.g., staff secretary reports that she observed father hitting boy in waiting room)
- The child's description of being abused or neglected
- The parent's own description of abusive or neglectful behavior (e.g., "Then I hit him upside the head.")
- Accounts of child maltreatment from partner or other family members (e.g., partner reports physically abusive behavior toward child)
- Peer or anyone else reports to you that child told him about physical abuse
- "Suspicious" injuries suggesting physical abuse (e.g., extensive and unexplained bruises, burns, lacerations, welts, human bite marks, bald spots, or abrasions)
- Injuries inconsistent with information provided by caregiver
- Newborns with medical evidence of fetal exposure to drugs or alcohol
- Munchausen syndrome by proxy (see Pasqualone & Fitzgerald, 1999)

SEXUAL ABUSE

- Evidence or reports of commercial exploitation through prostitution or the production of pornographic materials

- Child reports indecent exposure, fondling, penetration, oral sex, masturbation, or other sexual activity with an adult
- Peer or anyone else reports to you that child told him about sexual abuse
- Any sexual activity with a peer that was precipitated by force, threats, or coercion (depending on ages and specific state laws, an adult having sex with an adolescent may be statutory rape)
- If you are a medical professional: medical findings suggesting sexual abuse (e.g., pain, itching, bruising, or bleeding in the genitalia; venereal disease; frequent urinary tract or yeast infections; or pregnancy)

NEGLECT

- Newborns denied nutrition, life-sustaining care, or other medically indicated treatment
- Demonstrated parental inability to care for a newborn baby
- Young children left alone (e.g., 7-year-old left in charge of younger siblings all day)
- Parent or caretaker expels child or adolescent from home (e.g., parent is angered with 15-year-old girl returning home 20 minutes after curfew, refuses to let teen into home, and teen walks to friend's house alone and in the dark and stays there overnight)
- Abandoned children (e.g., 8-year-old left with neighbor for 2 days, parents' whereabouts unknown)
- Demonstrated parental disabilities (e.g., mental illness or retardation or alcohol or drug abuse) severe enough to make child abuse or child neglect likely (e.g., parent is out abusing drugs with friends most evenings, leaving 12-year-old alone at home)
- Signs of physical deprivation suggesting child neglect (e.g., child is notably too thin)
- Consistent hunger, sometimes resulting in stealing or begging for food
- Inappropriate dress, poor hygiene, or lice
- Severe dirt and disorder in the home
- Children in physically dangerous situations (e.g., parent is unconcerned that child is often found exploring a construction site in the evening)
- Apparently untreated physical injuries, illnesses, or impairments suggesting medical neglect (e.g., child is not taken to the emergency room promptly after breaking bone in foot)

- "Accidental" injuries suggesting gross inattention to the child's need for safety
- Apparent parental indifference to a child's severe psychological or developmental problems (e.g., parent doesn't bother to enroll previously suicidal child in psychotherapy)
- Chronic and unexplained absences from school suggesting parental responsibility for the nonattendance
- Parent drives while intoxicated with child in car
- Parent keeps child out of school to work or care for siblings

EMOTIONAL ABUSE
(NOT REQUIRED TO BE REPORTED IN ALL STATES)

- Apparent parental condoning of or indifference to a child's misbehavior suggesting improper ethical guidance (e.g., parent seems pleased that child has stolen small items from the local grocery store or parent encourages child to use substances)
- Habitual belittling, humiliating, insulting, hostile, or rejecting statements (e.g., "You're stupid" or "You'll never amount to anything")
- Child is routinely ignored, and parent is unconcerned about child's difficulties, which could include school, medical, or mental health problems, among others
- Child is locked in closets or rooms alone
- Child is threatened with harm or exposed to violence
- Violation of parental visitation rights
- Exposure to domestic violence

Note: No list can be complete or appropriate to every state's specific laws; use your judgment and consult appropriately to make a determination whether to report child maltreatment, given the details of each specific case.

References: Besharov and Laumann (1996); Kalichman (1999); Lambie (2005); Renninger, Veach, and Bagdade (2002); Rodriguez-Strednicki and Twaite (2004a, 2004b).

Examples and Signs of Elder Abuse

PHYSICAL ABUSE

- Caretaker slaps, hits, bites, pinches, pulls hair, burns, or scalds elder
- Caretaker force-feeds elder, sometimes resulting in choking
- Caretaker overmedicates elder as a chemical restraint, giving more of psychotropic medication than was prescribed
- Caretaker withholds pain medications
- Caretaker improperly uses physical restraint: inappropriate restraint type or forceful application, prolonged positioning, or the use of restraints to ensure isolation or unnecessary immobility
- Caretaker's report of injury not consistent with physical findings
- Multiple injuries in various states of healing
- Injuries to the eye, nose, or mouth are suspect
- Bruising to the head or neck is suspect

SEXUAL ABUSE

- Unexplained vaginal or anal bleeding
- Bruises around the breasts or genital area
- Unexplained venereal disease/genital infections

NEGLECT

- Caretaker deprives elder of needed assistance in activities of daily living, such as getting meals and drinks, washing, and toileting

- Evidence of malnutrition, starvation, or dehydration
- Poor hygiene, dirty clothes or bedding, or inadequate clothing

MEDICAL NEGLECT OR ABUSE

- Caretaker does not bring elder for needed medical treatment, delays in seeking treatment, or does not provide needed care for the elder's diseases in the home
- Presence of bedsores
- Needed eyeglasses, hearing aids, or dentures are withheld
- Caretaker undermedicates elder or administers medication improperly
- Medical professional may note multiple unused medications
- Munchausen syndrome by proxy

EMOTIONAL ABUSE

- Yelling, swearing, verbal, or nonverbal insults or humiliation
- Threats to institutionalize or abandon the elder
- Caretaker socially isolates elder

FINANCIAL ABUSE

- Theft or misappropriation of money, property, or valuables
- Abrupt changes in or sudden establishment of wills or changing of deeds
- Elder lacks amenities, (e.g., television) that elder should be able to afford
- Shortage of money or unpaid bills despite adequate income or funds
- Reluctance of caretaker to pay for needed clothes and other necessities
- Signed checks when the older person is unable to write
- Forged signatures on legal documents
- The signing of legal documents (wills, deeds, or trusts) by a cognitively impaired individual
- Caretaker neglects elder in the home yet refuses placement because of financial dependence on elder
- Financial abusers can be individuals outside the family, such as contractors, salespeople, attorneys, caregivers, insurance agents, clergy, accountants, bookkeepers, and friends

References: K. A. Collins (2006); Cooney, Howard, and Lawlor (2006); D. Harris (2006); Jayawardena and Liao (2006); Kemp and Mosqueda (2005); Loue (2001); Neno and Neno (2005); Thompson and Priest (2005).

Appendix Twenty-Three

Challenging Emotions in Therapy: Case Studies

It is impossible to take a cookbook approach to understanding transference and countertransference, as each therapist–client dyad is affected by unique personal histories on the part of both participants. Nonetheless, this appendix will provide a few examples of common transference and countertransference situations in therapy so that you can see how the clinician might interpret and use these feelings in the therapy. For some of these situations, I make a few comments on the therapeutic management of the situation. For other situations, I supply the vignette and some information and leave the management of the therapy for class discussion.

THE FEARFUL, DISTRUSTING CLIENT

Kathleen Gibson sees a new client for an intake session. She is frustrated that the client will not reveal anything about his history. "You have to trust me," she insists. The client then describes a history of repeated sexual trauma from age 5 to age 15. He cries uncontrollably at times and hyperventilates. At the end of the session, Kathleen gives him an appointment for a follow-up appointment, but he never comes back.

Elena Hernandez is a 27-year-old single woman who has come in for psychotherapy. She is being seen by Patrick Kelly, a mental health trainee. Patrick is trying to get a social history and an understanding of any symptoms she might be having. She works for a travel agency but feels that her boss treats her with contempt. She is single and has a

3-year-old daughter. She appears to be estranged from most of her family. She has one friend who lives in the same apartment building as she does, but her attitude is a bit negative toward the friend since the friend is on disability for mental illness. She doesn't go to church and doesn't appear to have any other friends. In response to his questions about symptoms, Elena's responses are vague and evasive. At times, she appears suspicious of his motives. She denies having any experiences of sexual trauma but in a manner that makes Patrick wonder if she is being honest. Patrick hypothesizes that Elena's distrust and avoidance of closeness developed for a good reason—that might have been childhood abuse or other maltreatment. He sees that she is not ready to talk to him about anything that leaves her too vulnerable. He says, "I see that you have been a little vague when I asked you questions. Perhaps you are uncertain whether you are ready to trust me with this information. Is this right? [Elena nods her agreement] I'm sure you have a good reason for that. Can you tell me what your concerns are?" Elena starts to talk tentatively about her fear that Patrick will hurt her if he knows too much about her. At the end of the session, Patrick assures her that he will not press her for information that she is not comfortable telling him. Near the end of the session, he assesses risk issues: "Before we stop today, I would like to ask you just a few questions that have to do with your safety. Can you see if you can try to answer them for me?" Elena is cooperative with a brief assessment of suicidality and homicidality. When Patrick talks with his supervisor later, he talks about his understanding that Elena needs to develop a trusting relationship with him and that this will not happen quickly. He and his supervisor agree that it may be weeks before he knows much more about her history but that establishing a strong therapeutic alliance and keeping Elena in therapy is more important.

Comment: Distrust can be a confusing and distressing reaction from a new client who does not even know you well. Clearly, Elena's distrust of Patrick in the second of the previous vignettes is a transference reaction. Addressing her distrust is an important first stage in therapy. These two vignettes illustrate effective (Patrick) and ineffective (Kathleen) ways to address this distrust. Patrick understands that his client has developed her suspiciousness and distrust for a good reason. She has almost certainly been or felt mistreated by someone important to her. For example, Berenson and Andersen (2006) found that female undergraduates with a history of physical or emotional abuse had a predisposition to transference feelings of mistrust, expecting rejection, emotional indifference, and desire to avoid closeness. These feelings must be an early focus of therapy.

THE NEEDY CLIENT AND THE
PARENTAL/PROTECTIVE-FEELING THERAPIST

Jamie Gutierrez is mental health trainee working in a large medical center. He is assigned a new client to monitor while she is in the partial hospitalization program, a 35-year-old woman who has post-traumatic stress disorder (PTSD), borderline personality traits, and recurrent major depression. The client talks to him about her problems, including her concerns about her therapist, who she has seen weekly for 2 months. The client describes her therapist as harsh, cold, and demanding. She says that she has difficulty attending her therapy sessions. Jamie sympathizes with her and suggests that the client work with him in long-term psychotherapy instead. He tells her to call the therapist and cancel her future appointments. Later, talking to his supervisor, he discovers that the previous therapist is the medical center's foremost expert in treating borderline personality disorder. The supervisor advises him that, additionally, this therapist is known to be warm and helpful to clients and staff. With the supervisor's help, Jamie realizes that he has taken the client's transference as reality and that he has some personal countertransference issues around rescuing people who are helpless. He realizes that soon the client will see him as harsh, cold, and demanding as well and describe him in this way to other staff.

Jeff Chung is a mental health trainee at a medical center. He has a client with PTSD who tells him that she can't trust him. He wants to help her, so he goes above and beyond with his efforts to place her in appropriate housing, get benefits, and so on. In fact, the client doesn't lift a finger; Jeff does all the work for her. He hopes that this will show her that he is on her side and can be trusted.

Comment: Being overly gratifying in response to the client's transference issues is a common therapeutic mistake according to research by Gelso, Hill, Mohr, Rochlen, and Zack (1999). Here, Jamie has risked alienating other mental health staff by going out of his way to protect a client, not understanding that her reaction to the original therapist could be based in transference. Just because the client feels needy and helpless, this does not mean that Jamie must be protective in return. This vignette also illustrates a common clinical phenomenon in mental health agencies called *splitting*. Here, the client has (unconsciously) split her therapists into two opposing camps since they have not been in good communication about her care, and thus one of them mistook the client's transference for reality.

The second vignette is another example of being overly gratifying to the client; Jeff is taking far too many steps to help her rather than addressing her transference reaction of distrust and neediness as a therapeutic issue. Getting overinvolved with the client is a one form of problematic countertransference behavior (Hayes & Gelso, 2001). Here are some other examples of being overinvolved:

- Trying to rescue a client while ignoring the client's need to develop own coping skills
- Pushing confrontation of an abuse perpetrator or urging legal action against an abuse perpetrator without regard to the client's wishes or to the likely ineffectiveness of these actions to satisfy the client's emotional needs
- Insisting on the client becoming total estranged from an abusive family

THE BORING CLIENT AND THE DISENGAGED THERAPIST

Miriam Weinstein has a client who keeps talking about the same marital problems over and over. He is boring her with this repetition. She is frustrated that he is not following through on getting marital counseling, which is obviously needed. Miriam says to the client, "I'm realizing that we've talked about this issue on a number of occasions before. Somehow it must be helping you to go over this again, or perhaps you may want to get something out of our discussion that you haven't gotten yet. What do you think? Can you give me some feedback about this?" The client's response indicates that he has been ruminating incessantly about these issues between sessions, trying to figure out a way to address them, but not coming up with any new insights. Miriam then asks, "I'm noticing that you continue to be upset about these marital problems but that something is holding you back from calling to make an appointment for marital therapy. Do you have any idea what that is?"

Comment: Being bored by a client is something that happens occasionally to every therapist. However, therapists often feel guilty about being bored and blame themselves for not attending more closely. Or they get frustrated with the client and insist on behavior change that the client does not pursue. Actually, if you are bored by a client, this is important information about the treatment that you need to consider carefully. There are many reasons why a client might be boring you and many possible interventions for addressing this.

Perhaps your countertransference response of boredom is telling you something about the client. When you think this may be the case, Yalom (2002) suggests the following intervention:

> For the last several minutes, I notice that I've been feeling disconnected from you, somewhat distanced. I'm not sure why, but I know I'm feeling different now than at the beginning of the session, when you were describing your feelings . . . or last session, when you spoke from the heart.

Note that the word "boring" appears nowhere in this intervention. Yalom doesn't hypothesize why the client is boring him, but he offers his reaction to the client as a genuine observation of her behavior and encourages further exploration. Brown (2001) tells about a course of psychotherapy in which she was bored by a client who she actually liked very much. She hypothesized that the client had some way of interacting with others that deflected attention from herself. When Brown shared these observations with the client, the client was able to be in touch with her ambivalence about closeness. One final consideration is that you may be bored because the client is talking about ruminations and, in essence, is ruminating verbally. In that case, you may need to discuss and target the symptom of rumination therapeutically.

Alternatively, your countertransference response of boredom could be telling you something about yourself. Pope, Sonne, and Greene (2006) suggest that boredom might be "a clue that the therapist is on some level fighting against awareness of taboo topics or acutely uncomfortable feelings or impulses" (p. 82). Perhaps in the vignette, Miriam may be avoiding talking about the client's problems with sexual functioning, his history of sexual abuse and how that affects his marriage, or other possible uncomfortable topics. Similarly, Hayes and Gelso (2001) suggest that being bored in a therapy session might mean that you are distancing yourself from the client because some of your unresolved personal issues are being stimulated by what the client is talking about. This might be the case if Miriam, herself, were having marital problems but did not want to think about them.

THE BORDERLINE CLIENT AND THE
IRRITATED/FRUSTRATED THERAPIST

Belinda Brown is a 42-year-old psychotherapy client recently assigned to Cliff Yakamura, a mental health trainee. Cliff sees her in a community mental health clinic. Belinda has been treated by various students for a year each, and in his review of Belinda's chart, Cliff sees that each student made a diagnosis of borderline personality disorder. Cliff calls her to schedule her first appointment. Belinda makes sarcastic comments to him over the phone and calls him "another little newbie" and "fresh meat." During her first session, she talks about how fantastic her previous student therapist is and how she is sure that Cliff will never be able to live up to that standard. She insists that he print out his progress notes for her to review on a weekly basis, grumbling vaguely that "errors have been made in the past." Cliff responds, "I'm sorry, but I don't have the time to print out your progress notes for your review on a weekly basis, and, frankly, I don't think it would be the most effective use of your therapy hour. I understand that you have a right to see the notes, but we will need to work out something else. Before we discuss that, could you tell me how you feel that it would help you to see these notes?" Belinda changes the subject, then insists that Cliff give her his personal cell phone number because "all of my other student therapists did." Cliff states, "I'm sorry, but I have a strict policy not to give out my cell phone number to clients. This is because there is a 24-hour hotline available to you in an emergency and also because you can leave a message for me on my voice mail at the clinic anytime. But I am curious, how do you feel it would have helped you to have my cell phone number?" Belinda tells him that he's too rigid, and then she spends the rest of the session complaining about how her family has been treating her lately. It is time to schedule the next appointment. Even though she is on disability and has few scheduled activities, Belinda wants an appointment in the last hour of the day since she says that is most convenient for her. Cliff does not want to see her then, as he would prefer to spend that time to do his progress notes and consult with his supervisor about any emergent issues. He firmly states, "I'm sorry, but I'm not available to see you at the last hour that the clinic is open. Here are the times when I could see you: 2:00 P.M. Monday or 3:00 P.M. Thursday. Which would you prefer?"

Comment: We can imagine that Cliff must feel angry and frustrated with Belinda. Coping with the angry/entitled client is challenging because of the intense emotions provoked. In a study using vignettes of three different clients, Brody and Farber (1996) found that psychotherapists indicated that they would feel especially angry and irritable when working with a borderline client and that this client would be especially difficult to like and to feel nurturing and compassionate toward.

Two common reactions are to behave angrily in return or to try to mollify the client and accede to demands, hoping that the client will calm down, feel nurtured, and like you. Neither of these approaches is effective. Behaving in an angry manner will result in a therapeutic impasse. Mollifying the client will just lead to increased demands and further violation of therapeutic boundaries. Do your best to react to the client in an appropriate professional manner instead.

However, there will be moments when your irritation with the client is obvious. Gabbard (2001a) suggests the following intervention in this situation:

> I feel like we've entered familiar territory here. You seem to resent my efforts and make accusations against me. I get irritated and defensive and make things worse. Then we reach a stalemate where I feel frustrated and impotent and you feel you're not getting any help. How do you understand this pattern, and what do you think we can do about it? (p. 987).

He is making a transference interpretation and simultaneously encouraging the client to think about more adaptive ways of relating. Note that even a highly experienced therapist such as Gabbard can find himself reenacting relationship patterns with clients; he shows in this quote how to address that therapeutically.

Like Cliff, you must patiently and firmly set appropriate limits and provide the client with an opportunity to discuss emotional reactions to this limit setting. Do not make extra allowances for the client, such as offering an appointment time that does not work for you; the client will not appreciate your extra effort and instead will demand even more. The client's dependency needs cannot and should not be fulfilled by you, the therapist. If you accede to too many demands, you will feel increasingly resentful and abused, decreasing your ability to be therapeutic (Kernberg Selzer, Koenigsberg, Carr, & Appelbaum, 1989).

THE PSYCHOTIC CLIENT AND THE
HELPLESS/INADEQUATE-FEELING THERAPIST

Yuri Petrovich is in treatment for schizophrenia. He was recently discharged from the hospital and is assigned to Andrea Mason, a mental health trainee. Yuri says that he wants to get a job and that he is lonely and wants a girlfriend. Andrea worries that he is too mentally ill to maintain a job and wonders about how he would find and maintain a healthy relationship with a girlfriend. Yuri tells Andrea that he hears his neighbors talking about him through the wall. He says that the neighbors are commenting on his movements and criticizing him with foul language. He is thinking about telling them off. Andrea feels anxiety that Yuri might get into trouble by acting on these symptoms and suggests that he shouldn't. Yuri accuses Andrea of not believing him. Clearly, Yuri doesn't have any insight that he is having hallucinations. Andrea makes the following intervention: "Yuri, I understand that you are hearing the voices of the neighbors, and it sounds like that is very distressing for you. I'd like to tell you my perspective on this, and I hope you'll hear me out. We might have a disagreement on this, but if we do, I hope that we can agree to disagree. I don't doubt at all that you are actually hearing voices. However, I think that what you are experiencing is what's called a hallucination. A hallucination is a sensory experience that your brain generates within itself. So, if you're hearing a voice, your brain is generating a voice in the same exact area that it processes voices that you hear through your ears. So these voices, even though they are generated in the brain, seem just as real as actual voices you hear. Do you have any questions about this? Now I understand that this is a lot to take in, and you might not be sure that I am right. That's okay. Can we agree to keep discussing this issue as we go along? I'd like to suggest that we both try to keep an open mind about this. If you find that the voices decrease when you take your medicine, I'd like you to consider that they might be hallucinations, okay?"

Comment: Horowitz (2002) eloquently described the emotional devastation of schizophrenia:

> Trying to comprehend the magnitude of loss that they endure is beyond imagination. Life prospects change forever. Social circles contract; vocational choices narrow if not vanish; once celebrated accomplishments fade into the past. The onset of illness deals not only a harsh blow to self-esteem but to the very core of identity. The grief that attends a wound to the self differs markedly from grief that accompanies the loss of a loved one. With the former, the object of loss—the self—is ever present, an eternal reminder of what once was. Remnants of the past linger like a haunting legacy that awakens remembrances of an unlived life. Even though pain may ebb for extended periods, there is always the risk that the wound to the self is reopened again whenever the limitations imposed by the illness hamper the realization of some long-cherished goal and the disappointment of unmet expectations surges anew. (pp. 236–237)

Clearly, no empathetic psychotherapist can remain untouched by this. In a study using vignettes of three different clients, Brody and Farber (1996) found that psychotherapists indicated that they would feel especially anxious and hopeless when working with a schizophrenic client and that this client would be especially challenging.

Early in treatment, clients with psychotic disorders may still be having prominent *positive symptoms*—hallucinations, delusions, and thought disorder. The clients often have enough insight to realize that the therapist doesn't believe in the hallucinations and delusions but not enough insight to realize that these are symptoms. The client's friends and relatives may have been telling him that these things aren't really happening, but he knows what his experience is. The severity of the client's illness can make both him (Nordentoft et al., 2002) and you feel hopeless, and depression is indeed an important comorbid concern with schizophrenic clients (Dixon et al., 2001).

It is normal to feel uncomfortable and hopeless about psychotic symptoms at first. Most clinicians do. However, these clients can be very fulfilling to the knowledgeable therapist; they can make great improvements, and their potential has historically been grossly underestimated and undertreated. If your clients have psychotic disorders, attempt to educate yourself and the rest of the staff about effective interventions for improving their functioning and quality of life, including medication management, psychoeducation, living skills training (for information on all three of these, see Falloon, Held, Roncome, Coverdale, & Laidlaw, 1998), cognitive therapy (Butler, Chapman, Forman, & Beck, 2006), social skills training (Bellack, Mueser, Gingerich, & Agresta, 1997), family group psychoeducation (Hogarty et al., 1986), cognitive training (Twamley, Jeste, & Bellack, 2003), and vocational rehabilitation (Twamley, Jeste, & Lehman, 2003). This knowledge will increase your comfort level and hopefulness with this population.

Clients with psychotic disorders often are paranoid and suspicious. These feelings are related to their paranoid delusions, but you may have countertransference responses to them nonetheless. One response would be to placate the individual in order to build rapport, such as by agreeing that the neighbors are indeed talking to him. However, you don't really believe this, so it would be a therapeutic error that might lead to inappropriate client behavior. Another response would be to be evasive; however, this will just reinforce the client's paranoia. Remember that ample research supports the value of psychoeducation in schizophrenia (Hogarty et al., 1986). It is helpful to take a nonconfrontative psychoeducational approach, as Andrea does.

SEXUAL FEELINGS AND BEHAVIOR IN THE CLIENT

Harry Gray is a 32-year-old psychotherapy client assigned to Melissa Paul, a mental health trainee. He often comments on Melissa's outfits, initially telling her that she looks "lovely," but in the most recent session, he said that she looks "hot." Melissa has the uncomfortable feeling that he is looking at her breasts at times during the therapy session. He has remarked that he wishes he had met her socially instead and states that he feels that they could have been "very close special friends," emphasizing his point with a wink.

Kim Fisher, a mental health trainee, is talking with a new client in her office. The client is low functioning and has severe mental illness. As the session progresses, she notices that the client is wearing loose shorts, that his penis is poking out of one of the legs of the shorts, and that he is rubbing his penis through the cloth. Kim tells the client that she sees him touching himself and that the session will have to end for today. The client protests that he wasn't doing anything, but she insists that the session is over anyway. She then finds her supervisor and talks the situation over. They explore whether Kim should keep the client or whether the client should be transferred to a male therapist.

Comment: A survey of psychologists found that almost three-fourths had been told by a client that the client was sexually attracted to the therapist, and nearly 90% felt that a client had flirted with them (Pope & Tabachnick, 1993). In addition, the survey found that nearly one-fifth of the psychologists had experienced a client touching his or her genitals during a session, as in the second of the previous vignettes.

In response to a client's sexual feelings or behavior toward you, you might feel anxiety, embarrassment, or anger (Hillman & Stricker, 2001), or you might have other feelings, including sexual ones, in return. One suggestion for managing a client's sexual transference is this: "[The student] therapist reinforced that although it was her responsibility to ensure that their sessions would always remain safe and professional, talking about and discussing these feelings could be important in helping him understand how he relates to [others]. . . . She added that feelings and behavior are two very different things" (Hillman & Stricker, 2001, p. 275). They note, additionally, that as the transference was explored verbally, the strength of the sexualized feelings lessened.

SEXUAL FEELINGS IN THE THERAPIST

Deepa Nair, a mental health trainee, has ambivalent feelings about her client, Ellen Hansen. Ellen is a lesbian and has been talking about her relationship problems with her partner, Patrice. Occasionally, she will talk about their sex life, which Deepa finds unexpectedly titillating. Deepa has always thought of herself as heterosexual, which increases her feelings of sexual confusion about the client.

[The intern therapist, Martin] noticed that he was sexually attracted to his client in about the second session, when he experienced an emotional and physical response to her presence. The client was not only physically attractive to Martin but also impressed him as articulate, sophisticated, and generally richer in interpersonal attributes than other clients. Martin had never been sexually attracted to a client before and was very distressed by the situation; he experienced a range of negative feelings. For example, he felt embarrassed that he was sexually attracted to someone who had numerous complex problems. He felt guilty that he was devoting more attention to this client than to others, and he felt "tortured" inside because he enjoyed being attracted to her and did not try to change his feelings. In fact, as the sessions progressed, Martin found himself looking forward to seeing the client each week. Thus, the sexual attraction created an emotional dilemma that he struggled to manage. (Ladany et al., 1997, p. 420)

Comment: A therapist often feels ashamed of being sexually attracted to a client even when the therapist is not at risk of having sex with the client. Research has shown that most therapists have occasional sexual attractions to clients (Bernson, Tabachnick, & Pope, 1994; Pope, Sonne, & Greene, 2006). However, there is profound ambivalence and shame about this as well; most therapists also believed that simply feeling sexually attracted by a client is unethical (Pope, Tabachnick, & Keith-Spiegel, 1987), probably because, as we all know, sex with a client is always inappropriate. In a qualitative study with psychology interns, Ladany et al. (1997) found that sexual feelings on the part of the therapist led to being more invested in and attentive to the client but also (understandably) to feeling distracted. The student therapists also struggled with boundaries with these clients, some by distancing themselves, while others struggled with being overly giving and protective.

It may help to consider the types of countertransference we already talked about. Here are some possibilities (the first two are adapted from Pope & Tabachnick, 1993). Perhaps the client is projecting a particularly sexy image, wearing short skirts, high heels, low-cut blouses, and so on. Or perhaps he or she is being flirtatious. In this case, your reaction reflects a common reaction among others who encounter the client. Perhaps the client just happens to be your "type," and your sexual interest is the normal response you would have had if you met the client under other circumstances. Perhaps the client was abused as a child and thinks that her sexuality is the only thing that others value about her. Perhaps the client gets sexual and other close feelings confused. Coping with these feelings is a delicate and complex issue. Experts agree that telling the client about these sexual feelings is rarely therapeutic (Gutheil & Gabbard, 1998; Jorstad, 2002). When this comes up for you, consider discussing the feelings with peers, supervisors, or your own therapist. And if you have any concerns that you might act on them, you are ethically obligated to seek assistance, such as consultation and psychotherapy.

THE LIKED CLIENT AND THE CHALLENGED THERAPIST

[I am challenged by] those clients about whom I think, "I wish I had met you outside of therapy." These are people who could be my friends, I think, if only I had not been their therapist. In one such instance, with a woman I'll call Joyce, I responded to those emotions by becoming extremely distant and formal with her as a somewhat conscious strategy to insure that nothing resembling a friendly interaction would happen in the course of the therapy. I became the boundaries queen, keeping every single rule of therapist disengagement that I could think of. I usually self-disclose; I shut that down. I normally respond straightforwardly to client questions about my inner state; I became the master of deflected "and what do you think I'm feeling?" Of course, since I was quite right that Joyce would have made a lovely friend for me if I'd met her under different circumstances, she was intuitive and emotionally attuned, and knew that there was something very wrong. She expressed her genuine affection and concern for me, which I responded to by becoming even more formal and distant. This, in turn, wounded her in some very core places, where she had been punished and rejected for her ability to see just how few clothes the emperors in her family were wearing. The process went on for nearly a year, during which therapy became less and less productive for her. The boundaries were impeccable, but that's about all. She finally became angry enough with me to let me know clearly what she was experiencing. And I was finally able to see how my attempts to avoid my grief and feelings of loss about never being able to have this woman as my friend, as well as my fears of losing control and pursuing a friendship if I allowed myself to experience the warmth and care I had for her, were translating into distance, indifference, and lack of engagement. Having been able to get more honest with myself about what was going on, I began the slow and difficult process of mending the relationship, which included my acknowledging that she was special to me in this way even though I knew that a friendship would never occur. (Brown, 2001, p. 1011)

I realized that two things sparked my extreme countertransference with Elly. First, I liked her too much—for her personal beauty and competence, and for her taking so readily to my theory and practice of REBT. You could say I liked her for herself and for appreciating me and my therapeutic theory. Second, I was afraid to uncomfortably confront Elly about her LFT [low frustration tolerance—in this case with boyfriends] problems. I was afraid, I realized, that I would have a difficult time convincing her and thought that I might lose her as a client. I would never put myself down if this happened, but I might consider it too uncomfortable and too interruptive of the pleasure I had while seeing Elly. So, my LFT produced countertransference reactions in me that interfered with my helping Elly. Bad! It didn't make me a rotten therapist but did make me ineffective with Elly. I apologized to her for my mistake and went back to cultivating my garden. I learned my lesson and rarely made the same countertransference mistake again. (A. Ellis, 2001, p. 1003)

Comment: Two expert psychotherapists shared the previous vignettes. Both of these discuss some of the inherent pitfalls of working with the liked client. Brown talks about keeping too much distance for fear that if she didn't, she would have gotten too close. Ellis discusses placating the client to maintain the comfort and ease of the therapy.

THE ANXIOUS/DEPRESSED CLIENT
AND THE CONCERNED THERAPIST

Akbar Khan is a 19-year-old Pakistani American psychotherapy client recently assigned to Aiyana Reed, a mental health trainee. Aiyana sees Akbar in a student health clinic at a large state university. Akbar is an engineering major, and he has a few close friends from high school. He has not made any new friends at college and spends much of his time in his dorm room studying or playing video games. As she gets to know him, Aiyana notes that Akbar tends to answer her in monosyllables whenever possible. He demonstrates little spontaneity in what he reports to her and seems anxious and on edge. He readily admits that he is fearful of meeting others and believes that they will judge him negatively. Some fellow students have made insensitive comments and jokes to him as well about his ethnic background, reinforcing his fears.

Comment: In a study using vignettes of three different clients, Brody and Farber (1996) found that psychotherapists indicated that they would feel more depressed working with a depressed client but that this client would be especially likely to be gratifying to work with and to help. The depressed client was seen as most likable, and the therapists easily felt nurturing and compassionate toward the depressed client. However, the client in this vignette is anxious about interacting with others and may have a social phobia in addition to being depressed. He also struggles with experiences of racial discrimination that have contributed to his social avoidance and fears.

THE DISLIKED CLIENTS AND THE OVERWHELMED THERAPISTS

Guillermo Moreno is a mental health trainee working in an intake clinic. A client comes in for an intake and during the course of the interview reveals that he was incarcerated for sexually abusing his stepdaughter. The client was recently released into the community. Understandably, Guillermo finds this behavior repulsive and is disgusted with the client. He finds this behavior so creepy that he just wants the client to leave as soon as possible rather than finishing assessing him thoroughly and making an appropriate treatment plan.

Elizabeth Little is a mental health trainee working with Trisha Yates, a client who has PTSD and abuses alcohol periodically. Trisha leads a disorganized and chaotic life. She has physically abused her children in the past and is being monitored by the state. She has been hospitalized many times for suicidal behavior. Elizabeth notices that she has a feeling of dread every day she is scheduled to see Trisha. She finds the negative way that Trisha talks about her children to be abhorrent. She finds herself having fantasies that Trisha will drop out of treatment so that Elizabeth will no longer have any responsibility toward her. She finds that she tends to eat junk food for lunch when Trisha is coming in the afternoon.

Comment: Both of the clients in these vignettes are very difficult to like. Yet, clearly, both need help and are asking for help by coming to therapy. Sooner or later, we will all be confronted with disliked clients. Coping with them is a difficult task in managing countertransference.

THE NARCISSISTIC CLIENT AND THE DISTANCING THERAPIST

Anna Saunders is a mental health trainee who is doing supportive psychotherapy as an adjunctive treatment for pain patients. She is assigned a new patient who is a successful business executive. He had an injury and is now left with chronic pain. The patient spends much of the session bragging about his financial success, his forthcoming management book (although he has been looking unsuccessfully for a publisher for over a year), and his anticipated substantial speaking engagement fees. Anna finds him irritating despite working with her supervisor to consider some hypotheses about his underlying issues. After discussing the issue with her supervisor, Anna realizes that she tends to ignore the client when he is bragging instead of considering how to fruitfully address his maladaptive interpersonal behavior so that he can be more interpersonally effective one-on-one. After discussing the issue with her own psychotherapist, Anna realizes that the patient reminds her of her father, who also had some narcissistic traits. She realizes that she harbors resentment against both of them.

Comment: In the case of Anna in this vignette, it is likely that she is having more than one type of countertransference. Most therapists would probably find the client's behavior irritating and off-putting. However, even supervision is not helping Anna cope with this, so it is likely that she is having a personal reaction as well. This type of strong idiosyncratic reaction to a client will happen to every therapist sooner or later. This is one of the reasons why personal therapy is always wise for psychotherapists; it helps you in the process of understanding your emotional reactions to clients. To effectively treat this client, Anna will need awareness of her personal issues about her father and will need to be making progress in addressing these issues in her own personal therapy.

THE TERMINATING CLIENT AND THE ABANDONED THERAPIST

Vince Robertson is a mental health trainee working in a college counseling center. He has been working with a client, Evan Lucas, for almost a year. However, termination of therapy is coming up soon since Vince is moving on to another training site. In addition, Evan has made significant progress in therapy, so he does not plan to continue with another therapist. Vince finds himself feeling profoundly sad at the loss of the therapy relationship with Evan. He dreads the termination session and is starting to feel abandoned even though he is the one who is leaving. He finds himself tempted to encourage Evan to maintain contact with him, although he knows that this would be a boundary violation. Vince talks to his own therapist about the issue. Together, they discuss Vince's personal issues of loss.

Comment: Researchers on countertransference have pinpointed termination as one issue that is likely to trigger countertransference reactions (Hayes et al., 1998). This book is about starting therapy rather than ending it. However, I recommend reading Kaner and Prelinger (2005) for a helpful discussion of the process of termination.

References

Ackerly, G. D., Burnell, J., Holder, D. C., & Kurdek, L. A. (1988). Burnout among licensed psychologists. *Professional Psychology: Research and Practice, 19,* 624–631.

Agar, K., Read, J., & Bush, J. (2002). Identification of abuse histories in community mental health centre: The need for policies and training. *Journal of Mental Health, 11,* 533–543.

Alvarez, K. M., Donohue, B., Kenny, M. C., Cavanagh, N., & Romero, V. (2004). The process and consequences of reporting child maltreatment: A brief overview for professionals in the mental health field. *Aggression and Violent Behavior, 10,* 311–331.

Alvarez, K. M., Kenny, M. C., Donohue, B., & Carpin, K. M. (2004). Why are professionals failing to initiate mandated reports of child maltreatment, and are there any empirically based training programs to assist professionals in the reporting process? *Aggression and Violent Behavior, 9,* 563–578.

American Counseling Association. (2005). *ACA code of ethics.* Retrieved January 11, 2007, from http://www.counseling.org/Resources/CodeOfEthics/TP/Home/CT2.aspx.

American Lung Association. (2006). *What are asthma and allergy triggers?* Retrieved December 28, 2006, from http://www.lungusa.org/site/apps/s/content.asp?c=dvLUK9O0E&b=34706&ct=67442.

American Psychiatric Association. (2000). *Diagnostic and statistical manual of mental disorders* (4th ed., text revision). Washington, DC: Author.

American Psychiatric Association. (2006). *Principles of medical ethics: With annotations especially applicable to psychiatry.* Retrieved January 11, 2007, from http://www.psych.org/psych_pract/ethics/ppaethics.pdf.

American Psychological Association. (2002). *Ethical principles of psychologists and code of conduct 2002.* Retrieved January 4, 2007, from http://www.apa.org/ethics/code2002.pdf.

American Psychological Association Practice Organization. (2007, Winter). Putting HIPAA into Practice. In *Good practice: Topical edition.* Washington, DC: Author.

American Psychological Association Presidential Task Force on Evidence-Based Practice. (2006). Evidence-based practice in psychology. *American Psychologist, 61,* 271–285.

Andersen, S. M., & Berk, M. S. (1998). Transference in everyday experience: Implications of experimental research for relevant clinical phenomena. *Review of General Psychology, 2,* 81–120.

Andersen, S. M., & Chen, S. (2002). The relational self: An interpersonal social-cognitive theory. *Psychological Review, 109,* 619–645.

Anderson, A. (1999). "Don't scream, Miss Annie, don't scream." *American Family Physician, 59,* 213–215.

Anderson, K. L. (2002). Perpetrator or victim? Relationships between intimate partner violence and well-being. *Journal of Marriage and Family, 64,* 851–863.

Anderson, T. R., Bell, C. C., Powell, T. E., Williamson, J. L., & Blount, M. A. (2004). Assessing psychiatric patients for violence. *Community Mental Health Journal, 40,* 379–399.

Angst, J., & Cassano, G. (2005). The mood spectrum: Improving the diagnosis of bipolar disorder. *Bipolar Disorders, 7,* 4–12.

Appleby, L., Shaw, J., Amos, T., McDonnell, R., Harris, C., McCann, K., et al. (1999). Suicide within 12 months of contact with mental health services: National clinical survey. *British Medical Journal, 318,* 1235–1239.

Arthur, G. L., Brende, J. O., & Quiroz, S. E. (2003). Violence: Incidence and frequency of physical and psychological assaults affecting mental health providers in Georgia. *Journal of General Psychology, 130,* 22–45.

Ashton, V. (2004). The effect of personal characteristics on reporting child maltreatment. *Child Abuse and Neglect, 28,* 985–997.

Astin, M. C. (1997). Traumatic therapy: How helping rape victims affects me as a therapist. *Women and Therapy, 20,* 101–109.

Aubry, T. D., Hunsley, J., Josephson, G., & Vito, D. (2000). Quid pro quo: Fee for services delivered in a psychology training clinic. *Journal of Clinical Psychology, 56,* 23–31.

Azikiwe, N., Wright, J., Cheng, T., & D'Angelo, L. J. (2005). Management of rape victims (regarding STD treatment and pregnancy prevention): Do academic emergency departments practice what they preach? *Journal of Adolescent Health, 36,* 446–448.

Bachelor, A. (1995). Clients' perception of the therapeutic alliance: A qualitative analysis. *Journal of Counseling Psychology, 42,* 323–337.

Baerger, D. R. (2001). Risk management with the suicidal patient: Lessons from case law. *Professional Psychology: Research and Practice, 32,* 359–366.

Baethge C., Baldessarini R. J., Freudenthal K., Streeruwitz A., Bauer M., & Bschor T. (2005). Hallucinations in bipolar disorder: Characteristics and comparison to unipolar depression and schizophrenia. *Bipolar Disorders, 7,* 136–145.

Baker, F. M., & Bell, C. C. (1999). Issues in the psychiatric treatment of African Americans. *Psychiatric Services, 50,* 362–368.

Balsam, K. F., & Mohr, J. J. (2007). Adaptation to sexual orientation stigma: A comparison of bisexual and lesbian/gay adults. *Journal of Counseling Psychology, 54,* 306–319.

Barber, J. P., Connolly, M. B., Crits-Christoph, P., Gladis, L., & Siqueland, L. (2000). Alliance predicts patients' outcome beyond in-treatment change in symptoms. *Journal of Consulting and Clinical Psychology, 68,* 1027–1032.

Barlow, K., Grenyer, B., & Ilkiw-Lavalle, O. (2000). Prevalence and precipitants of aggression in psychiatric inpatient units. *Australian and New Zealand Journal of Psychiatry, 34,* 967–974.

Baron, J. (1996). Some issues in psychotherapy with gay and lesbian clients. *Psychotherapy, 33,* 611–616.

Beach, K., & Power, M. (1996). Transference: An empirical investigation across a range of cognitive-behavioural and psychoanalytic therapies. *Clinical Psychology and Psychotherapy, 3,* 1–14.

Beahrs, J. O., & Gutheil, T. G. (2001). Informed consent in psychotherapy. *American Journal of Psychiatry, 158,* 4–10.

Beck, A. T., Brown, G., & Steer, R. A. (1989). Prediction of eventual suicide in psychiatric inpatients by clinical ratings of hopelessness. *Journal of Consulting and Clinical Psychology, 57,* 309–310.

Beck, J. S. (1995). *Cognitive therapy: Basics and beyond.* New York: Guilford Press.

Beck, J. S. (2005). *Cognitive therapy for challenging problems: What to do when the basics don't work.* New York: Guilford Press.

Beeman, D. G., & Scott, N. A. (1991). Therapists' attitudes toward psychotherapy informed consent with adolescents. *Professional Psychology: Research and Practice, 22,* 230–234.

Bellack, A. S., Mueser, K. T., Gingerich, S., & Agresta, J. (1997). *Social skills training for schizophrenia: A step-by-step guide.* New York: Guilford Press.

Bender, S., & Messner, E. (2003). *Becoming a therapist: What do I say, and why?* New York: Guilford Press.

Berenson, K. R., & Andersen, S. M. (2006). Childhood physical and emotional abuse by a parent: Transference effects in adult interpersonal relations. *Personality and Social Psychology Bulletin, 32,* 1509–1522.

Berg, A. Z., Bell, C. C., & Tupin, J. (2000). Clinician safety: Assessing and managing the violent patient. *New Directions for Mental Health Services, 86,* 9–28.

Berger, S. S., & Buchholz, E. S. (1993). On becoming a supervisee: Preparation for learning in a supervisory relationship. *Psychotherapy, 30,* 86–92.

Bergeron, L. R., & Gray, B. (2003). Ethical dilemmas of reporting suspected elder abuse. *Social Work, 48,* 96–105.

Bernsen, A., Tabachnick, B. G., & Pope, K. S. (1994). National survey of social workers' sexual attraction to their clients: Results, implications, and comparison to psychologists. *Ethics and Behavior, 4,* 369–388.

Bernstein, D. A., Borkovec, T. D., & Hazlett-Stevens, H. (2000). *New directions in progressive relaxation training: A guidebook for helping professionals.* Westport, CT: Praeger Paperback.

Besharov, D. J., & Laumann, L. A. (1996). Child abuse reporting. *Society, 33,* 40–46.

Betan, E., Heim, A. K., Conklin, C. Z., & Westen, D. (2005). Countertransference phenomena and personality pathology in clinical practice: An empirical investigation. *American Journal of Psychiatry, 162,* 890–898.

Beyerstein, B. L. (1997). Why bogus therapies often seem to work. *Skeptical Inquirer, 21*, 29–34. Retrieved August 12, 2007, from http://www.csicop.org/si/9709/beyer.html.

Bienen, M. (1990). The pregnant therapist: Countertransference dilemmas and willingness to explore transference material. *Psychotherapy, 27*, 607–612.

Bonati, M., & Clavenna, A. (2005). The epidemiology of psychotropic drug use in children and adolescents. *International Review of Psychiatry, 17*, 181–188.

Borum, R., & Reddy, M. (2001). Assessing violence risk in *Tarasoff* situations: A fact-based model of inquiry. *Behavioral Sciences and the Law, 18*, 375–385.

Bowden, C. (2001). Strategies to reduce misdiagnosis of bipolar depression. *Psychiatric Services, 52*, 51–55.

Bowden, C. (2005). A different depression: Clinical distinctions between bipolar and unipolar depression. *Journal of Affective Disorders, 84*, 117–125.

Braaten, E. B., Otto, S., & Handelsman, M. M. (1993). What do people want to know about psychotherapy? *Psychotherapy, 30*, 565–570.

Bradley, R., Heim, A. K., & Westen, D. (2005). Transference patterns in the psychotherapy of personality disorders: Empirical investigation. *British Journal of Psychiatry, 186*, 342–349.

Brase, G. L., & Richmond, J. (2004). The white-coat effect: Physician attire and perceived authority, friendliness and attractiveness. *Journal of Applied Social Psychology, 34*, 2469–2481.

Brendel, R. W., & Bryan, E. (2004). HIPAA for psychiatrists. *Law and Psychiatry, 12*, 177–183.

Brent, D. A., Oquendo, M., Birmaher, B., Greenhill, L., Kolko, D., Stanley, B., et al. (2002). Familial pathways to early-onset suicide attempt: Risk for suicidal behavior in offspring of mood-disordered suicide attempters. *Archives of General Psychiatry, 59*, 801–807.

Briere, J., & Gil, E. (1998). Self-mutilation in clinical and general samples: Prevalence, correlates and functions. *American Journal of Orthopsychiatry, 68*, 609–620.

Brody, E. M., & Farber, B. A. (1996). The effects of therapist experience and patient diagnosis on countertransference. *Psychotherapy, 3*, 372–380.

Brooks, J., Holttum, S., & Lavender, A. (2002). Personality style, psychological adaptation and expectations of trainee clinical psychologists. *Clinical Psychology and Psychotherapy, 9*, 253–270.

Brown, L. S. (2001). Feelings in context: Countertransference and the real world in feminist therapy. *Journal of Clinical Psychology/In session: Psychotherapy in Practice, 57*, 1005–1012.

Burckell, L. A., & Goldfried, M. R. (2006). Therapist qualities preferred by sexual-minority individuals. *Psychotherapy: Theory, Research, Practice, Training, 43*, 32–49.

Burgess, H. J., Fogg, L. F., Young, M. A., & Eastman, C. I. (2004). Bright light therapy for winter depression—Is phase advancing beneficial? *Chronobiology International, 21*, 759–775.

Burkard, A. W., Johnson, A. J., Madson, M. B., Pruitt, N. T., Contreras-Tadych, D. A., Kozlowski, J. M., et al. (2006). Supervisor cultural responsiveness and unresponsiveness in cross-cultural supervision. *Journal of Counseling Psychology, 53*, 288–301.

Burkard, A. W., Knox, S., Groen, M., Perez, M., & Hess, S. A. (2006). European American therapist self-disclosure in cross-cultural counseling. *Journal of Counseling Psychology, 53,* 15–25.

Burkard, A. W., Ponterotto, P. G., Reynolds, A. L., & Alfonso, V. C. (1999). White counselor trainees' racial identity and working alliance perceptions. *Journal of Counseling and Development, 77,* 324–329.

Burns, J., Dudley, M., Hazell, P., & Patton, G. (2005). Clinical management of deliberate self-harm in young people: The need for evidence-based approaches to reduce repetition. *Australian and New Zealand Journal of Psychiatry, 39,* 121–128.

Butler, A. C., Chapman, J. E., Forman, E. M., & Beck, A. T. (2006). The empirical status of cognitive-behavioral therapy: A review of meta-analyses. *Clinical Psychology Review, 26,* 17–31.

Cameron, S., & turtle-song, i. (2002). Learning to write case notes using the SOAP format. *Journal of Counseling and Development, 80,* 286–292.

Campbell, C. D., & Gordon, M. C. (2003). Acknowledging the inevitable: Understanding multiple relationships in rural practice. *Professional Psychology: Research and Practice, 34,* 430–434.

Campbell, R., Wasco, S. M., Ahrens, C. E., Sefl, T., & Barnes, H. E. (2001). Preventing the "second rape": Rape survivors' experiences with community service providers. *Journal of Interpersonal Violence, 16,* 1239–1259.

Carey, B. (2006, September 19). A psychiatrist is slain, and a sad debate deepens. *New York Times.* Retrieved June 22, 2006, from http://www.nytimes.com/2006/09/19/health/psychology/19slay.html?ex=1182657600&en=a823d23616a71c9a&ei=5070.

Centers for Disease Control and Prevention. (2007). *U.S. Public Health Service Syphilis Study at Tuskegee.* Retrieved May 18, 2007, from http://www.cdc.gov/nchstp/od/tuskegee/time.htm.

Challiner, V., & Griffiths, L. (2000). Electroconvulsive therapy: A review of the literature. *Journal of Psychiatric and Mental Health Nursing, 7,* 191–198.

Chemtob, C. M., Bauer, G. B., Hamada, R. S., Pelowski, S. R., & Muraoka, M. Y. (1989). Patient suicide: Occupational hazard for psychologists and psychiatrists. *Professional Psychology: Research and Practice, 20,* 294–300.

Choca, J. P., & Van Denburg, E. J. (1996). *Manual for clinical psychology trainees* (3rd ed.). New York: Brunner/Mazel.

Christensen, A., & Rudnick, S. (1999). A glimpse of Zen practice within the realm of countertransference. *American Journal of Psychoanalysis, 59,* 59–69.

Christopher, J. C., Christopher, S. E., Dunnagan, T., & Schure, M. (2006). Teaching self-care through mindfulness practices: The application of yoga, meditation and qigong to counselor training. *Journal of Humanistic Psychology, 46,* 494–509.

Clementson, L. (2007, February 4). The racial politics of speaking well. *New York Times.* Retrieved April 12, 2007, from http://www.nytimes.com/2007/02/04/weekinreview/04clemetson.html?ex=1328245200&en=b0c0215875608f7a&ei=5088&partner=rssnyt&emc=rss.

Cocco, K. M., & Carey, K. B. (1998). Psychometric properties of the Drug Abuse Screening Test in psychiatric outpatients. *Psychological Assessment, 10,* 408–414.

Collins, K. A. (2006). Elder maltreatment: A review. *Archives of Pathology and Laboratory Medicine, 130,* 1290–1296.

Collins, S., & Long, A. (2003). Working with the psychological effects of trauma: Consequences for mental health-care workers — A literature review. *Journal of Psychiatric and Mental Health Nursing, 10,* 417–424.

Comas-Diaz, L., & Jacobsen, F. M. (1991). Ethnocultural transference and countertransference in the therapeutic dyad. *American Journal of Orthopsychiatry, 61,* 392–402.

Compas, B. E., Haaga, D. A. F., Keefe, F. J., Leitenberg, H., & Williams, D. A. (1998). Sampling of empirically supported psychological treatments from health psychology: Smoking, chronic pain, cancer and bulimia nervosa. *Journal of Consulting and Clinical Psychology, 66,* 89–112.

Constantine, M. G. (2007). Racial microaggressions against African American clients in cross-racial counseling relationships. *Journal of Counseling Psychology, 54,* 1–16.

Constantine, M. G., & Sue, D. W. (2007). Perceptions of racial microaggressions among black supervisees in cross-racial dyads. *Journal of Counseling Psychology, 54,* 142–153.

Cooney, C., Howard, R., & Lawlor, B. (2006). Abuse of vulnerable people with dementia by their carers: Can we identify those most at risk? *International Journal of Geriatric Psychiatry, 21,* 564–571.

Cooper, P. C. (1999). Buddhist meditation and countertransference: A case study. *American Journal of Psychoanalysis, 59,* 71–85.

Courtois, C. (1993, Spring). Vicarious traumatization of the therapist. *NCP Clinical Newsletter,* 8–9.

Courtois, C. (1997). Healing the incest wound: A treatment update with attention to recovered-memory issues. *American Journal of Psychotherapy, 51,* 464–496.

Coyle, S. L. (2002). Physician-industry relations. Part 1: Individual physicians. *Annals of Internal Medicine, 136,* 396–402.

Craig, R. J. (Ed.). (2005). *Clinical and diagnostic interviewing.* New York: Jason Aronson.

Cramer, J. A., & Rosenheck, R. (1998). Compliance with medication regimens for mental and physical disorders. *Psychiatric Services, 49,* 196–201.

Crits-Christoph, P., Gibbons, M. B. C., & Hearon, B. (2006). Does the alliance cause good outcome? Recommendations for future research on the alliance. *Psychotherapy: Theory, Research, Practice, Training, 43,* 280–285.

Csikszentmihalyi, M. (1999). If we are so rich, why aren't we happy? *American Psychologist, 10,* 821–827.

Cuellar, A. K., Johnson, S. L., & Winters, R. (2005). Distinctions between bipolar and unipolar depression. *Clinical Psychology Review, 25,* 307–339.

Cuijpers, P., van Straten, A., & Warmerdam, L. (2007). Behavioral activation treatments of depression: A meta-analysis. *Clinical Psychology Review, 27,* 318–326.

Cybulska, B., & Forster, G. (2005). Sexual assault: Examination of the victim. *Medicine, 33,* 23–28.

Dalenberg, C. (2000). *Countertransference and the treatment of trauma.* Washington, DC: American Psychological Association.

Davidson, R. J., Kabat-Zinn, J., Schumacher, J., Rosenkranz, M., Muller, D., San-torelli, S. F., et al. (2003). Alterations in brain and immune function produced by mindfulness meditation. *Psychosomatic Medicine, 65,* 564–570.

Davies, T. (2001). Informed consent in psychiatric research. *British Journal of Psychiatry, 178,* 397–398.

Dawson, D. A. (2003). Methodological issues in measuring alcohol use. *Alcohol Research and Health, 27,* 18–29.

Dearing, R. L., Maddux, J. E., & Tangney, J. P. (2005). Predictors of psychological help seeking in clinical and counseling psychology graduate students. *Professional Psychology: Research and Practice, 36,* 323–329.

Deffenbacher, J. L., Oetting, E. R., & DiGiuseppe, R. A. (2002). Principles of empirically supported interventions applied to anger management. *The Counseling Psychologist, 30,* 262–280.

DePaulo, B. M., Lindsay, J. J., Malone, B. E., Muhlenbruck, L., Charlton, K., & Cooper, H. (2003). Cues to deception. *Psychological Bulletin, 129,* 74–118.

Devine, P. G. (1989). Stereotypes and prejudice: Their automatic and controlled components. *Journal of Personality and Social Psychology, 56,* 5–18.

De Wilde, L. (1996). *Monk.* New York: Marlowe.

Dhalla, S., & Kopec, J. (2007). The CAGE questionnaire for alcohol misuse: A review of reliability and validity studies. *Clinical and Investigative Medicine, 30,* 33–41.

Diamond, T., & Muller, R. T. (2004). The relationship between witnessing parental conflict during childhood and later psychological adjustment among university students: Disentangling confounding risk factors. *Canadian Journal of Behavioural Science, 36,* 295–309.

Diaz, E., Woods, S. W., & Rosenheck, R. A. (2005). Effects of ethnicity on psychotropic medications adherence. *Community Mental Health Journal, 41,* 521–537.

Diener, E., & Seligman, M. E. P. (2005). Beyond money: Toward an economy of well-being. *Psychological Science in the Public Interest, 5,* 1–31.

DiLorenzo, T. M., Bargman, E. P., Stucky-Ropp, R., Brassington, G. S., Frensch, P. A., & LaFontaine, T. (1999). Long-term effects of aerobic exercise on psychological outcomes. *Preventive Medicine, 28,* 75–86.

Dixon, L., Green-Paden, L., Delahanty, J., Lucksted, A., Postrado, L., & Hall, J. (2001). Variables associated with disparities in treatment of patients with schizophrenia and comorbid mood and anxiety disorders. *Psychiatric Services, 52,* 1216–1222.

Donoghue, J., & Hylan, T. R. (2001). Antidepressant use in clinical practice: Efficacy v. effectiveness. *British Journal of Psychiatry, 879,* s9–s17.

Dutton, M. A., Green, B. L., Kaltman, S. I., Roesch, D. M., Zeffiro, T. A., & Krause, E. D. (2006). Intimate partner violence, PTSD, and adverse health outcomes. *Journal of Interpersonal Violence, 21,* 955–968.

Easterlin, R. A. (2003). Explaining happiness. *Proceedings of the National Academy of Sciences of the United States of America, 100,* 11176–11183.

Ehrensaft, M. K., Cohen, P., Brown, J., Smailes, E., Chen, H., & Johnson, J. G. (2003). Intergenerational transmission of partner violence: A 20-year prospective study. *Journal of Consulting and Clinical Psychology, 71,* 741–753.

Ekman, P., & O'Sullivan, M. (1991). Who can catch a liar? *American Psychologist, 46,* 913–920.

Elbogen, E. B., Tomkins, A. J., Pothuloori, A. P., & Scalora, M. J. (2003). Documentation of violence risk information in psychiatric hospital patient charts: An empirical examination. *Journal of the American Academy of Psychiatry and the Law, 31,* 58–64.

Ellis, A. (2001). Rational and irrational aspects of countertransference. *Journal of Clinical Psychology, 57,* 999–1004.

Ellis, M. V. (2001). Harmful supervision, a cause for alarm: Comment on Gray et al. (2001) and Nelson and Friedlander (2001). *Journal of Counseling Psychology, 48,* 401–406.

Epley, N., & Kruger, J. (2005). When what you type isn't what they read: The perseverance of stereotypes and expectancies over e-mail. *Journal of Experimental Social Psychology, 41,* 414–422.

Epstein, M. (1998). *Going to pieces without falling apart: A Buddhist perspective on wholeness.* New York: Broadway Books.

Evans, J. (2000). Interventions to reduce repetition of deliberate self-harm. *International Review of Psychiatry, 12,* 44–47.

Evans, R. W. (2006). *Precipitating factors.* Retrieved December 28, 2006, from http://www.migraines.org/treatment/pdfs/migraine-1.pdf.

Ewing, J. A. (1984). Detecting alcoholism: The CAGE questionnaire. *Journal of the American Medical Association, 252,* 1905–1907.

Eyler, L. T., & Jeste, D. V. (2006). Enhancing the informed consent process: A conceptual overview. *Behavioral Sciences and the Law, 24,* 553–568.

Falloon, I. R. H., Held, T., Roncone, R., Coverdale, J. H., & Laidlaw, T. M. (1998). Optimal treatment strategies to enhance recovery from schizophrenia. *Australian and New Zealand Journal of Psychiatry, 32,* 43–49.

Fauth, J. (2006). Toward more (and better) countertransference research. *Psychotherapy: Theory, Research, Practice, Training, 43,* 16–31.

Feldhaus, K. M., Koziol-McLain, J., Amsbury, H. L., Norton, I. M., Lowensteine, S. R., & Abbot, J. T. (1997). Accuracy of 3 brief screening questions for detecting partner violence in the emergency room. *Journal of the American Medical Association, 277,* 1357–1361.

Feldman-Summers, S., & Pope, K. S. (1994). The experience of "forgetting childhood abuse": A national survey of psychologists. *Journal of Consulting and Clinical Psychology, 62,* 636–639.

Felton, J. S. (1998). Burnout as a clinical entity—Its importance in health care workers. *Occupational Medicine, 48,* 237–250.

Finder, A. (2006, June 11). For some, online personal undermines a resume. *New York Times.* Available at http://www.nytimes.com.

Finlayson, L. M., & Koocher, G. P. (1991). Professional judgment and child abuse reporting in sexual abuse cases. *Professional Psychology: Research and Practice, 22,* 464–472.

First, M. B., Spitzer, R. L., Gibbon, M., & Williams, J. B. W. (2002). *Structured Clinical Interview for DSM-IV-TR Axis I Disorders, Research Version, Patient Edition (SCID-I/P).* New York: Biometrics Research, New York State Psychiatric Institute.

Flannery, R. B. (2005). Precipitants to psychiatric patient assaults on staff: Review of empirical findings, 1990–2003, and risk management implications. *Psychiatric Quarterly, 76*, 317–326.

Flannery, R. B., Schuler, A. P., Farley, E. M., & Walker, A. P. (2002). Characteristics of assaultive psychiatric patients: Ten year analysis of the assaulted staff action program (ASAP). *Psychiatric Quarterly, 73*, 59–69.

Fox, K. R. (1999). The influence of physical activity on mental well-being. *Public Health Nutrition, 2*, 411–418.

Franklin, C. L., Sheeran, T., & Zimmerman, M. (2002). Screening for trauma histories, posttraumatic stress disorder (PTSD), and subthreshold PTSD in psychiatric outpatients. *Psychological Assessment, 14*, 467–471.

Freeman, A., Pretzer, J., Fleming, B., & Simon, K. M. (1990). *Clinical applications of cognitive therapy.* New York: Plenum Press.

Friedman, R. A. (2006). Violence and mental illness—How strong is the link? *New England Journal of Medicine, 355*, 2064–2066.

Gabbard, G. O. (1994). Psychotherapists who transgress sexual boundaries with patients. *Bulletin of the Menninger Clinic, 58*, 124–135.

Gabbard, G. O. (1996). Lessons to be learned from the study of sexual boundary violations. *American Journal of Psychotherapy, 50*, 311–322.

Gabbard, G. O. (2000a). Disguise or consent: Problems and recommendations concerning the publication and presentation of clinical material. *International Journal of Psychoanalysis, 81*, 1071–1086.

Gabbard, G. O. (2000b). A neurobiologically informed perspective on psychotherapy. *British Journal of Psychiatry, 177*, 117–122.

Gabbard, G. O. (2001a). A contemporary psychoanalytic model of countertransference. *Journal of Clinical Psychology/In Session, 57*, 983–991.

Gabbard, G. O. (2001b). Editorial: Preserving confidentiality in the writing of case reports. *International Journal of Psychoanalysis, 82*, 1067–1068.

Gabbard, G. O. (2004a). *Long-term psychodynamic psychotherapy: A basic text.* Arlington, VA: American Psychiatric Publishing.

Gabbard, G. O. (2004b). The illusion of safety. *American Journal of Psychiatry, 161*, 427–428.

Gabbard, G. O., Lazar, S. G., Hornberger, J., & Spiegel, D. (1997). The economic impact of psychotherapy: A review. *American Journal of Psychiatry, 154*, 147–155.

Gabbard, G. O., & Westen, D. (2003). Rethinking therapeutic action. *International Journal of Psychoanalysis, 84*, 823–841.

Gans, J. S., & Counselman, E. F. (1996). The missed session: A neglected aspect of psychodynamic psychotherapy. *Psychotherapy, 33*, 43–50.

Garb, H. N. (1997). Race bias, social class bias, and gender bias in clinical judgment. *Clinical Psychology: Science and Practice, 4*, 99–120.

Garman, A. N., Corrigan, P. W., & Morris, S. (2002). Staff burnout and patient satisfaction: Evidence of relationships at the care unit level. *Journal of Occupational Health Psychology, 7*, 235–241.

Gellerman, D. M., & Suddath, R. (2005). Violent fantasy, dangerousness, and the duty to warn and protect. *Journal of the American Academy of Psychiatry and the Law, 33*, 484–495.

Gelles, R. J. (2006). Child maltreatment and foster care. *Gender Issues, 23,* 36–47.

Gelso, C. J., Fassinger, R. E., Gomez, M. J., & Latts, M. G. (1995). Countertransference reactions to lesbian clients: The role of homophobia, counselor gender, and countertransference management. *Journal of Counseling Psychology, 42,* 356–364.

Gelso, C. J., & Hayes, J. A. (2001). Countertransference management. *Psychotherapy, 38,* 418–422.

Gelso, C. J., Hill, C. E., Mohr, J. J., Rochlen, A. B., & Zack, J. (1999). Describing the face of transference: Psychodynamic therapists' recollections about transference in cases of successful long-term therapy. *Journal of Counseling Psychology, 46,* 257–267.

Gelso, C. J., Latts, M. G., Gomez, M. J., & Fassinger, R. E. (2002). Countertransference management and therapy outcome: An initial evaluation. *Journal of Clinical Psychology, 58,* 861–867.

Gilbert, D. (2006). *Stumbling on happiness.* New York: Knopf.

Glass, L. I. (2003). The gray areas of boundary crossings and violations. *American Journal of Psychotherapy, 57,* 429–444.

Glick, P., Larsen, S., Johnson, C., & Branstiter, H. (2005). Evaluations of sexy women in low- and high-status jobs. *Psychology of Women Quarterly, 29,* 389–395.

Glinkauf-Hughes, C., & Mehlman, E. (1995). Narcissistic issues in therapists: Diagnostic and treatment considerations. *Psychotherapy, 32,* 213–221.

Goldner, E. M., Hsu, L., Waraich, P., & Somers, J. M. (2002). Prevalence and incidence studies of schizophrenic disorders: A systematic review of the literature. *Canadian Journal of Psychiatry, 47,* 833–843.

Goldstein, W. N. (2000). The transference in psychotherapy: The old vs. the new, analytic vs. dynamic. *American Journal of Psychotherapy, 54,* 167–171.

Gonzalez, F. (1995). Working with Mexican-American clients. *Psychotherapy, 32,* 696–706.

Gonzalez-Figueroa, E., & Young, A. M. (2005). Ethnic identity and mentoring among Latinas in professional roles. *Cultural Diversity and Ethnic Minority Psychology, 11,* 213–226.

Gossop, M., Harris, J., Best, D., Man, L., Manning, V., Marshall, J., et al. (2003). Is attendance at Alcoholics Anonymous meetings after inpatient treatment related to improved outcomes? A 6-month follow-up study. *Alcohol and Alcoholism, 38,* 421–426.

Gratz, K. L. (2003). Risk factors for and functions of deliberate self-harm: An empirical and conceptual review. *Clinical Psychology: Science and Practice, 10,* 192–205.

Gray, A. (1994). *An introduction to the therapeutic frame.* London: Routledge.

Gray, L. A., Ladany, N., Walker, J. A., & Ancis, J. R. (2001). Psychotherapy trainees' experience of counterproductive events in supervision. *Journal of Counseling Psychology, 48,* 371–383.

Gutheil, T. G. (1980). Paranoia and progress notes: A guide to forensically informed psychiatric record-keeping. *Hospital and Community Psychiatry, 31,* 479–482.

Gutheil, T. G. (2001). Moral justification for *Tarasoff*-type warnings and breach of confidentiality: A clinician's perspective. *Behavioral Sciences and the Law, 19,* 345–353.

Gutheil, T. G. (2005). Boundary issues and personality disorders. *Journal of Psychiatric Practice, 11*, 88–96.

Gutheil, T. G., & Gabbard, G. O. (1993). The concept of boundaries in clinical practice: Theoretical and risk-management dimensions. *American Journal of Psychiatry, 150*, 188–196.

Gutheil, T. G., & Gabbard, G. O. (1998). Misuses and misunderstandings of boundary theory in clinical and regulatory settings. *American Journal of Psychiatry, 155*, 409–414.

Gutheil, T. G., & Hilliard, J. T. (2001). "Don't write me down": Legal, clinical and risk-management aspects of patients' requests that therapists not keep notes or records. *American Journal of Psychotherapy, 55*, 157–165.

Gutheil, T. G., & Simon, R. I. (2005). E-mails, extra-therapeutic contact, and early boundary problems: The internet as a "slippery slope." *Psychiatric Annals, 35*, 952–960.

Hage, S. M. (2006). A closer look at the role of spirituality in psychology training programs. *Professional Psychology: Research and Practice, 37*, 303–310.

Hahn, W. K. (1998). Gifts in psychotherapy: An intersubjective approach to patient gifts. *Psychotherapy, 1*, 78–86.

Haidt, J. (2005). *The happiness hypothesis: Finding modern truth in ancient wisdom.* New York: Basic Books.

Hamer, F. M. (2006). Racism as a transference state: Episodes of racial hostility in the psychoanalytic context. *Psychoanalytic Quarterly, 75*, 197–214.

Hamilton-Giachritsis, C. E., & Browne, K. D. (2005). A retrospective study of risk to siblings in abusing families. *Journal of Family Psychology, 19*, 619–624.

Handelsman, M. M., & Galvin, M. D. (1988). Facilitating informed consent for outpatient psychotherapy: A suggested written format. *Professional Psychology: Research and Practice, 19*, 223–225.

Harris, D. (2006). Elder abuse. *Update, 73*.

Harris, E. C., & Barraclough, B. (1997). Suicide as an outcome for mental disorders. A meta-analysis. *British Journal of Psychiatry, 170*, 205–228.

Harris, M. (2005, August). *What your supervisees want you to know about racial diversity.* Paper presented at the annual meeting of the American Psychological Association, Washington, DC.

Harstall, C., & Ospina, M. (2003). How prevalent is chronic pain? *Pain: Clinical Updates, 11*, 1–4.

Harvey, A. G., & Tang, N. K. Y. (2003). Cognitive behavior therapy for primary insomnia: Can we rest yet? *Sleep Medicine Reviews, 7*, 237–262.

Hayes, J. A. (2004). The inner world of the psychotherapist: A program of research on countertransference. *Psychotherapy Research, 14*, 21–36.

Hayes, J. A., & Gelso, C. J. (2001). Clinical implications of research on countertransference: Science informing practice. *Journal of Clinical Psychology/In Session: Psychotherapy in Practice, 57*, 1041–1051.

Hayes, J. A., McCracken, J. E., McClanahan, M. K., Hill, C. E., Harp, J. S., & Carozzoni, J. S. (1998). Therapist perspectives on countertransference: Qualitative data in search of a theory. *Journal of Counseling Psychology, 45*, 468–482.

Herbert, P. B. (2002). The duty to warn: A reconsideration and critique. *Journal of the American Academy of Psychiatry and the Law, 30,* 417–424.

Herbert, P. B., & Young, K. A. (2002). *Tarasoff* at twenty-five. *Journal of the American Academy of Psychiatry and the Law, 30,* 275–281.

Hesse, A. (2002). Secondary trauma: How working with trauma survivors affects therapists. *Clinical Social Work Journal, 30,* 293–309.

Hettema, J. M., Neale, M. C., & Kendler, K. S. (2001). A review and meta-analysis of the genetic epidemiology of anxiety disorders. *American Journal of Psychiatry, 158,* 1568–1578.

Hiday, V. A. (2003). Outpatient commitment: The state of empirical research on its outcomes. *Psychology, Public Policy and Law, 9,* 8–32.

Hill, M. (1999). For love and money. *Women and Therapy, 22,* 1–3.

Hillman, J., & Stricker, G. (2001). The management of sexualized transference and countertransference with older adult patients: Implications for practice. *Professional Psychology: Research and Practice, 32,* 272–277.

Hirschfeld, R. M. A., Williams, J. B. W., Spitzer, R. L., Calabrese, J. R., Flynn, L., Keck, P. E., et al. (2000). Validity of the mood disorder questionnaire: A general population study. *American Journal of Psychiatry, 157,* 1873–1875.

Hobson, R. P., & Kapur, R. (2005). Working in the transference: Clinical and research perspectives. *Psychology and Psychotherapy: Theory, Research and Practice, 78,* 275–293.

Hogarty, G. E., Anderson, C. M., Reiss, D. J., Kornblith, S. J., Greenwald, D. P., Javna C. D., et al. (1986). Family psychoeducation, social skills training, and maintenance chemotherapy in the aftercare treatment of schizophrenia. I. One-year effects of a controlled study on relapse and expressed emotion. *Archives of General Psychiatry, 43,* 633–642.

Hoglend, P. (2004). Analysis of transference in psychodynamic psychotherapy: A review of empirical research. *Canadian Journal of Psychoanalysis, 12,* 280–300.

Hoglend, P., Johansson, P., Marble, A., Bogwald, K., & Amlo, S. (2007). Moderators of the effects of transference interpretations in brief dynamic psychotherapy. *Psychotherapy Research, 17,* 162–174.

Hopko, D. R., Lejuez, C. W., Ruggiero, K. J., & Eifert, G. H. (2003). Contemporary behavioral activation treatments for depression: Procedures, principles, and progress. *Clinical Psychology Review, 23,* 699–717.

Horn, P. J. (1994). Therapists' psychological adaptation to client suicide. *Psychotherapy, 31,* 190–195.

Horowitz, J. (2007, February 4). Biden unbound: Lays into Clinton, Obama, Edwards. *New York Observer.* Retrieved May 29, 2008, from http://www.observer.com/node/36658.

Horowitz, R. (2002). Psychotherapy and schizophrenia: The mirror of countertransference. *Clinical Social Work Journal, 30,* 235–244.

Horvitz-Lennon, M., Normand, S. T., Gaccione, P., & Frank, R. G. (2001). Partial versus full hospitalization for adults in psychiatric distress: A systematic review of the published literature (1957–1997). *American Journal of Psychiatry, 158,* 676–685.

Hudenko, W. (n.d.). *The relationship between PTSD and suicide.* National Center for PTSD. Retrieved January 27, 2008, from http://ncptsd.kattare.com/ncmain/ncdocs/fact_shts/fs_ptsd_and_suicideprof.html?opm=1&rr=rr1367&srt=d&echorr=true.

Hunt, G. E., Bergen, J., & Bashir, M. (2002). Medication compliance and comorbid substance abuse in schizophrenia: Impact on community survival 4 years after a relapse. *Schizophrenia Research, 54,* 253–264.

Hunt, H. A. (2005). *Essentials of private practice: Streamlining costs, procedures, and policies for less stress.* New York: Norton.

Independent Practitioner. (2007, Winter). Opening lines in therapy—Div 42 members share their favorites. *Independent Practitioner, 27,* 22.

Institute of Medicine. (2002). *Reducing suicide: A national imperative.* Washington, DC: Author.

Jackson, H., & Nuttall, R. L. (2001). A relationship between childhood sexual abuse and professional sexual misconduct. *Professional Psychology: Research and Practice, 32,* 200–204.

Jacobs, D. G., & Brewer, M. L. (2006). Application of the APA Practice Guidelines on Suicide to clinical practice. *CNS Spectrums, 11,* 447–454.

Jain, S., Shapiro, S. L., Swanick, S., Roesch, S. C., Mills, P. J., Bell, I., et al. (2007). A randomized controlled trial of mindfulness meditation versus relaxation training: Effects on distress, positive states of mind, rumination and distraction. *Annals of Behavioral Medicine, 33,* 11–21.

Jayaratne, S., Croxton, T. A., & Mattison, D. (2004). A national survey of violence in the practice of social work. *Families in Society: The Journal of Contemporary Social Services, 85,* 445–453.

Jayawardena, K. M., & Liao, S. (2006). Elder abuse at end of life. *Journal of Palliative Medicine, 9,* 127–136.

Jenkins, S. R., & Baird, S. (2002). Secondary traumatic stress and vicarious traumatization: A validational study. *Journal of Traumatic Stress, 15,* 423–432.

Jogerst, G. J., Daly, J. M., Brinig, M. F., Dawson, J. D., Schmuch, G. A., & Ingram, J. G. (2003). Domestic elder abuse and the law. *American Journal of Public Health, 93,* 2131–2136.

Joiner, T. E., Conwell, Y., Fitzpatrick, K. K., Witte, T. K., Schmidt, N. B., Berlim, M. T., et al. (2005). Four studies on how past and current suicidality relate even when "everything but the kitchen sink" is covaried. *Journal of Abnormal Psychology, 114,* 291–303.

Joiner, T. E, Walker, R. L., Rudd, M. D., & Jobes, D. A. (1999). Scientizing and routinizing the assessment of suicidality in outpatient practice. *Professional Psychology Research and Practice, 30,* 447–453.

Jorstad, J. (2002). Erotic countertransference: Hazards, challenges and therapeutic potentials. *Scandinavian Psychoanalytic Review, 25,* 117–134.

Kahn, N. E. (2003). Self-disclosure of serious illness: The impact of boundary disruptions for patient and analyst. *Contemporary Psychoanalysis, 39,* 51–74.

Kahneman, D., Krueger, A. B., Schkade, D., Schwarz, N., & Stone, A. A. (2006). Would you be happier if you were richer? A focusing illusion. *Science, 312,* 1908–1910.

Kalichman, S. C. (1999). *Mandated reporting of suspected child abuse: Ethics, law, and policy.* Washington, DC: American Psychological Association.

Kaner, A., & Prelinger, E. (2005). *The craft of psychodynamic psychotherapy.* New York: Jason Aronson.

Kawachi, I., & Berkman, L. F. (2001). Social ties and mental health. *Journal of Urban Health: Bulletin of the New York Academy of Medicine, 78,* 458–467.

Keck, P. E., McElroy, S. L., Strakowski, S. M., West, S. A., Sax, K. W., Hawkins, J. M., et al. (1998). 12-month outcome of patients with bipolar disorder following hospitalization for a manic or mixed episode. *American Journal of Psychiatry, 5,* 646–652.

Keefe, F. J., Dunsmore, J., & Burnett, R. (1992). Behavioral and cognitive-behavioral approaches to chronic pain: Recent advances and future directions. *Journal of Consulting and Clinical Psychology, 60,* 528–536.

Kemp, B. J., & Mosqueda, L. A. (2005). Elder financial abuse: An evaluation framework and supporting evidence. *Journal of the American Geriatrics Society, 53,* 1123–1127.

Kernberg, O. F., Selzer, M. A., Koenigsberg, H. W., Carr, A. C., & Appelbaum, A. H. (1989). *Psychodynamic psychotherapy of borderline patients.* New York: Basic Books.

Kessler, L. E., & Waehler, C. A. (2005). Addressing multiple relationships between clients and therapists in lesbian, gay, bisexual, and transgender communities. *Professional Psychology: Research and Practice, 36,* 66–72.

Kessler, R. C., Adler, L. A., Ames, M., Barkley, R., Birnbaum, H., Greenberg, P., et al. (2005). The prevalence and effects of adult attention deficit/hyperactivity disorder on work performance in a nationally representative sample of workers. *Journal of Occupational and Environmental Medicine, 47,* 565–572.

Kessler, R. C., Adler, L. A., Barkley, R., Biederman, J., Conners, K. C., Faraone, S. V., et al. (2005). Patterns and predictors of attention-deficit/hyperactivity disorder persistence into adulthood: Results from the National Comorbidity Survey Replication. *Biological Psychiatry, 57,* 1442–1451.

Kessler, R. C., Berglund, P., Demler, O., Jin, R., & Walters, E. E. (2005). Lifetime prevalence and age-of-onset distributions of *DSM-IV* disorders in the National Comorbidity Survey Replication. *Archives of General Psychiatry, 62,* 593–602.

Kessler, R. C., Chiu, W. T., Demler, O., & Walters, E. (2005). Prevalence, severity and comorbidity of the 12-month DSM-IV disorders in the National Comorbidity Survey Replication. *Archives of General Psychiatry, 62,* 617–627.

Kibbe, D. C. (2005). *10 steps to HIPAA security compliance.* Retrieved January 19, 2007, from http://www.aafp.org/fpm/20050400/43tens.html.

Kiesler, D. J. (2001). Therapist countertransference: In search of common themes and empirical referents. *Journal of Clinical Psychology/In Session, 57,* 1053–1063.

Kim, E. Y., & Miklowitz, D. J. (2002). Childhood mania, attention deficit hyperactivity disorder and conduct disorder: A critical review of diagnostic dilemmas. *Bipolar Disorders, 4,* 215–225.

Kimerling, R., Trafton, J. A., & Nguyen, B. (2006). Validation of a brief screen for post-traumatic stress disorder with substance use disorder patients. *Addictive Behaviors, 31,* 2074–2079.

Kirkwood, G., Rampes, H., Tuffrey, V., Richardson, J., & Pilkington, K. (2005). Yoga for anxiety: A systematic review of the research evidence. *British Journal of Sports Medicine, 39,* 884–891.

Kirsch, I., Moore, T. J., Scoboria, A., & Nicholls, S. S. (2002). The emperor's new drugs: An analysis of antidepressant medication data submitted to the U.S. Food and Drug Administration. *Prevention and Treatment, 5,* n.p. Retrieved May 17, 2007, from http://www.journals.apa.org/prevention/volume5/pre00500 23a.html.

Kitzmann, K. M., Gaylord, N. K., Holt, A. R., & Kenny, E. D. (2003). Child witnesses to domestic violence: A meta-analytic review. *Journal of Consulting and Clinical Psychology, 71,* 339–352.

Kleespies, P. M. (1993). The stress of patient suicidal behavior: Implications for interns and training programs in psychology. *Professional Psychology: Research and Practice, 24,* 477–482.

Kleespies, P.M., Penk, W. E., & Forsyth, J. P. (1993). The stress of patient suicidal behavior during clinical training: Incidence, impact and recovery. *Professional Psychology Research and Practice, 24,* 293–303.

Kleespies, P. M., Smith, M. R., & Becker, B. R. (1990). Psychology interns as patient suicide survivors: Incidence, impact and recovery. *Professional Psychology: Research and Practice, 21,* 257–263.

Knickerbocker, L., Heyman, R. E., Slep, A. M. S., Jouriles, E. N., & McDonald, R. (2007). Co-occurrence of child and partner maltreatment: Definitions, prevalence, theory and implications for assessment. *European Psychologist, 12,* 36–44.

Knox, K. L., Conwell, Y., & Caine, E. D. (2004). If suicide is a public health problem, what are we doing to prevent it? *American Journal of Public Health, 94,* 37–46.

Knox, S., Burkard, A. W., Jackson, J. A., Schaack, A. M., & Hess, S. (2006). Therapists-in-training who experience a client suicide: Implications for supervision. *Professional Psychology: Research and Practice, 37,* 547–557.

Knox, S., Hess, S. A., Peterson, D. A., & Hill, C. E. (1997). A qualitative analysis of client perceptions of the effects of helpful therapist self-disclosure in long-term therapy. *Journal of Counseling Psychology, 44,* 274–283.

Knox, S., Hess, S. A., Williams, E. N., & Hill, C. E. (2003). "Here's a little something for you": How therapists respond to client gifts. *Journal of Consulting Psychology, 50,* 199–210.

Knox, S., & Hill, C. E. (2003). Therapist self-disclosure: Research-based suggestions for practitioners. *Journal of Clinical Psychology, 59,* 529–539.

Koocher, G. (2006). On being there. *Monitor on Psychology, 37,* 5. Retrieved October 18, 2006, from http://www.apa.org/monitor/apr06/pc.html.

Kopp, S. (1977). *Back to one: A practical guide for psychotherapists.* Palo Alto, CA: Science and Behavior Books.

Kottler, J. A. (2003). *On being a therapist* (3rd ed.). San Francisco: Jossey-Bass.

Krakowski, M. I., & Czobor, P. (2004). Psychosocial risk factors associated with suicide attempts and violence among psychiatric inpatients. *Psychiatric Services, 55,* 1414–1419.

Kruger, J., Epley, N., Parker, J., & Ng, Z. (2005). Egocentrism over e-mail: Can we communicate as well as we think? *Journal of Personality and Social Psychology, 89*, 925–936.

Kumar, S., & Simpson, A. I. F. (2005). Application of risk assessment for violence methods to general adult psychiatry: A selective literature review. *Australian and New Zealand Journal of Psychiatry, 39*, 328–335.

Kuyken, W., Peters, E., Power, M. J., & Lavender, T. (2003). Trainee clinical psychologists' adaptation and professional functioning: A longitudinal study. *Clinical Psychology and Psychotherapy, 10*, 41–54.

Laboratory Corporation of America. (2007). *Drugs of abuse reference guide*. Retrieved September 7, 2007, from http://www.labcorpsolutions.com/images/Drugs_of_Abuse_Reference_Guide_Flyer_3166.pdf.

Ladany, N., O'Brien, K. M., Hill, C. E., Melincoff, D. S., Knox, S., & Peterson, D. A. (1997). Sexual attraction toward clients, use of supervision, and prior training: A qualitative study of predoctoral psychology interns. *Journal of Counseling Psychology, 44*, 413–424.

Lalonde, J. K., Hudson, J. I., Gigante, R. A., & Pope, H. G. (2001). Canadian and American Psychiatrists' attitudes toward dissociative disorders diagnoses. *Canadian Journal of Psychiatry, 46*, 407–412.

Lam, R. W., & Levitan, R. D. (2000). Pathophysiology of seasonal affective disorder: A review. *Journal of Psychiatry Neuroscience, 25*, 469–480.

Lambie, G. W. (2005). Child abuse and neglect: A practical guide for professional school counselors. *Professional School Counseling, 8*, 249–258.

Lancer, R., Motta, R., & Lancer, D. (2007). The effect of aerobic exercise on obsessive-compulsive disorder, anxiety, and depression: A preliminary investigation. *The Behavior Therapist, 30*, 53, 57–62.

Laszloffy, T. A., & Hardy, K. V. (2000). Uncommon strategies for a common problem: Addressing racism in family therapy. *Family Process, 39*, 35–51.

Lauder, W., Anderson, I., & Barclay, A. (2005). Housing and self-neglect: The responses of health, social care and environmental health agencies. *Journal of Interprofessional Care, 19*, 317–325.

Lawoko, S., Soares, J. J. F., & Nolan, P. (2004). Violence towards psychiatric staff: A comparison of gender, job and environmental characteristics in England and Sweden. *Work and Stress, 18*, 39–55.

Leiter, M. P., & Harvie, P. L. (1996). Burnout among mental health workers: A review and a research agenda. *International Journal of Social Psychiatry, 42*, 90–101.

Levitt, A. J., & Boyle, M. H. (2002). The impact of latitude on the prevalence of seasonal depression. *Canadian Journal of Psychiatry, 47*, 361–367.

Levy, K. N., Clarkin, J. F., Yeomans, F. E., Scott, L. N., Wasserman, R. H., & Kernberg, O. F. (2006). The mechanisms of change in the treatment of borderline personality disorder with transference focused psychotherapy. *Journal of Clinical Psychology, 62*, 481–501.

Lewis, C. A., & Cruise, S. M. (2006). Religion and happiness: Consensus, contradictions, comments and concerns. *Mental Health, Religion and Culture, 9*, 213–225.

Liappas, J., Paparrigopoulos, T., Tzavellas, E., & Christodoulou, G. (2002). Impact of alcohol detoxification on anxiety and depressive symptoms. *Drug and Alcohol Dependence, 68,* 215–220.

Lill, M. M., & Wilkinson, T. J. (2005). Judging a book by its cover: Descriptive survey of patients' preferences for doctors' appearance and mode of address. *British Medical Journal, 331,* 1524–1527.

Lin, E. H. B., Katon, W. J., Simon, G. E., Von Korff, M., Bush, T. M., Walker, E. A., et al. (2000). Low-intensity treatment of depression in primary care: Is it problematic? *General Hospital Psychiatry, 22,* 78–83.

Lin, K., & Cheung, F. (1999). Mental health issues for Asian Americans. *Psychiatric Services, 50,* 774–780.

Linehan, M. M. (1993). *Cognitive-behavioral treatment of borderline personality disorder.* New York: Guilford Press.

Linehan, M. M., Comtois, K. A., Murray, A. M., Brown, M. Z., Gallop, R. J., Heard, H. L., et al. (2006). Two-year randomized controlled trial and follow-up of dialectical behavior therapy vs therapy by experts for suicidal behaviors and borderline personality disorder. *Archives of General Psychiatry, 63,* 757–766.

Linehan, M. M., Goodstein, J. L., Nielsen, S. L., & Chiles, J. A. (1983). Reasons for staying alive when you are thinking of killing yourself: The Reasons for Living Inventory. *Journal of Clinical and Consulting Psychology, 51,* 276–286.

Ling, C. W. (1997). Crossing cultural boundaries. *Nursing, 27,* 32d–32f.

Little, L., & Hamby, S. L. (1996). Impact of a clinician's sexual abuse history, gender, and theoretical orientation on treatment issues related to childhood sexual abuse. *Professional Psychology: Research and Practice, 27,* 617–625.

Loue, S. (2000). Intimate partner violence: Bridging the gap between law and science. *Journal of Legal Medicine, 21,* 1–34.

Loue, S. (2001). Elder abuse and neglect in medicine and law: The need for reform. *Journal of Legal Medicine, 22,* 159–209.

Louma, J. B., & Pearson, J. L. (2002). Suicide and marital status in the United States, 1991–1996: Is widowhood a risk factor? *American Journal of Public Health, 92,* 1518–1522.

Lukens, E. P., & McFarlane, W. R. (2004). Psychoeducation as evidence-based practice: Considerations for practice, research, and policy. *Brief Treatment and Crisis Intervention, 4,* 205–225.

Maher, M. J., Rego, S. A., & Asnis, G. M. (2006). Sleep disturbances in patients with post-traumatic stress disorder: Epidemiology, impact and approaches to management. *CNS Drugs, 20,* 567–590.

Maislin, G., Pack, A. I., Kribbs, N. B., Smith, P. L., Schwartz, A. R., Kline, L. R., et al. (1995). A survey screen for prediction of apnea. *Sleep, 18,* 158–166.

Maslach, C. (2001). What have we learned about burnout and health? *Psychology and Health, 16,* 607–611.

Maslach, C. (2003). Job burnout: New directions in research and intervention. *Current Directions in Psychological Science, 12,* 189–192.

Maslach, C., Schaufeli, W. B., & Leiter, M. P. (2001). Job burnout. *Annual Review of Psychology, 52,* 397–422.

Maxie, A. C., Arnold, D. H., & Stephenson, M. (2006). Do therapists address ethnic and racial differences in cross-cultural psychotherapy? *Psychotherapy: Theory, Research, Practice, Training, 43,* 85–98.

McAdams, C. R., & Foster, V. A. (2000). Client suicide: Its frequency and impact on counselors. *Journal of Mental Health Counseling, 22,* 107–121.

McAndrew, S., & Warne, T. (2005). Cutting across boundaries: A case study using feminist praxis to understand the meanings of self-harm. *International Journal of Mental Health Nursing, 14,* 172–180.

McCann, I. L., & Pearlman, L. A. (1990). Vicarious traumatization: A framework for understanding the psychological effects of working with victims. *Journal of Traumatic Stress, 3,* 131–149.

McCarthy, A., Lee, K., Itakura, S., & Muir, D. W. (2006). Cultural display rules drive eye gaze during thinking. *Journal of Cross-Cultural Psychology, 37,* 717–722.

McGough, J. J., & Barkley, R. A. (2004). Diagnostic controversies in adult attention deficit hyperactivity disorder. *American Journal of Psychiatry, 161,* 1948–1956.

McKenry, P. C., Serovich, J. M., Mason, T. L., & Mosack, K. (2006). Perpetration of gay and lesbian partner violence: A disempowerment perspective. *Journal of Family Violence, 21,* 233–243.

McLaughlin, J. K., Wise, T. N., & Lipworth, L. (2004). Increased risk of suicide among patients with breast implants: Do the epidemiologic data support psychiatric consultation? *Psychosomatics: Journal of Consultation Liaison Psychiatry, 45,* 277–280.

McNiel, D. E., Eisner, J. P., & Binder, R. L. (2000). The relationship between command hallucinations and violence. *Psychiatric Services, 51,* 1288–1292.

McWilliams, N. (2004). *Psychoanalytic psychotherapy: A practitioner's guide.* New York: Guilford Press.

MedlinePlus. (2007). *Sleep disorders.* Retrieved April 6, 2007, from http://www.nlm.nih.gov/medlineplus/sleepdisorders.html.

Menahem, S., & Schvartzman, P. (1998). Is our appearance important to our patients? *Family Practice, 15,* 391–397.

Merikangas, K., & Yu, K. (2002). Genetic epidemiology of bipolar disorder. *Clinical Neuroscience Research, 2,* 127–141.

Miller, L. (1994). Biofeedback and behavioral medicine: Treating the symptom, the syndrome or the person? *Psychotherapy, 31,* 161–169.

Miller, W. R., & Rollnick, S. (2002). *Motivational interviewing: Preparing people for change* (2nd ed.). New York: Guilford Press.

Moline, M. E., Williams, G. T., & Austin, K. M. (1998). *Documenting psychotherapy: Essentials for mental health practitioners.* Thousand Oaks, CA: Sage.

Monahan, J. (1993). Limiting therapist exposure to *Tarasoff* liability. *American Psychologist, 48,* 242–250.

Montross, C. (2007). *Body of work: Meditations on mortality from the human anatomy lab.* New York: Penguin.

Morgan, J. F., Reid, F., & Lacey, J. H. (1999). The SCOFF questionnaire: Assessment of a new screening tool for eating disorders. *British Journal of Medicine, 319,* 1497–1498.

Morrison, J. (1995). *The first interview: Revised for DSM-IV.* New York: Guilford Press.

Morrison, J. (1997). *When psychological problems mask medical disorders: A guide for psychotherapists.* New York: Guilford Press.

Morrison, J. (2007). *Diagnosis made easier: Principles and techniques for mental health clinicians.* New York: Guilford Press.

Mort, J. R., & Aparasu, R. R. (2002). Prescribing of psychotropics in the elderly: Why is it so often inappropriate? *CNS Drugs, 16,* 99–109.

Mossman, D. (2004). How a rabbi's sermon resolved my *Tarasoff* conflict. *Journal of the American Academy of Psychiatry and the Law, 32,* 359–363.

Mroczek, D. K. (2001). Age and emotion in adulthood. *Current Directions in Psychological Science, 10,* 87–90.

National Association of Social Workers. (1999). *Code of ethics of the National Association of Social Workers.* Retrieved January 11, 2007, from http://www.socialwork.msu.edu/ethics/nasweth.html#103.

National Committee for the Prevention of Elder Abuse & National Adult Protective Services Association. (2007). *The 2004 Survey of State Adult Protective Services: Abuse of Vulnerable Adults 18 Years of Age and Older.* Washington, DC: National Center on Elder Abuse. Retrieved December 17, 2007, from http://www.ncea.aoa.gov/NCEAroot/Main_Site/pdf/APS_2004NCEASurvey.pdf.

National Institute of Mental Health. (1999, December). *Frequently asked questions about suicide.* Retrieved July 4, 2007, from http://www.nimh.nih.gov/suicideprevention/suicidefaq.cfm

National Institute of Mental Health. (2004, April). *Suicide facts and statistics.* Retrieved October 19, 2006, from http://www.nimh.nih.gov/suicideprevention/suifact.cfm.

National Institute on Alcohol Abuse and Alcoholism. (2007). *Online materials for clinicians and patients.* Retrieved September 7, 2007, from http://pubs.niaaa.nih.gov/publications/Practitioner/CliniciansGuide2005/clinicians_guide24_cp_mats.htm.

National Sleep Foundation. (2007). *Topics A to Zzzzs.* Retrieved April 6, 2007, from http://www.sleepfoundation.org/site/c.huIXKjM0IxF/b.2450839/k.BA4F/Topics_A_to_Zzzzs/apps/nl/newsletter2.asp.

Neighbors, H. W., Trierweiler, S. J., Ford, B. C., & Muroff, J. R. (2003). Racial differences in DSM diagnosis using a semi-structured instrument: The importance of clinical judgment in the diagnosis of African Americans. *Journal of Health and Social Behavior, 44,* 237–256.

Nelson-Gardell, D., & Harris, D. (2003). Childhood abuse history, secondary traumatic stress, and child welfare workers. *Child Welfare, 82,* 5–26.

Neno, R., & Neno, M. (2005). Identifying abuse in older people. *Nursing Standard, 20,* 43–47.

Nesbit, R. E. (2003). *The geography of thought: How Asians and Westerners think differently . . . and why.* New York: Free Press.

Newman, A. W., Wright, S. W., Wrenn, K. D., & Bernard, A. (2005). Should physicians have facial piercings? *Journal of General Internal Medicine, 20,* 213–218.

Newsome, S., Christopher, J. C., Dahlen, P., & Christopher, S. (2006). Teaching counselors self-care through mindfulness practices. *Teachers College Record, 108,* 1881–1900.

Nhat Hanh, T. (1975). *The miracle of mindfulness: A manual on meditation.* Boston: Beacon Press.

Nock, M. K., & Kessler, R. C. (2006). Prevalence of and risk factors for suicide attempts versus suicide gestures: Analysis of the National Comorbidity Survey. *Journal of Abnormal Psychology, 115,* 616–623.

Norcross, J. C. (2000). Psychotherapist self-care: Practitioner-tested, research-informed strategies. *Professional Psychology: Research and Practice, 31,* 710–713.

Norcross, J. C. (2005). The psychotherapist's own psychotherapy: Educating and developing psychologists. *American Psychologist, 60,* 840–850.

Norcross, J. C. (2006). Integrating self-help into psychotherapy: 16 practice suggestions. *Professional Psychology: Research and Practice, 37,* 683–693.

Norcross, J. C., & Guy, J. D. (2007). *Leaving it at the office: A guide to psychotherapist self-care.* New York: Guilford Press.

Norcross, J. C., Koocher, G. P., & Garofalo, A. (2006). Discredited psychological treatments and tests: A Delphi poll. *Professional Psychology: Research and Practice, 37,* 515–522.

Nordentoft, M., Jeppesen, P., Abel, M., Kassow, P., Petersen, L., Thorup, A., et al. (2002). OPUS study: Suicidal behaviour, suicidal ideation and hopelessness among patients with first-episode psychosis: One-year follow-up of a randomised controlled trial. *British Journal of Psychiatry, 181*(Suppl. 43), s98–s106.

Norris, D. M., Gutheil, T. G., & Strasburger, L. H. (2003). This couldn't happen to me: Boundary problems and sexual misconduct in the psychotherapy relationship. *Psychiatric Services, 54,* 517–522.

Occupational Safety and Health Administration. (2004). *Guidelines for preventing workplace violence for health care and social service workers.* Retrieved July 3, 2007, from http://www.osha.gov/Publications/osha3148.pdf.

Ohayon, M. M., & Roth, T. (2002). Prevalence of restless legs syndrome and periodic limb movement disorder in the general population. *Journal of Psychosomatic Research, 53,* 547–554.

O'Leary, B. J., & Norcross, J. C. (1998). Lifetime prevalence of mental disorders in the general population. In G. P. Koocher, J. C. Norcross, & S. S. Hill (Eds.), *Psychologists' desk reference* (pp. 3–5). New York: Oxford University Press.

Osterberg, L., & Blaschke, T. (2005). Adherence to medication. *New England Journal of Medicine, 353,* 487–497.

Otis, H. G., & King, J. H. (2006). Unanticipated psychotropic medication reactions. *Journal of Mental Health Counseling, 28,* 218–240.

Owens, D., Horrocks, J., & House, A. (2002). Fatal and non-fatal repetition of self-harm: Systematic review. *British Journal of Psychiatry, 181,* 193–199.

Packman, W. L., Marlitt, R. E., Bongar, B., & Pennuto, T. O. (2004). A comprehensive and concise assessment of suicide risk. *Behavioral Sciences and the Law, 22,* 667–680.

Packman, W. L., Pennuto, T. O., Bongar, B., & Orthwein, J. (2004). Legal issues of professional negligence in suicide cases. *Behavioral Sciences and the Law, 22,* 697–713.

Pasqualone, G. A., & Fitzgerald, S. M. (1999). Munchausen by proxy syndrome: The forensic challenge of recognition, diagnosis, and reporting. *Critical Care Nursing, 22,* 52–64.

Patel, S. (2007, June 12). "Been there?" Sometimes that isn't the point. *New York Times*. Retrieved July 1, 2007, from http://www.nytimes.com/2007/06/12/health/psychology/12essa.html?ex=1183435200&en=5c3585d1807ad6b9&ei=5070.

Pearlman, L. A., & Mac Ian, P. S. (1995). Vicarious traumatization: An empirical study of the effects of trauma work on trauma therapists. *Professional Psychology: Research and Practice, 26*, 558–565.

Peterson, A. M., Takiya, L., & Finley, R. (2003). Meta-analysis of trials of interventions to improve medication adherence. *American Journal of Health-System Pharmacy, 60*, 657–665.

Petit, J. (2005). Management of the acutely violent patient. *Psychiatric Clinics of North America, 28*, 701–711.

Philip, C. E. (1993). Dilemmas of disclosure to patients and colleagues when a therapist faces life-threatening illness. *Health and Social Work, 18*, 13–19.

Pieters, G., Speybrouck, E., De Gucht, V., & Joss, S. (2005). Assaults by patients on psychiatric trainees: Frequency and training issues. *Psychiatric Bulletin, 29*, 168–170.

Pinals, D. A., & Gutheil, T. G. (2001). Sanctity, secrecy and silence: Dilemmas in clinical confidentiality. *Psychiatric Annals, 31*, 113–118.

Piper, A., & Merskey, H. (2004). Dissociative identity disorder. Part 1. The excesses of an improbable concept. *Canadian Journal of Psychiatry, 49*, 592–600.

Pomerantz, A. M., & Handelsman, M. M. (2004). Informed consent revisited: An updated written question format. *Professional Psychology: Research and Practice, 35*, 201–205.

Pope, K. S., & Feldman-Summers, S. (1992). National survey of psychologists' sexual and physical abuse history and their evaluation of training and competence in these areas. *Professional Psychology: Research and Practice, 23*, 353–361.

Pope, K. S., Sonne, J. L., & Greene, B. (2006). *What therapists don't talk about and why: Understanding taboos that hurt us and our clients*. Washington, DC: American Psychological Association.

Pope, K. S., & Tabachnick, B. G. (1993). Therapists' anger, hate, fear, and sexual feelings: National survey of therapist responses, client characteristics, critical events, formal complaints, and training. *Professional Psychology: Research and Practice, 24*, 142–152.

Pope, K. S., Tabachnick, B., & Keith-Spiegel, P. C. (1987). The ethics of practice: Beliefs and behaviors of psychologists as therapists. *American Psychologist, 42*, 993–1006.

Postolache, T. T., Hardin, T. A., Myers, F. S., Turner, E. H., Yi, L. Y., Barnett, R. L., et al. (1998). Greater improvement in summer than with light treatment in winter in patients with seasonal affective disorder. *American Journal of Psychiatry, 155*, 1614–1616.

Pressly, P. K., & Heesacker, M. (2001). The physical environment and counseling: A review of theory and research. *Journal of Counseling and Development, 79*, 148–160.

Prins, A., Ouimette, P., Kimerling, R., Camerond, R. P., Hugelshofer, D. S., Shaw-Hegwer, J., et al. (2004). The primary care PTSD screen (PC–PTSD): Development and operating characteristics. *Primary Care Psychiatry, 9*, 9–14.

Prochaska, J. O., & Norcross, J. C. (2001). Stages of change. *Psychotherapy, 38*, 443–448.

Puetz, T. W., O'Connor, P. J., & Dishman, R. K. (2006). Effects of chronic exercise on feelings of energy and fatigue: A quantitative synthesis. *Psychological Bulletin, 132,* 866–876.

Purcell, R., Powell, M. B., & Mullen, P. E. (2005). Clients who stalk psychologists: Prevalence, methods and motives. *Professional Psychology: Research and Practice, 36,* 537–543.

Putney, M. W., Worthington, E. L., & McCullough, M. E. (1992). Effects of supervisor and supervisee theoretical orientation and supervisor-supervisee matching on interns' perceptions of supervision. *Journal of Counseling Psychology, 39,* 258–265.

RachBeisel, J., Scott, J., & Dixon, L. (1999). Co-occurring severe mental illness and substance use disorders: A review of recent research. *Psychiatric Services, 50,* 1427–1434.

Ramel, W., Goldin, P. R., Carmona, P. E., & McQuaid, J. R. (2004). The effects of mindfulness meditation on cognitive processes and affect in patients with past depression. *Cognitive Therapy and Research, 28,* 433–455.

Ramsay, J. R., & Rostain, A. L. (2005). Adapting psychotherapy to meet the needs of adults with attention-deficit/hyperactivity disorder. *Psychotherapy: Theory, Research, Practice, Training, 42,* 72–84.

Raquepaw, J. M., & Miller, R. S. (1989). Psychotherapist burnout: A componential analysis. *Professional Psychology: Research and Practice, 20,* 32–36.

Recupero, P. R., & Rainey, S. E. (2005). Informed consent to e-therapy. *American Journal of Psychotherapy, 59,* 319–331.

Renninger, S. M., Veach, P. M., & Bagdade, P. (2002). Psychologists' knowledge, opinions, and decision-making processes regarding child abuse and neglect reporting laws. *Professional Psychology: Research and Practice, 33,* 19–23.

Resnick, R. J. (2007). ADHD in adults: It's not just a kid thing anymore. *Independent Practitioner, 27,* 75–78.

Resnick, S. G., Bond, G. R., & Mueser, K. T. (2003). Trauma and posttraumatic stress disorder in people with schizophrenia. *Journal of Abnormal Psychology, 112,* 415–423.

Richter, K. P., Surprenant, Z. J., Schmelzle, K. H., & Mayo, M. S. (2003). Detecting and documenting intimate partner violence: An intake form question is not enough. *Violence Against Women, 9,* 458–465.

Rivas-Vasquez, R. A., Blais, M. A., Rey, G. J., & Rivas-Vasquez, A. A. (2001). A brief reminder about documenting the psychological consultation. *Professional Psychology: Research and Practice, 32,* 194–199.

Robertiello, G. (2006). Common mental health correlates of domestic violence. *Brief Treatment and Crisis Intervention, 6,* 111–121.

Robiner, W. N., Bearman, D. L., Berman, M., Grove, W. M., Colon, E., Armstrong, J., et al. (2002). Prescriptive authority for psychologists: A looming health hazard? *Clinical Psychology: Science and Practice, 9,* 231–248.

Robinson, D. G., Woerner, M. G., Delman, H. M., & Kane, J. M. (2005). Pharmacological treatments for first-episode schizophrenia. *Schizophrenia Bulletin, 31,* 705–722.

Robinson, D. G., Woerner, M. G., McMeniman, A., Mendelowitz, A., & Bilder, R. M. (2004). Symptomatic and functional recovery from a first episode of schizophrenia or schizoaffective disorder. *American Journal of Psychiatry, 161,* 473–479.

Rodriguez-Srednicki, O., & Twaite, J. A. (2004a). Understanding and reporting child abuse: Legal and psychological perspectives: Part one: Physical abuse, sexual abuse and neglect. *Journal of Psychiatry and the Law, 32,* 315–359.

Rodriguez-Srednicki, O., & Twaite, J. A. (2004b). Understanding and reporting child abuse: Legal and psychological perspectives: Part two: Emotional abuse and secondary abuse. *Journal of Psychiatry and the Law, 32,* 443–481.

Rogers, R. (Ed.). (1997). *Clinical assessment of malingering and deception* (2nd ed.). New York: Guilford Press.

Rogers, R., Sewell, K. W., Martin, M. A., & Vitacco, M. J. (2003). Detection of feigned mental disorders: A meta-analysis of the MMPI-2 and malingering. *Assessment, 10,* 160–177.

Rose, D., Fleischmann, P., & Wykes, T. (2004). Consumers' views of electroconvulsive therapy: A qualitative analysis. *Journal of Mental Health, 13,* 285–293.

Rosenthal, N. E. (1998). *Winter blues: Seasonal affective disorder, what it is and how to overcome it.* New York: Guilford Press.

Roth, T., & Roehrs, T. (2003). Insomnia: Epidemiology, characteristics and consequences. *Clinical Cornerstone, 5,* 5–15.

Rothschild, B. (2004). The physiology of empathy. *Counseling and Psychotherapy Journal, 15,* n.p.

Royal Australian and New Zealand College of Psychiatrists Clinical Practice Guidelines Team for Depression. (2004). Australian and New Zealand clinical practice guidelines for the treatment of depression. *Australian and New Zealand Journal of Psychiatry, 38,* 389–407.

Rudman, L. A., Ashmore, R. D., & Gary, M. L. (2001). "Unlearning" automatic biases: The malleability of implicit prejudice and stereotypes. *Journal of Personality and Social Psychology, 81,* 856–868.

Rudolph, M. N., & Hughes, D. H. (2001). Emergency assessments of domestic violence, sexual dangerousness, and elder and child abuse. *Psychiatric Services, 52,* 281–306.

Rupert, P. A., & Morgan, D. J. (2005). Work setting and burnout among professional psychologists. *Professional Psychology: Research and Practice, 36,* 544–550.

Rusch, N., & Corrigan, P. W. (2002). Motivational interviewing to improve insight and treatment adherence in schizophrenia. *Psychiatric Rehabilitation Journal, 26,* 23–32.

Sabin-Farrell, R., & Turpin, G. (2003). Vicarious traumatization: Implications for the mental health of health workers? *Clinical Psychology Review, 23,* 449–480.

Saletu-Zyhlarz, G. M., Anderer, P., Arnold, O., & Saletu, B. (2003). Confirmation of the neurophysiologically predicted therapeutic effects of trazodone on its target symptoms depression, anxiety and insomnia by postmarketing clinical studies with a controlled-release formulation in depressed outpatients. *Neuropsychobiology, 48,* 194–208.

Salmon, P. (2003). Anxiety, depression and sensitivity to stress: A unifying theory. *Clinical Psychology Review, 21,* 33–61.

Samuelson, S. L., & Clark, C. D. (2005). Screening for domestic violence: Recommendations based on a practice survey. *Professional Psychology: Research and Practice, 36,* 276–282.

Schachter, D. C., & Kleinman, I. (2004). Psychiatrists' attitudes about and informed consent practices for antipsychotics and tardive dyskinesia. *Psychiatric Services, 55,* 714–717.

Schauben, L. J., & Frazier, P. A. (1995). Vicarious trauma: The effects on female counselor of working with sexual trauma survivors. *Psychology of Women Quarterly, 19,* 49–64.

Schoenen, J. (2001). Migraine. *Pain: Clinical Updates, 9*(3), 1–9.

Schultz-Ross, R. A., & Gutheil, T. G. (1997). Difficulties in integrating spirituality into psychotherapy. *Journal of Psychotherapy Practice and Research, 6,* 130–138.

Schwartz, T. L., & Park, T. L. (1999). Assaults by patients on psychiatric residents: A survey and training recommendations. *Psychiatric Services, 50,* 381–383.

Segall, B. (2006). *Hundreds of patient records found in pharmacy dumpster.* Channel 13, WTHR, Indianapolis. Retrieved January 1, 2007, from http://www.wthr.com/Global/story.asp?S=5207597.

Seligman, M. E. P., Steen, T. A., Park, N., & Peterson, C. (2005). Positive psychology progress: Empirical validation of interventions. *American Psychologist, 60,* 410–421.

Sharkin, B. S., & Birky, I. (1992). Incidental encounters between therapists and their clients. *Professional Psychology: Research and Practice, 23,* 326–328.

Sheehan, D. V., Lecrubier, Y., Sheehan, K. H., Amorim, P., Janavs, J., Weiller, E., et al. (1998). The Mini-International Neuropsychiatric Interview (M.I.N.I.): The development and validation of a structured diagnostic psychiatric interview for the DSM-IV and ICD-10 [Online]. *Journal of Clinical Psychiatry, 59*(Suppl. 20), 22–33. Abstract from http://www.pubmed.gov.

Sheeran, T., & Zimmerman, M. (2002). Screening for posttraumatic stress disorder in a general psychiatric outpatient setting. *Journal of Consulting and Clinical Psychology, 70,* 961–966.

Shinn, M., Rosario, M., Morch, H., & Chestnut, D. E. (1984). Coping with job stress and burnout in the human services. *Journal of Personality and Social Psychology, 46,* 864–876.

Shugarman, L. R., Fries, B. E., Wolf, R. S., & Morris, J. N. (2003). Identifying older people at risk of abuse during routine screening practices. *Journal of the American Geriatrics Society, 51,* 24–31.

Simon, R. I. (1988). *Concise guide to clinical psychiatry and the law.* Washington, DC: American Psychiatric Press.

Simon, R. I. (1992). *Clinical psychiatry and the law* (2nd ed.). Washington, DC: American Psychiatric Publishing.

Simon, R. I. (1995). Deviant billing is risky business. *Psychotherapy Letter, 7,* n.p.

Simon R. I. (2004). *Assessing and managing suicide risk: Guidelines for clinically based risk management.* Washington, DC: American Psychiatric Publishing.

Simon, R. I. (2006). Imminent suicide: The illusion of short-term prediction. *Suicide and Life-Threatening Behavior, 36,* 296–301.

Simon, R. I., & Gutheil, T. G. (2004). Clinician factors associated with increased risk for patient suicide. *Psychiatric Annals, 34,* 750–754.

Singh, G. K., & Siahpush, M. (2002). Increasing rural-urban gradients in US suicide mortality, 1970–1997. *American Journal of Public Health, 92,* 1161–1167.

Skeem, J. L., Miller, J. D., Mulvey, E., Tiemann, J., & Monahan, J. (2005). Using a five-factor lens to explore the relation between personality traits and violence in psychiatric patients. *Journal of Consulting and Clinical Psychology, 73*, 454–465.

Skeem, J. L., Monahan, J., & Mulvey, E. P. (2002). Psychopathy, treatment involvement and subsequent violence among civil psychiatric patients. *Law and Human Behavior, 26*, 577–603.

Small, M. A., Lyons, P. M., & Guy, L. S. (2002). Liability issues in child abuse and neglect reporting statutes. *Professional Psychology: Research and Practice, 33*, 13–18.

Small, R. F. (1994). How can I legally and ethically avoid abandoning my client? *Psychotherapy Letter, 6*, n.p.

Smith, M. (2006). What do university students who will work professionally with children know about maltreatment and mandated reporting? *Children and Youth Services Review, 28*, 906–926.

Somberg, D. R., Stone, G. L., & Claiborn, C. D. (1993). Informed consent: Therapists' beliefs and practices. *Professional Psychology: Research and Practice, 24*, 153–159.

Spiegel, P. B. (1990). Confidentiality endangered under some circumstances without special management. *Psychotherapy, 27*, 636–643.

Spotswood, S. (2006, July). DoD personnel info part of VA data theft. *U.S. Medicine*. Retrieved January 1, 2007, from http://www.usmedicine.com/article.cfm?articleID=1346&issueID=89.

Stanton, M. D. (2004). Getting reluctant substance abusers to engage in treatment/self-help: A review of outcomes and clinical options. *Journal of Marital and Family Therapy, 30*, 165–182.

Statland, B. E., & Demas T. J. (1980). Serum caffeine half-lives. Healthy subjects vs. patients having alcoholic hepatic disease. *American Journal of Clinical Pathology, 73*, 390–393.

Steinberg, K. L., Levine, M., & Doueck, H. J. (1997). Effects of legally mandated child-abuse reports on the therapeutic relationship: A survey of psychotherapists. *American Journal of Orthopsychiatry, 67*, 112–122.

Stockman, A. F., & Green-Emrich, A. (1994). Impact of therapist pregnancy on the process of counseling and psychotherapy. *Psychotherapy, 31*, 456–462.

Strakowski, S. (2003). How to avoid ethnic bias when diagnosing schizophrenia. *Current Psychiatry, 2*(6), n.p.

Stuart, G. L., Moore, T. M., Gordon, K. C., Ramsey, S. E., & Kahler, C. W. (2006). *Journal of Interpersonal Violence, 21*, 376–389.

Sue, S., & Zane, N. (1987). The role of culture and cultural techniques in psychotherapy: A critique and reformulation. *American Psychologist, 42*, 37–45.

Sullivan, P. F. (2005). The genetics of schizophrenia. *PLoS Medicine, 2*, 614–618.

Sullivan, P. F., Neale, M. C., & Kendler, K. S. (2000). Genetic epidemiology of major depression: Review and meta-analysis. *American Journal of Psychiatry, 157*, 1552–1562.

Sullivan, T., Martin, W. L., & Handelsman, M. M. (1993). Practical benefits of an informed-consent procedure: An empirical investigation. *Professional Psychology: Research and Practice, 24*, 160–163.

Swanger, N. (2006). Visible body modification (VBM): Evidence from human resource managers and recruiters and the effects on employment. *International Journal of Hospitality Management, 25,* 154–158.

Swanson, J. W., Swartz, M. S., Essock, S. M., Osher, F. C., Wagner, R., Goodman, L.
A., et al. (2002). The social-environmental context of violent behavior in persons
treated for severe mental illness. *American Journal of Public Health, 92,* 1523–1531.

Symreng, I., & Fishman, S. M. (2004). Anxiety and pain. *Pain: Clinical Updates, 12,*
1–6.

Tan, S., & Leucht, C. (1997). Cognitive-behavioral therapy for clinical pain control:
A 15-year update and its relationship to hypnosis. *International Journal of Clinical
and Experimental Hypnosis, 45,* 396–416.

Taylor, D. J., Lichstein, K. L., Weinstock, J., Sanford, S., & Temple, J. R. (2007). A
pilot study of cognitive-behavioral therapy of insomnia in people with mild depression. *Behavior Therapy, 38,* 49–57.

Teaster, P. (2000). *A response to the abuse of vulnerable adults: The 2000 Survey of
State Adult Protective Services.* Washington, DC: National Center on Elder Abuse.
Retrieved December 17, 2007, from http://www.ncea.aoa.gov/NCEAroot/Main_
Site/pdf/research/apsreport030703.pdf.

Thompson, H., & Priest, R. (2005). Elder abuse and neglect: Considerations for mental health practitioners. *Adultspan Journal, 4,* 116–128.

Tinsley, J. A. (2000). Pregnancy of the early-career psychiatrist. *Psychiatric Services,
51,* 105–110.

Tucker, E. (2006, December 1). *Report sparks changes at pharmacy chains.* Associated
Press. Retrieved January 1, 2007, from http://www.mercurynews.com/mld/mercury
news/living/health/16136806.htm.

Turk, D. C., & Burwinkle, T. M. (2005). Clinical outcomes, cost effectiveness, and
the role of psychology in treatments for chronic pain sufferers. *Professional Psychology: Research and Practice, 36,* 602–610.

Twamley, E. W., Jeste, D. V., & Bellack, A. S. (2003). A review of cognitive training
in schizophrenia. *Schizophrenia Bulletin, 29,* 359–382.

Twamley, E. W., Jeste, D. V., & Lehman, A. F. (2003). Vocational rehabilitation in schizophrenia and other psychotic disorders: A literature review and meta-analysis of randomized controlled trials. *Journal of Nervous and Mental Disease, 191,* 515–523.

U.S. Department of Health and Human Services. (2003). *Summary of the HIPAA Privacy Rule.* Retrieved January 19, 2007, from http://www.hhs.gov/ocr/privacysum-
mary.pdf.

U.S. Department of Health and Human Services. (2005a). *Dietary guidelines for Americans.* Retrieved September 7, 2007, from http://www.health.gov/dietaryguidelines/
dga2005/document/default.htm.

U.S. Department of Health and Human Services. (2005b, September). *Results from the
2005 National Survey on Drug Use and Health: National findings.* Retrieved January 25, 2008, from http://www.oas.samhsa.gov/nsduh/2k5nsduh/2k5Results.pdf.

Valera, E. M., & Berenbaum, H. (2003). Brain injury in battered women. *Journal of
Consulting and Clinical Psychology, 71,* 797–804.

van der Kolk, B. A. (2002). In terror's grip: Healing the ravages of trauma. *Cerebrum,
4,* 34–50.

VanDeusen, K. M., & Way, I. (2006). Vicarious trauma: An exploratory study of the impact of providing sexual abuse treatment on clinician's trust and intimacy. *Journal of Child Sexual Abuse, 15,* 69–85.

Vasquez, M. J. T. (1992). Psychologist as clinical supervisor: Promoting ethical practice. *Professional Psychology: Research and Practice, 23,* 196–202.

Vasquez, M. J. T., Lott, B., Garcia-Vasquez, E., Grant, S. K., Iwamasa, G. Y., Molina, L. E., et al. (2006). Personal reflections: Barriers and strategies in increasing diversity in psychology. *American Psychologist, 61,* 157–172.

Verona, E., Sachs-Ericsson, N., & Joiner, T. E. (2004). Suicide attempts associated with externalizing psychopathology in an epidemiological sample. *American Journal of Psychiatry, 161,* 444–451.

Wachtel, P. L. (1993). *Therapeutic communication: Knowing what to say when.* New York: Guilford Press.

Walcott, D. M., Cerundolo, P., & Beck, J. C. (2001). Current analysis of the *Tarasoff* duty: An evolution towards the limitation of the duty to protect. *Behavioral Sciences and the Law, 19,* 325–343.

Walker, M., & Jacobs, M. (2004). *Supervision questions and answers for counsellors and therapists.* London: Whurr Publishers.

Warden, D. (2006). Military TBI during Iraq and Afghanistan wars. *Journal of Head Trauma Rehabilitation, 5,* 398–402.

Weaver, T., Madden, P., Charles, V., Stimson, G., Renton, A., Tyrer, P., et al. (2003). Comorbidity of substance misuse and mental illness in community mental health and substance misuse services. *British Journal of Psychiatry, 183,* 304–313.

Weinstein, B., Levine, M., Kogan, N., Harkavy-Friedman, J. M., & Miller, J. M. (2001). Therapist reporting of suspected child abuse and maltreatment: Factors associated with outcome. *American Journal of Psychotherapy, 55,* 219–233.

Weiss, M., & Murray, C. (2003). Assessment and management of attention-deficit hyperactivity disorder in adults. *Canadian Medical Association Journal, 168,* 715–722.

Welfel, E. R., Danzinger, P. R., & Santoro, S. (2000). Mandated reporting of abuse/maltreatment of older adults: A primer for counselors. *Journal of Counseling and Development, 78,* 284–292.

Wendler, D., & Rackoff, J. E. (2001). Informed consent and respecting autonomy: What's a signature got to do with it? *IRB: Ethics and Human Research, 23,* 1–4.

Westen, D. (2005). Implications of research in cognitive neuroscience for psychodynamic psychotherapy. In G. O. Gabbard, J. S. Beck, & J. Holmes (Eds.), *Oxford textbook of psychotherapy* (pp. 447–454). New York: Oxford University Press.

Weston, R., Temple, J. R., & Marshall, L. L. (2005). Gender symmetry and asymmetry in violent relationships: Patterns of mutuality among racially diverse women. *Sex Roles, 53,* 553–571.

Whaley, A. L. (2001). Cultural mistrust and the clinical diagnosis of paranoid schizophrenia in African American patients. *Journal of Psychopathology and Behavioral Assessment, 23,* 93–100.

Williams, S. L., & Frieze, I. H. (2005). Patterns of violent relationships, psychological distress, and marital satisfaction in a national sample of men and women. *Sex Roles, 52,* 771–784.

Wittenberg, K. J., & Norcross, J. C. (2001). Practitioner perfectionism: Relationship to ambiguity tolerance and work satisfaction. *Journal of Clinical Psychology, 57,* 1543–1550.

Wiwanitkit, V. (2005). Male rape, some notes on the laboratory investigation. *Sexuality and Disability, 23,* 41–46.

Woody, R. H. (1999). Domestic violations of confidentiality. *Professional Psychology: Research and Practice, 30,* 607–610.

Woolf, C. J., & Salter, M. W. (2000). Neuronal plasticity increasing the gain in pain. *Science, 2000,* 1765–1768.

Work Group on Eating Disorders, American Psychiatric Association. (2006). *Practice guideline for the treatment of patients with eating disorders* (3rd ed.). Retrieved January 25, 2008, from http://www.psych.org/psych_pract/treatg/pg/EatingDisorders3ePG_04-28-06.pdf.

Worz, R. (2003). Pain in depression; Depression in pain. *Pain: Clinical Updates, 11*(5), 1–4.

Yalom, I. (2002). *The gift of therapy: An open letter to a new generation.* New York: HarperPerennial.

Yeager, K. R., Saveanu, R., Roberts, A. R., Reissland, G., Mertz, D., Cirpili, A., et al. (2005). Measured response to identified suicide risk and violence: What you need to know about psychiatric patient safety. *Brief Treatment and Crisis Intervention, 5,* 121–141.

Young, T., Peppard, P. E., & Gottlieb, D. J. (2002). Epidemiology of obstructive sleep apnea: A population health perspective. *American Journal of Respiratory and Critical Care Medicine, 165,* 1217–1239.

Yufit, R. I. (2005). Assessment of suicide potential. In R. J. Craig (Ed.), *Clinical and diagnostic interviewing* (2nd ed., pp. 385–400). Lanham, MD: Rowman & Littlefield.

Zane, N., Sue, S., Chang, J., Huang, L., Huang, J., Srinvasan, S., Chun, K., Kurasaki, K., & Lee, E. (2005). Beyond ethnic match: Effects of client-therapist cognitive match in problem perception, coping orientation, and therapy goals on treatment outcomes. *Journal of Community Psychology, 33,* 569–585.

Zimmerman, M., & Mattia, J. L. (1999). Is posttraumatic stress disorder underdiagnosed in routine clinical settings? *Journal of Nervous and Mental Disease, 187,* 420–428.

Zuckerman, E. (2003). *The paper office* (3rd ed.). New York: Guilford Press.

Index

AA. *See* Alcoholics Anonymous

abandonment by therapist, of client, 38

abandonment-issue clients: therapist pregnancy and, 59; therapist vacations and, 36

abuse. *See* specific abuse/maltreatment topics

abuse reporting: confidentiality and, 93; mandated, 297–98; in progress notes, 172–73

abusive partner, staying with, 185

ACTION acronym, 281, 294

activities: appropriate client-initiated, 188–89; normalizing, 186–88

ADD. *See* attention deficit disorder

addiction: client, 66; physical, 224

ADHD. *See* attention deficit hyperactivity disorder

adjustment disorder, 113; in suicidality assessment, 254

adult ADHD. *See* attention deficit hyperactivity disorder, adult

affect, client: blunted, 105; clinical observations of, 105–7; depression and, 105; inappropriate, 106; labile, 106; mood and, 105–6

African Americans: diagnosing clients and, 122; medication adherence and, 207–8; Tuskegee study of, 208

agenda setting: client, 189; in starting psychotherapy, 181–82

age, therapist-client differences in, 66

agitation, client, 136

agoraphobia, 113

akathesia, 103

alcohol: abuse/dependence, 113, 148, 409–11; diagnosing clients and, 120–21; screening use of, 409–11; in suicidality assessment, 255

Alcoholics Anonymous (AA), 224

Alcohol Use Disorders Identification Test (AUDIT), 411

ambivalence, toward therapy, 31, 32

American Psychiatric Association, 116; ethics of case material usage, 94, 95

American Psychological Association: ethics of case material usage, 94; psychotropic medication and, 195

Andersen, S. M., 319

anger, client, 74

antianxiety medications, 200

antidepressants: bipolar disorder and, 115, 197; sexual side effects of, 198

antipsychotic medications: client motor activity and, 103; side effects of, 198

anxiety, client, 118; therapist anxiety and, 7–8; about therapy, 31

About the Author

Jan Willer is an adjunct faculty member at DePaul University in Chicago. As a former psychology internship training director, she has lectured, taught, and published on mental health training. She has a private practice in Chicago. Her website is www.drwiller.com.